Neurospeech Therapy for the Cerebral Palsied

A Neuroevolutional Approach

Neurospeech Therapy for the Cerebral Palsied

A Neuroevolutional Approach

THIRD EDITION

Edward D. Mysak

Professor of Speech Pathology
Chairman, Department of Speech Pathology and Audiology
Teachers College, Columbia University
Fellow of the American Speech-Language-Hearing Association

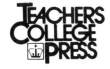

Teachers College
Columbia University
New York and London   *1980*

Library of Congress Cataloging in Publication Data

Mysak, Edward Damien, 1930–
    Neurospeech therapy for the cerebral palsied.

    First ed. published in 1963 under title: Principles of a reflex therapy approach to cerebral palsy; 2d ed. (1968) published under title: Neuro-evolutional approach to cerebral palsy and speech.
    1. Cerebral palsied children—Rehabilitation.
2. Cerebral palsied children—Language. 3. Speech therapy for children. 4. Developmental neurology.
I. Title. [DNLM: 1. Cerebral palsy—Rehabilitation.
2. Reflex. 3. Speech therapy. WS342 M998n]
RJ496.CM97   1980   618.92'836   80-18392

ISBN: 0-8077-2612-5

Manufactured in the United States of America

  2   3   4   5   6   7   8   9   88   87   86   85   84   83   82   81

To my wife Terri
and
my sons Damien and Blaise

Contents

PART II. Principles and Methods of Neurotherapy

Preface

CORRESPONDING TO THE evolutionary theme of the book, the book itself has undergone three cardinal evolutionary stages—the 1963, 1968, and 1980 stages. Central to all three versions of the book has been the application of developmental neurophysiology to the care and development of the child with cerebral palsy.

The current version incorporates pertinent information and findings in basic and applied developmental neurophysiology since the 1968 edition. The book is reorganized so as to reflect the belief that (a) the highest level of human evolution is the speech level, (b) the highest form of human behavior is speech behavior, and (c) the highest goal in cerebral palsy habilitation is speech habilitation. Toward this end, the book presents a major expansion of material regarding concepts and techniques of neurospeech therapy.

The book should hold special value for students as well as practitioners of speech pathology and audiology who seek to understand, evaluate, and care for the speech and hearing problems of the child with cerebral palsy. Physicians, physical and occupational therapists, special teachers, social workers, psychologists, and all others concerned with the speech communication problems of the cerebral palsied child and with finding their role in contributing to their alleviation should also find the book informative and useful.

I want to acknowledge again my indebtedness to many individuals for their important and continuing influences on the development of this latest edition of the book. Among these people are a long list of neurophysiologists who are identified in the text, the late and renowned Hughlings Jackson, Bertha and Karel Bobath, the late Temple Fay, Herman Kabat, and Margaret Rood.

I also want to acknowledge my sincere appreciation to all those who contributed directly and indirectly to the preparation and completion of this work. To my wife Terri and my sons Damien and Blaise, to whom the book is dedicated, I owe deep gratitude for all their love and support throughout the writing and rewriting period. To my brothers and sisters, Wanda, Frank, Clara, Bru, Joe, and Charlie, who have always been a great source of wisdom, happiness, and love for me, I express my warmest appreciation. Special thanks are also due to Mary Clark and Robert Tucker for their excellent typing of drafts of the original manuscript, to my brother Joe for his expert illustrations, and to Christine Guarino for her important contributions to the photographs of the book. And, finally, I want to thank all the children who agreed to contribute important photographs to the book.

E. D. M.
1980

Introduction

INTRODUCTORY MATERIAL THAT should contribute to reader orientation to the text includes a brief personal history on the application of developmental neurophysiology to the understanding and care of children with cerebral palsy; some comments pertaining to other treatment approaches and to the plan of the book; and, finally, a summary review of general information on cerebral palsy.

Neuroevolutional Orientation

At least by the early 1940s, signs of discontent appeared among some workers concerning the narrowness of approaching the neurophysiological disorder that is cerebral palsy from basically a musculoskeletal standpoint. The time appeared ripe to begin applying knowledge of developmental neurophysiology to the formation of habilitation programs for these children. My interest in neurotherapy grew in the following way:

In 1954, I had a concentrated experience with brain-impaired children in a summer camp, and it was there that I was struck with what appeared to be contradictions in management. Most of the children had obvious problems in movement and yet were strapped, braced, or supported in one way or another in fixed positions. I tried to appreciate at least the goal of prevention of deformities, although, at the same time, some of the devices and treatment plans used appeared to be contributing to deformities as well.

1

Also, I could appreciate the goal of attempting to match expected body posture with chronological age, but I noticed that many children who were prematurely placed into sitting positions (e.g., by strapping) appeared to develop "round shoulders" and that many who were prematurely placed into standing positions (e.g., via braces and crutches) appeared to develop "sway back." Further, because of concern for factors such as bodily safety, ease of transportation, and more ideal learning positions in classrooms and therapy rooms, children were positioned in specially constructed chairs, wheelchairs, and standing tables even though they did not manifest appropriate head, trunk, sitting, or standing balance.

Granted there might be psychological, perceptual, and practical benefits to be derived from the imposition of neurophysiologically premature postures, but there were structural and functional costs that did not always appear to be well understood by those involved with the management of the child, including the parents. In short, the "hurry-up," "fix-it," "gadget," "cosmetic" or "practical" approaches often exacted high neurophysiological costs from the child. A need existed for the vigorous pursuit of the "let's make sure all unmanifested brain function has been tapped" or the developmental neurophysiological approach. I, like so many workers before me, believed that at least a better balance between traditional and neurophysiological approaches was needed.

From that time, and especially since I began work at Newington Children's Hospital in Connecticut in 1957, I began to study literature in applied neurophysiology, especially the writings of Bertha and Karel Bobath and Herman Kabat.

In 1958, I developed a film showing reflexive maturation of children and examples of my interpretation of general and speech techniques found in the Bobath literature (Mysak, 1958). The film was based on reading and personal experiences since there was no opportunity to take a course on the subject at that time. Motivation for the film project stemmed from my own and my health colleagues' limited knowledge of neurological approaches to therapy and from my interest in acquainting colleagues with the approach.

In 1959, I attended what I believe was the first short course offered by the Bobaths in this country. At that time, I showed my film to the Bobaths and made revisions based on their reactions and comments. Also, in 1959, I published an article contrasting traditional and neurophysiological approaches to the management of cerebral palsy, pointing up the significance of the orientation to speech disorders and therapy (Mysak, 1959).

In 1960 and 1962, film reports of the results of two studies of the application of a neurotherapy orientation were released (Mysak, 1960, 1962). The majority of the children responded to the procedures and techniques with interesting and good progress. (Written descriptions of their progress were presented in a previous version of this book [Mysak, 1968]).

In 1961, M. R. Fiorentino, my associate in the Newington studies, and I published an article on neurophysiologic considerations in occupational therapy for the cerebral palsied (Mysak and Fiorentino, 1961). The focus of the article was on basic arm-hand activities.

In 1963, the first version of this book, entitled *Principles of a Reflex Therapy Approach to Cerebral Palsy,* was published. As is apparent by the title, the concentration was on reflexes and their contribution to therapy. Also in 1963, an article was published that reviewed oropharyngeal reflexology and its significance to speech development, disorders, and therapy among the cerebral palsied (Mysak, 1963).

Finally, a chapter (Mysak, 1965) and the second version of the book, entitled *Neuroevolutional Approach to Cerebral Palsy and Speech,* revealing my growing concern with evolutionary concepts, appeared. Since the last publication in 1968, and right up to the writing of the present book, I have continued to develop the theory and techniques of neurospeech therapy.

Other Orientations

At least three approaches to the management of human diseases and disorders are recognized: symptomatic, causal, and preventive. Various combinations of these three approaches may be used during the treatment history of any one disease. Whichever approach or combination of approaches is being used at any one time is related to (a) the amount of knowledge available relative to the particular disease process, (b) the treatment methods and techniques available, and (c) the number of trained specialists available to employ the treatment methods and techniques. So whenever a disease and its cause are well understood, a good chance exists for the emergence of the highest form of management, that is, prevention. The discovery and isolation of polio viruses and the subsequent development of vaccines is a good example of such preventive medicine. Prior to polio preventive measures, however, polio was treated symptomatically. During the acute stage, there were attempts to reduce the fever; and when a chronic paralytic stage remained, physical therapy and braces were usually prescribed. Such symptomatic treatment rarely relieved the paralytic symptoms to any significant extent.

A similar treatment history exists for the form of cerebral palsy arising from incompatible bloods between mother and child, for example, Rh factor incompatibility. Before the disease process was well understood, certain mothers would deliver infants who, within 24 hours or so, displayed symptoms of jaundice and who later on might show symptoms of athetosis and hearing disorder. Such children were also treated symptomatically at first, receiving any required orthopedic attention, physical therapy, and aural habilitation work. Then, as more was learned about such disease processes, a causal approach to treatment evolved in the form of massive replacement of the affected blood of the child at birth with normal blood. When all went well, the child might be rendered asymptomatic for all practical purposes. Finally, preventive measures became available in the form of (a) counseling of Rh-negative females concerning the consequences of marrying Rh-positive males, (b) counseling of Rh-negative mothers regarding the possible consequences of conceiving second or third Rh-positive children, and (c) the use of RhoGAM to inhibit the buildup of antibodies within Rh-negative mothers following the birth of their first child.

If only more causes of cerebral palsy were as well understood and could be managed through causal and preventive approaches! But, alas, this is not the case, and the majority of cerebral palsies continue to receive primarily symptomatic treatment. Such treatment includes attention to secondary tendon, muscle, and bone anomalies via various orthopedic devices and special surgical techniques, and traditional forms of physical, occupational, and speech therapies.

Because symptom approaches frequently show such limited results, different forms of causal therapy have been pursued. Special forms of neurosurgery (e.g., Myers, 1956), drugs (e.g., Denhoff and Holden, 1961), electrical stimulation of the brain, that is, cerebellar implants (Cooper et al., 1976), and spinal cord stimulation (Waltz and Pani, 1978) have all been tried. Unfortunately, such causal therapy approaches are appropriate for only certain individuals and usually offer special and limited results.

The point of this section is not only to identify the range and types of treatments available to the cerebral palsied, but to make it clear that the author, in his presentation of the neuroevolutional approach, does not intend to imply that the neuroevolutional approach is always the one of choice. Rather, it is the position of the author that each child requires a thorough team evaluation followed by the development of a management program that is most appropriate for him or her. For the sake of each individual child with cerebral palsy, cerebral palsy teams should not reflect traditional vs. neurophysiological camps. Good teams are those that offer the possibility of the best approach or combinations of approaches for any one particular child. Type of involvement, age of the child, degree of secondary involvements, motivation of the child, and orientation of the parents are all factors that might dictate against one approach and for another. The all-important consideration is that therapy decisions should be made on the basis of what is best for any particular child and not on the biases of any group of health professionals.

The Plan

By the neuroevolutional approach to the understanding and care of children with cerebral palsy, the author wishes to convey his belief that the condition of the child with cerebral palsy is best understood through the application of knowledge concerning the neurophylogenesis of man and the neuro-ontogenesis of the individual. And, also, that it is through knowledge of neurophylo-ontogenesis that therapy plans and goals may best be formulated and therapy techniques may best be devised and developed. Further, it is intended that the neuroevolutional approach incorporates the concept that the highest form of human behavior is speech behavior and that the highest habilitation goal is speech habilitation.

Since the primary focus of the book is the habilitation of the child with cerebral palsy through a neuroevolutional approach, Chapters 1 and 2, devoted to the neurophylogenesis and neuro-ontogenesis of speech respectively, were designed not so much to provide general information on the phylogenesis and ontogenesis of speech, but to form the basis from which to make neurophysiological analyses of the speech disorder in cerebral palsy and to formulate neurophysiologically based speech therapy. Correspondingly, the neurocommunicative disorder in cerebral palsy described in Chapter 3 is discussed from the standpoint of disorders of basic movements involved in listening, speech postures, hand movements, and speech movements and in skilled movements involved in listening, speech, and expressive communication. Devoted to the analysis and comparison of four major orientations to neurotherapy—the paleoreflex, motor unit, sensory receptor, and postural patterns orientations—Chapter 4 is designed not necessarily to present these orientations faithfully and completely but, more importantly, to provide a store of information and concepts upon which a substantial part of the eclectic approach called neurospeech therapy is based. Chapters 5 through 8 comprise the chapters on neurospeech therapy per se. Chapter 5 includes certain general information on neurospeech therapy such as goals and definitions, program requirements, and bases and principles of treatment. Chapter 6 describes a way of evaluating the child's basic and skilled speech movements through the use of a newly developed Neurophysiological Speech Index. The index is intended to serve as a means of estimating the neurophysiological speech age of the child and of assisting in the development of a plan of therapy for the child. Finally, Chapters 7 and 8 present procedures and techniques for stimulating basic and skilled speech movements.

General Information

This last section of the introduction presents a summary review of general information on cerebral palsy. It provides a general orientation to cerebral palsy before the reader becomes immersed in the neuroevolutional approach to the problem. Areas of cerebral palsy to be reviewed are its definition, history, and medical diagnosis; its incidence, classification, and etiology; and its associated problems. For those who desire additional and more detailed general information, older sources (e.g., Crothers and Paine, 1959; Cardwell, 1965; and Denhoff and Robinault, 1960) as well as newer ones (e.g., Connor, Williamson, and Siepp [Eds.], 1978; Cruickshank [Ed.], 1976; Marks, 1974; and Pearson and Williams [Eds.], 1972) are available.

DEFINITION

A clinically useful definition of cerebral palsy should include the factors of onset, whether prenatal, natal, postnatal, or during the period of infancy; brain involvement, whether cortical, subcortical, cerebellar, and so on; chronicity, whether acute, static, or progressive; severity, whether mild, moderate, or severe; and functions involved, whether sensory, motor, and so on.

For purposes of this book, cerebral palsy refers to the full range of chronic, childhood brain syndromes—all the way from mild, isolated dysarthria to severe sensorimotor involvements. More specifically, cerebral palsies are viewed as disease complexes whose onset occurs between conception and two years of age or so; that reflect static damage to any part of the brain; and that appear in various forms and combinations of sensorimotor, perceptual, behavioral, and speech disorders.

HISTORY

Childhood brain dysfunction was suffered by humans from earliest recorded time. Asymmetrical figures suggesting postural abnormalities associated with CNS involvement have been found carved on ancient monuments. Crippled individuals are referred to in ancient Hebrew and Greek scriptures and in the Bible. Some of these were certainly of nervous system origin; others may have had various musculoskeletal origins. Medical descriptions of symptoms of brain dysfunction may be found in pediatric textbooks of the latter half of the 15th century. A classic paper on the connection between abnormal birth histories and childhood brain dysfunctions appeared in 1861 (Little, 1861). Finally, interest in helping these children grew in the United States in the early 1940s, and Phelps (1940, 1941, 1948, 1950) is credited with organizing one of the earliest systematic programs of therapy for the cerebral palsied.

One thing is clear from the little we know about the history of what is now referred to as cerebral palsy, and that is that childhood brain dysfunction in various forms has been with us for a very long time. Another thing that is clear is that, in comparison, attempts at organizing neurotherapies based on developmental neurophysiology have been going on for a very short time.

MEDICAL EVALUATION

The organismic nature of cerebral palsy is acknowledged by the recommendation of a planned comprehensive evaluation of the problem involving various medical and other health specialists (Denhoff and Robinault, 1960).

Histories

Such an evaluation includes a careful study of family history of cerebral palsy, prenatal history (e.g., bleeding, infection, anesthesia, accidents, irradiation), natal history (e.g., precipitate or prolonged delivery, forceps manipulation, placental cord abnormalities, jaundice, trauma), neonatal and postnatal histories (e.g., birth distress, irritability, feeding, sleeping, and respiratory problems), and developmental history (e.g., problems with head balance, reaching, crawling and creeping, sitting, standing, walking, and talking).

Examinations

Recommended studies include a physical examination (e.g., fontanels, height and weight, and so on), psychological examination (e.g., intelligence, emotional), physical and occupational therapy examinations, laboratory work-ups (e.g., EEG, PEG), and a speech and hearing examination.

Such a comprehensive evaluation allows for a more definitive diagnosis, helps determine the full scope of the problem, and contributes to the development of the therapy plan.

Incidence

The accuracy of the rate of occurrence of a disease or disorder is dependent on a number of factors such as agreement on the definition of the disease, accuracy of diagnostic procedures, and consistency in reporting the disease. Because of these and other reasons, incidence figures on many diseases are no more than rough estimates.

Because of the range of cerebral dysfunctions that may be subsumed under the term *cerebral palsy* and the divergence of opinion on what should and should not be called cerebral palsy, the true incidence of cerebral palsy is difficult to establish. Rates that have been reported range from 1 to 6 per 1,000. A rather detailed review of studies of incidence was presented by Cruickshank (1976, Ch. 1).

CLASSIFICATION

Those who attempt to classify a disease and its various forms seek terminology that will carry information on clinical findings, anatomical location, and etiology of the disease. Many diseases do not allow for such a neat system of classification. A term for one form of cerebral palsy—the Rh-athetotic—does carry all the desired information. Rh-athetosis describes athetotic symptoms arising from damage to the basal nuclei due to Rh-blood incompatability. Because the other forms of the problem are not so nicely classified, terminology in cerebral palsy reflects basically its clinical signs. Terms that describe various forms of cerebral palsy and that are in current use are spasticity, athetosis, ataxia, rigidity, tremor, atonia, and mixed. Most of these terms comprise a system of classification proposed by Phelps (1950). Various subclinical forms should also be recognized such as isolated dysarthrias, or forms of congenital suprabulbar paresis.

Subclinical

The term *subclinical* is used to identify oligosymptomatic children or those who do not manifest obvious sensorimotor problems or who show limited involvement.

Characteristics of children with nonobvious sensorimotor signs may include various degrees and combinations of irregularity of intellectual profile; refractive errors and problems in binocular balance; chewing and swallowing problems; hyperreflexia (gag and patellar, hyperacusis); difficulty in regularization of toilet habits; retarded dextralization or an ambisinistrous condition; bilaterally symmetrical sensorineural hearing loss; torticollis-scoliosis; toe walking; behavioral fugues; delayed onset of speech and dysrhythmic speech.

Characteristics of a relatively specific central condition called congenital suprabulbar paresis was described by Worster-Drought (1968). The complete syndrome is manifested by paralysis or paresis of lips, tongue, velum, larynx, and swallowing difficulty; the incomplete syndrome is manifested by isolated paralysis or paresis of the velum or tongue.

Spasticity

Spasticity refers to a spasmogenic condition that is traditionally attributed to involvement of the pyramidal tract in the cortical or subcortical areas and sometimes to lesions in the brain stem and upper spinal cord. In general, it is manifested by hypertonic movements or by consistent limitations in directions and ranges of movements. The neurodynamics of spasticity may be described as the lack of constant and automatic inhibition by the cerebrum of one or more of the various levels of the CNS from which basic muscle tonus is controlled. Simply put, individuals are unable to inhibit muscles whose antagonists they need to contract. More specifically, symptoms of spasticity include exaggerated stretch reflexes, clasp-knife hypertonicity, hyperreflexia, Babinski's reflex, diminished superficial reflexes (abdominal, cremasteric), associated movements, clonus, greater involvement of antigravity muscles, and the tendency to contracture in characteristic postures.

Athetosis

Athetosis literally means without a fixed base, and the condition is traditionally attributed to involvement of the basal nuclei and their connections. In general, it is manifested by involuntary movements or inconsistency in movements in appropriate directions and of appropriate ranges. The neurodynamics of athetosis may be described as an alternating shift of tonus from one muscle group to another. More specifically, symptoms of athetosis include involuntary movements preceding voluntary movements or preemptive movements, vermiform or writhing movements, and variable tonus.

Ataxia

Ataxia literally means a lack of order. The condition is traditionally attributed to involvement of the cerebellum, and, therefore, it is manifested by cerebellar dyscoordination. The neurodynamics of ataxia may be described as a failure of the CNS to receive appropriate feedback concerning the progress of movements at any one time due to disturbance in general and/or special proprioception. More specifically, symptoms of cerebellar involvement include dyssynergia, dysmetria, dysdiadochokinesia, intention tremor, expressionless facies, disturbance of stance and festinating gait, ocular and head nystagmus, and vertigo.

Rigidity

Rigidity literally means stiff or inflexible, and the condition is traditionally attributed to widespread involvement of inhibitory centers of the brain. In general, it is manifested by a lack of, or extremely limited, movements. The neurodynamics of rigidity may be described similarly to those of spasticity except that resistance to passive motion occurs in both the agonist and antagonist muscle groups. Other characteristics that distinguish rigidity from spasticity are that in rigidity resistance is greater to slow rather than rapid passive motion, that the antagonists to the antigravity muscles are more involved, and that there are no clonus or stretch reflexes. Among the forms of rigidity are cogwheel rigidity, where resistance to passive motion gives way in a jerky fashion, and lead-pipe rigidity, where resistance to passive motion is plastic or steady.

Tremor

Tremor literally means trembling or shaking, and action or intention tremor is traditionally attributed to cerebellar involvement, while passive or nonintention tremor is attributed to basal nuclei involvement. Like athetosis alternating tremor is a form of hyperkinesis, but unlike the vermiform movements of athetosis, it is characterized by regular and symmetrical, or pendular, movements produced by alternating contraction of muscles and their antagonists.

Atonia

Atonia literally means relaxed, flaccid, without tone or tension, and the condition is traditionally attributed to involvement of the cerebellum. The neurodynamics of atonia may be described as a failure of muscles to respond to volitional stimulation. Symptoms include weak or absent stretch reflexes, loss of positive supporting reflexes, and possible Babinski's sign, clonus, and increased tendon reflexes. Atonia is frequently prodromic to spasticity or athetosis.

Mixed

Pure forms of tremor or atonia are rare and are more likely to appear as part of the symptom complexes of other forms of cerebral palsy. Contrarily, mixed types of cerebral palsy are common but usually any one case is classified according to its predominant symptomatology.

From the standpoint of neuroevolutional evaluation and therapy, the traditional classification of cerebral palsy just described has little function, and, hence, little reference is made to the various types in the book. Twitchell (1965) expressed well the view held by this writer when he said that "from the neurophysiological view, the separation of patients into various categories—such as spasticity, rigidity, athetosis, tremor—is wholly artificial." He believes that regardless of classification the same physiological substrata for the different cerebral palsies can be demonstrated in all patients. "Strict adherence to the various classifications of cerebral palsy are artificial and based on unphysiologic tenets." And from the viewpoint of management he urged that "more attention be paid to the physiological basis for the motor deficit in each individual patient so that treatment could be oriented to that individual patient rather than to some arbitrary group." This is a thought that resonates with the neuroevolutional approach to the problem.

ETIOLOGY

Like many other diseases, the causes of cerebral palsy can be divided broadly into familial and environmental categories.

Familial

A small percentage of congenital cerebral palsies appear related to familial tendencies for certain cranial malformations, degenerative diseases such as progressive spastic paraplegia, and static conditions such as familial athetosis, paraplegia, and tremor. Clinicians usually exclude conditions such as cranial malformations and degenerative diseases from their definition of cerebral palsy.

Environmental

The majority of conditions that eventually are diagnosed as cerebral palsy result from lesions incurred during the perinatal period, or from conception to about one month following birth. A wide range of causes exists for these lesions.

Prenatal etiological factors include maternal bleeding; infection, such as mumps, rubella, influenza; blood incompatibilities, such as the Rh-negative factor; toxemia; anesthesia and irradiation; placental and cord disturbances; and accidents. Embryonal and fetal CNS malformations are also factors.

Natal etiological factors include precipitate or prolonged delivery, breech or caesarean deliveries, prematurity, placenta praevia, forceps manipulation and trauma, jaundice, and syphilis, meningitis, and other infections.

Postnatal etiological factors include infections (e.g., meningitis, encephalitis, roseola, measles, whooping cough, respiratory infections), trauma, poisoning (e.g., lead, alcohol), anoxia, and neoplasms of the brain.

It is also possible that, in any one case, a combination of factors may be found.

ASSOCIATED PROBLEMS

Because of the great number of possible etiologic factors, it should be expected that, in addition to the more obvious neuromuscular symptoms, children with cerebral palsy would display a wide range of associated problems, in addition to those of speech and hearing. Among them are convulsions, mental retardation, emotional problems, sensory disturbances, and perceptual problems.

Convulsions

Seizures of all forms may be found among the cerebral palsied, even migraine and abdominal seizures. Included among the various forms of seizures are grand mal, characterized by aura and generalized involvement; Jacksonian, characterized by progressive involvement of adjacent areas of the body as reflected in the motor cortex; masticatory, characterized by chewing, swallowing, smacking, and salivation behaviors; adversive, characterized by eye and head roll prior to generalized seizure; tonic postural, characterized by tonic without clonic involvement; sensory, characterized by local or widespread disturbances; somatosensory, characterized by vertigo, visual, auditory, or olfactory symptoms; petit mal, characterized by sudden and fleeting moments of staring; minor motor, characterized by a brief or abortive generalized seizure; akinetic, characterized by a sudden loss of postural tone, often only of the head and neck; and psychic equivalent, characterized by organized behavior patterns of which the child is not aware.

The incidence of convulsive disorder among the cerebral palsied varies widely depending on the reporter. Among athetotics, figures of about 2 percent, 10 percent, and 30 percent have been reported; among spastics, figures as high as 50 percent, 60 percent, and 80 percent have been reported. Here, too, incidence figures are influenced greatly by the investigator's definition of seizure disorder and the accuracy of diagnosis of the wide range of possible symptoms.

Mental Retardation

Given all the possible problems that children with cerebral palsy may show, it is not surprising that a large number of them do not do well on formal tests of intelligence. The accuracy of intellectual assessment of these children is confounded by their motor, sensory, perceptual, experiential, and speech and hearing limitations. Testers must have experience with these children, be aware of all their possible problems, be ready to test for available information in novel ways, and learn how to recognize nonobvious responses from these children.

Incidence figures of children who score below 70 on intelligence tests range from about 30 percent up to about 70 percent with most around 50 percent. Because of all the problems mentioned relative to testing these children, and because of all the opportunities for secondary-factor influence on intellectual development, incidence figures on mental retardation in this population must be interpreted with caution.

Emotional Problems

Again, given the multitude of possible sensorimotor, perceptual, and sociocommunicative problems of the child with cerebral palsy, it should not be surprising to find "emotional problems" of various kinds among them. Possible parental reactions of guilt and rejection and overprotection of the child further complicate his or her socioemotional development.

Emotional immaturity and instability, introversion, and depression are findings that appear in studies of these children.

Sensory Disturbances

Because the motor problems of these children are often so dramatic and obvious, their many possible sensory involvements may be overlooked. Also, difficulty in testing the various sensory modalities often masks the presence of problems in these areas.

Included among sensory disturbances found among children with cerebral palsy are problems in tactile sensation, two-point discrimination, position sense, pain and temperature, and visual acuity and visual fields.

Refractive errors have been observed in over 50 percent of these children and visual field defects in about 25 percent.

Perceptual Problems

Tactile, auditory, and visual perceptual problems are all possible among children with cerebral palsy.

Astereognosis describes the lack of ability of some children with cerebral palsy to perceive tactually objects that they grasp or have placed in their hands, for example, small toys, figures, or coins. Problems in oral stereognosis or problems in identifying forms placed in the mouth, for example, plastic forms representing various shapes, may also be found. Auditory perceptual problems such as in hearing the difference between certain sounds, synthesizing combinations of sounds, and memory span for sounds may be observed. Also, visual perceptual problems such as in seeing the whole pattern of a letter or the word pattern of a group of letters, or the ability to discriminate a visual figure on a background of other visual stimuli may be identified. Complicating visual perceptual problems are problems of oculomotor balance (strabismus) and ocular nystagmus. Oculomotor imbalances have been observed in over 50 percent of these children.

Because of the obvious motor manifestations of cerebral palsy and of past orientations in the training of various clinicians and therapists dealing with these children, less emphasis was placed on the development of habilitation procedures and techniques aimed at the learning, emotional, sensory, and perceptual problems of these children. It should now be widely accepted that, regardless of the specialty of the health professional, all who work with cerebral palsied children should be as concerned with the other-than-motor manifestations of the problem as they are with the motor manifestations.

Hopefully, this introduction has contributed to reader orientation to the central purpose of this book—the application of developmental neurophysiology to the understanding and care of children with cerebral palsy.

REFERENCES

Cardwell, V. E. *Cerebral palsy—advances in understanding and care.* New York: North River Press (1965).

Connor, F. P., Williamson, G. G., and Siepp, J. M. (Eds.), *Program guide for infants and toddlers with neuromotor and other developmental disabilities.* New York: Teachers College Press, Teachers College, Columbia University (1978).

Cooper, I. S., Riklan, M., Amin, I., Waltz, J. M., and Cullinan, T. Chronic cerebellar stimulation in cerebral palsy. *Neurology,* 26, 744–753 (1976).

Crothers, B., and Paine, R. S. *The natural history of cerebral palsy.* Cambridge, Mass.: Harvard University Press (1959).

Cruickshank, W. M. (Ed.), *Cerebral palsy: Its individual and community problems.* Syracuse, New York: Syracuse University Press (1976).

Denhoff, E., and Holden, R. H. Relaxant drugs in cerebral palsy, 1949-1960. *New England J. Med.,* 204, 475-480 (1961).

———and Robinault, I. *Cerebral palsy and related disorders.* New York: McGraw-Hill (1960).

Little, W. J. On the influence of abnormal parturition, difficult labor, premature birth, and asphyxia neonatorum on the mental and physical condition of the child, especially in relation to deformities. *Tr. Obst. Soc. London,* 3, 293 (1861).

Marks, N. C. *Cerebral palsied and learning disabled children.* Springfield, Ill.: Charles C Thomas (1974).

Myers, R. Results of bilateral intermediate midbrain crusotomy in seven cases of severe athetotic and dystonic quadriparesis. *Amer. J. Phys. Med.,* 35, 84-105 (1956).

Mysak, E. D. Dysarthria and oropharyngeal reflexology: A review. *J. Speech Hearing Dis.,* 28, 252-260 (1963).

———*Neuroevolutional approach to cerebral palsy and speech.* New York: Teachers College Press, Teachers College, Columbia University (1968).

———*Principles of a reflex therapy approach to cerebral palsy.* New York: Teachers College Press, Teachers College, Columbia University (1963).

———Reflex therapy and cerebral palsy habilitation. In W. T. Daley (Ed.), *Speech and language therapy with the cerebral palsied child.* Washington, D.C.: The Catholic University of America Press (1965).

———Significance of neurophysiological orientation to cerebral palsy habilitation. *J. Speech Hearing Dis.,* 24, 221-230 (1959).

———Study films of a neurophysiological approach to cerebral palsy habilitation: Parts I & II. Films released by Newington Children's Hospital, Newington, Conn. (1960, 1962).

———The Bobath approach to cerebral palsy habilitation. Film released by Newington Children's Hospital, Newington, Conn. (1958).

———and Fiorentino, M. R. Neurophysiological considerations in occupational therapy for the cerebral palsied. *Amer. J. Occup. Ther.,* 15, May-June (1961).

Pearson, P. H. and Williams, C. E. (Eds.). *Physical therapy services in the developmental disabilities.* Springfield, Ill.: Charles C Thomas (1972).

Phelps, W. M. Etiology and classification of cerebral palsy. In *Proceedings of the Cerebral Palsy Institute,* New York: Association for the Aid of Crippled Children, Inc. (1950).

———Factors influencing the treatment of cerebral palsy. *Physiother. Rev.,* 21, 136-138 (1941).

———Let's define cerebral palsy, *Cripp. Child,* 26, 3-5 (1948).

———The treatment of cerebral palsies. *J. Bone Joint Surg.,* 22, 1004-1012 (1940).

Twitchell, T. E. Variations and abnormalities of motor development. *J. Amer. Phys. Ther. Assoc.,* 45, 424-430 (1965).

Waltz, J. M., and Pani, K. C. Spinal cord stimulation in disorders of the motor system. Presented at the *Symposium on Advances in External Control of Human Extremities.* Dubrovnik, September (1978).

Worster-Drought, C. Speech disorders in children. *Dev. Med. Child Neurol.,* 10, 427–440 (1968).

Part I

NEUROGENESIS
OF SPEECH
AND ITS DISORDERS

1

Neurophylogenesis of Speech

THE NEUROEVOLUTION OF speech embraces both phylogenetic and on-togenetic concepts of speech development. Speech movements represent the highest level of human neuro-phylo-ontogenesis. Neuroevolution is viewed as the progressive integration and elaboration of lower sensorimotor integration centers by higher ones until the ultimate integration of integration centers results in bipedal standing, walking, and talking behavior.

This is the first of two chapters devoted to the neurogenesis of speech: this one emphasizes the phylogenetic aspects, the next, the ontogenetic aspects. In discussing speech neurogenesis, it is not possible to distinguish completely between the two aspects. Speech phylogenesis involved the de-velopment of the bipedal posture, manual dexterity, the liberation of the mouth from use in crude grasping and manipulative activities, and the development of the communisphere. Phyletic traces of this evolution are seen when observing speech development in the infant. True speech development co-occurs approximately with the development of bipedal head, neck, and trunk balance, the emergence of a preferred hand, the in-tegration of various cranio-oropharyngeal reflexes (protective, feeding, emotional), and the need to communicate.

The plan of the chapter is to discuss the general integration-elaboration concept of neuroevolution, bipedal evolution, the evolution of expressive communication, and, finally, the implications of the chapter for the understanding and care of children with cerebral palsy.

Integration-Elaboration Concept of Neuroevolution

The integration-elaboration concept of neuroevolution describes the progressive integration of lower sensorimotor integration centers of the CNS by higher centers until the grand integration of all lower centers by the highest center results in bipedal walking and in talking. Support for the concept may be drawn from a number of theories: the evolution and dissolution of the nervous system, recapitulation, the triune brain, and the reflexization of movement.

EVOLUTION AND DISSOLUTION OF THE NERVOUS SYSTEM

Jackson (1958), based on his studies and long experience with nervous diseases, developed theories of the evolution and dissolution of the nervous system and of duplex symptomatology in nervous diseases. Integration-elaboration implications are found in these early ideas of Jackson.

Evolution of the CNS

Jackson (1958, p. 46) described evolution as "an ascending development in a particular order." The progression is from CNS centers which are relatively well organized at birth, or the lowest centers, to those which are continually organizing through life, or the highest centers. This progression is from the most simple to the most complex, from the most automatic to the least automatic, and from the most organized to the least organized.

Dissolution of the CNS

According to Jackson (1958, p. 46) dissolution, or the "reverse of the process of evolution," is the reduction of CNS activity from least organized, most complex, and least automatic toward the most organized, most simple, and most automatic. In the case of neuropathology, therefore, dissolution represents reduction to a lower level of neuro-ontogenesis. Jackson also spoke of uniform and local dissolutions and also depths of dissolution. By uniform dissolution, he meant that the whole nervous system was relatively evenly reversed; by local dissolution, he meant that disease of a part of the nervous system caused a local reversal of evolution. "Disease may occur on any evolutionary level on one side or on both sides;

it may affect the sensory elements chiefly, or the motor elements chiefly" (p. 47).

On depth of dissolution, Jackson stated: "An injurious agency, such as alcohol, taken into the system, flows to all parts of it; but the highest centres, being least organized, 'give out' first and most; the middle centres, being more organized, resist longer; and the lowest centres, being most organized, resist longest" (p. 47).

Jackson also believed that the symptomatology of all nervous diseases is duplex, or characterized by both a positive and a negative element. Negative symptoms reflected loss or defect of function, while positive symptoms reflected involuntary activities. Because destructive lesions produce loss or defect of function, or negative symptoms, they could not be responsible for positive symptoms. Positive symptoms, or involuntary activities, result from released activity of lower brain centers due to the removal of some inhibitory mechanism by the lesion. In terms of the doctrine of dissolution, the negative element is the loss of the least organized, most complex, and least automatic functioning; the positive element is the release of more organized, less complex, and more automatic functioning.

Various examples may serve to illustrate the concept of duplex symptomatology (Jackson, 1958, pp. 48–49). In hemiplegia, "owing to destruction of a part of a plexus in the mid-region of the brain," he said there is "loss of more or fewer of the most voluntary movements of one side of the body; we find that the arm, the more voluntary limb, suffers the more and the longer; we find too, that the most voluntary part of the face suffers more than the rest of the face." On the matter of positive and negative elements, Jackson stated that "although the unilateral movements (the more voluntary) are lost, the more automatic, the bilateral, are retained."

Jackson offered "delirium in acute non-cerebral disease" as one example of duplex symptomatology at the highest center. "The patient's condition is partly negative and partly positive. Negatively, he ceases to know that he is in hospital, and ceases to recognize persons about him . . . he is defectively conscious . . . We may conveniently say that it shows loss of function of the topmost 'layer' of his highest centres . . . The other half of his condition is positive. Besides his not knowings, there are his wrong knowings. He imagines himself to be at home or at work, and acts, as far as practicable, as if he were."

Integration-Elaboration Concept

Jackson's concepts of evolution and dissolution of the nervous system and duplex symptomatology in neuropathology corresponds to the integration-elaboration concept of neuroevolution. Jackson's concept of evolution of the nervous system implies the progressive integration of sensorimotor integration centers by higher centers. His concept of dissolution shows that lower center activity is not inhibited or lost as a function of maturation, so to speak, but is incorporated and elaborated upon by higher centers, which, if disturbed, may release these patterns again in the form of positive symptoms.

RECAPITULATION

Recapitulation refers to the repetition in ontogeny of the evolutionary stages through which the species evolved. A number of quotes from different sources may also be seen to be supportive of the integration-elaboration concept of neuroevolution.

Travis (1931, p. 15) stated, "It is believed that each cardinal evolutionary step in nervous development is recorded as a more or less distinct level in the human nervous equipment." He goes on to say that higher centers assume a directive and regulatory control over the lower centers which continue to serve their basic functions (p. 22). Related comments by other writers include: "in the development of neuromotor activity, ontogeny may recapitulate phylogeny just as it does in the development of the pharynx" (Swinyard, 1967, p. 219); "there appears to be in the behavior repertoire of the newborn infant certain patterns which reflect a phyletic heritage" (McGraw, 1962, p. 11); and, finally, "during the first years of life the infant passes through the stage of the quadruped and thus repeats the phylogenetic pattern of man" (Peiper, 1963, p. 177).

Particularly apropos of the integration-elaboration concept is Travis' comment that higher centers assume a directive and regulatory control over the lower centers that continue to serve their basic functions. Although the comment was made in a book published in 1931, it could just as well have appeared in a book written in 1980.

TRIUNE BRAIN

MacLean's (1973) concept of brain evolution in terms of the triune brain (or the three-in-one brain) and Sagan's (1977, pp. 57–83) interpretation of it is particularly relevant to the integration-elaboration concept of neuroevolution. The brain, according to MacLean, is composed of three brains, only one of which—the neocortex—is responsible for human talking and walking behaviors. Each brain represents a major evolutionary stage and may be differentiated neuroanatomically and functionally.

The neural chassis, or the frame or foundation for the three brains, the oldest part of the brain, is composed of the spinal cord, medulla and pons (hindbrain), and the midbrain. Basic neural mechanisms for reproduction and self-preservation, including regulation of the heart, circulation, and respiration, are contained within the neural chassis. It represents almost all of the brain in a fish or amphibian.

According to MacLean, this neural chassis has three drivers: The most ancient of the three, the reptilian, or R-complex, surrounds the midbrain and is shared with humans by other mammals and reptiles. The limbic system, which, in turn, surrounds the R-complex, is the next oldest driver and is also shared by other mammals but not in its full form with the reptiles. The neocortex, the most recent evolutionary development, surrounds the rest of the brain and is the ultimate driver. Humans, primates, and higher mammals have a relatively massive neocortex.

Brain evolution may best be explained by the superimposition of new systems on old ones, or through the concept of recapitulation. In fact, intrauterine human development appears marked by preceding stages suggestive of fish, reptiles, and nonprimate mammals. The embryonic development of the human brain also appears to show sequential staging in development from neural chassis to R-complex, to limbic system, and, finally, to neocortex. "Thus evolution by addition and the functional preservation of the preexisting structure must occur for one of two reasons—either the old function is required as well as the new one, or there is no way of bypassing the old system that is consistent with survival" (Sagan, 1977, p. 61).

R-complex

According to MacLean, the R-complex (composed mostly of the olfactostriatum, corpus striatum, and globus pallidus) is important in aggressive behavior, territoriality, ritual, and in the establishment of social hierarchies. Sagan theorizes that the ritual aspects of hebephrenic schizophrenia may be the result of hyperactivity of a center in the R-complex. (In Jacksonian terms, such a symptom would be interpreted as a positive or release symptom.) He also theorizes that the frequent ritualistic behavior of young children may be reflective of incomplete development of the neocortex (in Jacksonian terms, a manifestation of the ascending development in a particular order of brain maturation).

Limbic System

The limbic system (including the olfactory cortex, thalamus, hypothalamus, amygdala, pituitary gland, hippocampus) is apparently involved in generating strong emotions (as opposed to the reptilian mind). Rage, fear, or sentimentality have been observed in malfunctions of the limbic system. The beginnings of altruistic behavior are believed to reside in the limbic system. Emotional aspects of smell (olfactory cortex), remembering and recall (hippocampus), oral and gustatory functions, and sexual functions are also related to limbic system functioning.

Neocortex

The neocortex (including frontal, parietal, temporal, occipital lobes) mediates characteristically human cognitive functions. The various subdivisions may have different functions and some may share functions. For example, the frontal lobe is apparently involved "with deliberation and the regulation of action; the parietal lobes, with spatial perception and the exchange of information between the brain and the rest of the body; the temporal lobes, with a variety of complex perceptual tasks; and the occipital lobes, with vision, the dominant sense in humans and other primates" (Sagan, 1977, p. 72).

Frontal lobes may also be involved in motor as well as cognitive anticipation and implicated in the connection between vision and erect bipedal posture. Also, of great importance to the concept of human neuroevolution in this chapter, the frontal lobes may have been responsible for the human bipedal posture, which, in turn, freed our hands and mouths. And, according to Penfield (1966), sections of the frontal lobes and the temporoparietal region in conjunction with various thalamic nuclei are responsible for spoken language.

In summing his discussion of MacLean's triune-brain model, Sagan (1977, p. 80, 81) warns that it would "be an oversimplification to insist upon perfect separation of function." Nevertheless, "it seems a useful first approximation to consider the ritualistic and hierarchical aspects of our lives to be influenced strongly by the R-complex and shared with our reptilian forebears; the altruistic, emotional and religious aspects of our lives to be localized to a significant extent in the limbic system and shared with our nonprimate mammalian forebears (and perhaps the birds); and reason to be a function of the neocortex, shared to some extent with the higher primates and such cetaceans as dolphins and whales." He goes on to say that, "While ritual, emotion and reasoning are all significant aspects of human nature, the most nearly unique human characteristic is the ability to associate abstractly and to reason."

Integration-Elaboration Concept

Again, the triune-brain model suggests the progressive incorporation of lower brains by higher ones and the subsequent control, modification, and elaboration of all behaviors associated with earlier or lower brains by the highest or latest to evolve brain. And of particular importance to the orientation of this book is the theory that the grand integration by the neocortex of the R-complex and limbic system was responsible for human walking and talking behaviors.

REFLEXIZATION OF MOVEMENT

It is not new or original to hypothesize that reflexes form the basis for voluntary movements. Fay (1954) wrote about eliciting primitive reflexes such as certain spinal automatisms (flexion, extension, cross reflexes) and tonic neck reflexes, such as the asymmetrical tonic neck reflex, in combination and in a prone position to form an early pattern of progression. The organizing of the reflexes into a movement pattern of an amphibian (homolateral crawling) or reptilian (cross-pattern) type was recommended not only to develop muscles and their activity, but also because such maneuvers might result in the emergence of partially controlled coordinated movements. Here Fay was speaking of organizing reflexes into larger patterns and hopefully stimulating higher center control over them—ideas that are in accord with the concept of reflexization of movement.

The author (Mysak, 1968, pp. 73-74) also discussed the basic respiratory activities of coughing, sobbing, sighing, and yawning; the laryngeal or glottic closing reflex; the rooting reflex; the lip reflex; the mouth-opening reflex; basic biting, suckling, chewing patterns; and suckling, swallowing, pharyngeal, palatal, and yawn reflexes, which may all be viewed as precursory patterns to prelinguistic phonatory and articulatory patterns, and, finally, to skilled speech movements. That is, from these basic reflexive movements emerge, respectively, skilled movements necessary for speech breathing; speech voicing; speaker-listener postural attitudes; labial sounds; mandibular sounds; linguadental, lingua-alveolar, linguapalatal, linguavelar sounds; and for producing nasal-nonnasal sound distinctions.

The concept of reflexization of voluntary movement is found in the writings of Rood and the Bobaths. (See Chapter 4.) Others (e.g., Denny-Brown, 1950; Twitchell, 1959) have also expressed ideas relating to "vertical integration" or the concept that willed movements are reflections of composed and integrated basic reflexes.

Reflexes as Components of Volitional Movement

Easton (1972) also hypothesized "that reflexes form the basic language of the motor program." Although the phenomenon of motor coordination has rarely been studied in an integrated fashion, Easton believed findings from studies that have been done on reflexes in pathological situations or special surgical preparations, for example, allow one "to infer that normal motor coordination is based to a huge extent on the reflexes" and that they "very probably underlie all or most volitional movements in man."

Reflexes are economical units with which to compose volitional movements, according to Easton. "Coordinative structure" (CS) is the term Easton uses for the word reflex to connote that the response involves one or more muscles acting together and that it underlies volitionally composed movements. Since the CNS appears designed to respond automatically to certain stimuli with basic reflexes or CSs, and since the CNS is considered to contain a "library" or set of such responses, "It would not be economical if this library of pre-arranged responses, this CS set, were ignored when volitional movements had to be composed. It would be both simpler and faster to choose and concatenate—perhaps orchestrate—elements of the CS set into one grand volitional coordinative structure than to compose such a structure out of individual muscle contractions or changes in joint angles."

Basic coordinative structures or reflexes may be observed in surgical preparations, intact animals, and in mammalian fetuses. For example, the spinal animal (only the cord or part of it is connected to the animal's musculature) shows, among others, the flexion reflex (limb flexion in response to noxious stimulation of the skin), the plantar reflex (plantar flexion of the toes when the sole of the foot is scratched), as well as shake and scratch reflexes. Decerebrate preparations (transection above cord) reveal, for example, a number of reflexes more integrated than spinal reflexes and among them are the tonic neck reflexes (head rotation or neck flexion causes postural changes in limbs that bias musculature toward movement in the direction of gaze), and the labyrinthine, body-on-head, neck, and body-on-body righting reflexes (all responsible for head righting, body aligning, and bringing the animal to its feet). Higher levels of decerebration may allow for stepping, standing, and even locomotion; a very high decerebrate or decorticate preparation may allow running and climbing patterns. The decorticate preparation may differ from the intact animal in its overall behavior only in terms of the behavior being stereotyped and lacking apparent initiative. Intact animals show, of course, the greatest integration in their actions. With functioning cerebral cortex, hopping reactions (reactions that keep the animals' legs beneath its body as seen in humans if the body is physically displaced in space) and placing reactions (as seen in humans when the toe, for example, strikes the curb of a sidewalk and humans automatically lift the foot and place it on the sidewalk to keep from tripping) are observed.

The "reflexive journey" up the neuraxis reveals that even at the spinal level there are CSs that resemble components of volitional movements, and centers capable of producing motor rhythms that contribute, for example, to shaking and scratching behaviors; at the decerebrate level are seen reflexes that coordinate larger groups of muscles and resemble more closely volitional movements; and at still higher levels may be seen reflexive standing, stepping, running, and climbing. This "journey" lends further support to the concept that volitional movements or volitional coordinative structures reflect the selection and concatenation or orchestration of CSs by the CNS.

Reflexes as "Tuners" of Volitional Movement

An associated hypothesis to the idea that reflexes form the "basic language of the motor program" (Easton, 1972) is the one that reflexes appear to be used as facilitators of certain volitional patterns, or as "tuning reflexes."

Reflex postures during "stylized" motor activities such as observed in sports and dancing were studied by Fukada (1961). For example, stances in archery, driving a golf ball, baseball pitching and batting, fencing, boxing, and rifle shooting are suggestive of the asymmetrical tonic neck reflex (head rotation causing postural changes in limbs, i.e., increased extensor tone in face limbs and increased flexor tone in skull limbs, which tend to influence musculature to favor movement in the direction of gaze). Preparatory postures in skiing and broad jumping suggest the use of the symmetrical tonic neck reflex, that is, neck flexion increasing flexor tone in the arms and extensor tone in the legs, and neck extension doing the reverse.

Reflex postures during more "natural" motor activities such as observed in work were studied by Hellebrandt, Schale, and Carnes (1962). For example, lifting a load via wrist flexion was facilitated by head ventroflexion (stimulus for the symmetrical tonic neck reflex), or head rotation away from the arm (stimulus for the asymmetrical tonic neck reflex)—both reflexes influencing the arm musculature in favor of flexor activity. Accordingly, lifting a load via wrist extension was facilitated by head dorsiflexion, or head rotation toward the arm, thus providing stimuli for the tonic neck reflexes that influence the arm musculature in favor of extensor activity.

Movements during free style swimming or during crawl stroke swimming patterns are also suggestive of the CNS using combinations of reflexes or engaging in reflex patterning, in terms of Fay. Crawl stroke swimming may be viewed as a pattern that combines spinal automatisms and the asymmetrical tonic neck reflexes, while breast and butterfly strokes appear to reflect the use of patterns that combine spinal automatisms and the symmetrical tonic neck reflexes.

Easton (1972) also reported the findings of a series of studies to determine whether "there are reflexes linking the extrinsic muscles of the eye (in cats) with the muscles of the rest of the body" or whether there are "eye tuning reflexes." Sensory information from stretch receptors in extrinsic muscles of the eye appeared to influence muscle tone and maybe even labyrinthine reflexes. "The principal effect of stretch of the horizontal eye muscles appears to be a pattern of inhibition tending to foster a turn of the head and neck away from the direction of gaze. The principal effects of stretch of the vertical muscles are on the forelimb muscles, such that downward directed gaze might foster forelimb extension and upward directed gaze forelimb flexion."

The observation of reflex postures during stylized and more natural movement patterns suggests that such reflexes as tonic neck, tonic labyrinthine, righting, and labyrinthine positional reflexes (Landau reflex) provide facilitatory influences for various voluntary movement patterns. It has not been determined whether the reflex pattern is evoked spontaneously as a result of the volitional effort (Hellebrandt, Schale, and Carnes, 1962)—for example, resistance during lifting reflexly regulates the posture of the head, thus stimulating the tonic neck reflex, which, in turn, facilitates the volitional effort—or whether the CNS, sensing the need for more effort, volitionally "recruits" (Easton, 1972) other reflexes (if, indeed, the CNS patterns complex reflexes and volitional movements from basic CSs) to facilitate the effort. Easton appears to favor the latter explanation.

(The concept of the continued use by the CNS of lower-center reflexes would not conflict with the neurotherapies of Fay and Kabat, but would with that of the Bobaths. Chapter 4 is devoted to the discussion of various neurotherapies including those of Fay, Kabat, and the Bobaths.)

In sum then, the observation of progressively more complex reflex activity concomitant with experimental preparations made at higher levels of the neuraxis and the observation of tuning reflexes during normal motor activities may be seen as good support for the concept that reflexes underlie normal motor activities.

Integration-Elaboration Concept

Reflexization of movement, or the progressive incorporation by the CNS of lower order reflex programs into more complicated ones, and the use of those patterns by the CNS to form and facilitate volitional motor activities is specifically supportive of the integration-elaboration concept.

Bipedal Evolution

Bipedal evolution is a specific example of the integration-elaboration concept of CNS development. The progressive integration and elaboration of three modes of human body progression is discussed here: the amphibiotic-reptilian mode, the mammalian-quadrupedal mode, and, finally, the mammalian-bipedal mode. It was this essential evolution that contributed to the appearance of human speech behavior.

Each mode of human body progression is analyzed from the standpoint of elemental versus tuning reflexes and reflex patterns. According to Greene (1969), reflexes may be divided into elemental and tuning reflexes. Elemental reflexes are those that appear like component parts of a particular motor pattern—for example, the spinal reflexes of flexion, extension, and cross reflexes could be viewed as components of a part of a locomotion pattern—or of primitive but complete motor acts like the scratch and righting reactions. Tuning reflexes are those that appear to influence musculature so as to facilitate particular volitional movements; such reflexes may be peripherally elicited during the period of the movement, or centrally recruited. For example, as previously discussed, tonic neck reflexes appear to facilitate particular stylized movements as well as particular natural work movements. Elemental and tuning reflexes are also referred to as phasic and tonic or as nonpostural and postural.

Reflex patterns were discussed by Fay (1954). Fay believed that when spinal automatisms and tonic neck reflexes were viewed separately and with the child in supine, they appeared to have little functional significance; however, with the child in prone, combining the asymmetrical tonic neck reflex with forms of spinal automatisms could produce an amphibian pattern of progression.

AMPHIBIOTIC-REPTILIAN MODE OF PROGRESSION

Fay (1954) described the amphibiotic and reptilian modes of progression, and these patterns were later described and pictorialized by Doman and Delacato (1960). The very early stage is marked by—

- limb movements that allow the child to roll over from prone to supine and back again (rolling over to prone is a critical movement for an overturned frog or salamander);
- primarily upper limb movements that move the child's body in circles or backward (approximately one to five months);
- patternless crawling (arms alone, arm and leg on one side more than the other side) that finally results in body progression toward a particular goal;
- frog-like homologous crawling marked by a push-pull pattern of upper limbs pulling and lower limbs pushing;
- homolateral crawling, also characterized by a push-pull pattern, but this time with the arm and leg of one side pushing while the arm and leg of the other side are pulling; and
- cross-pattern crawling, also characterized by a push-pull pattern, but this time with the right arm and left leg pushing while the left arm and right leg are pulling (two to ten months).

Not all children go through all phases of crawling. Homologous, homolateral, and cross-pattern crawling may be observed in frogs, salamanders, and lizards, respectively. In accord with the integration-elaboration concept is the overlapping of time in the development of the various stages of crawling. Also, the spinal and brainstem (medulla and pons) reflexes appear as the CSs of these crawling patterns.

The analysis of spinal and brainstem reflexes in terms of elemental and tuning reflexes follows.

Elemental Spinal Reflexes

Spinal reflexes, also referred to as Babinski's defensive reflexes and Sherrington's spinal automatisms, are mediated by areas of the CNS up to the base of the fourth ventricle. They are elemental movement reflexes and coordinate the muscles of the limbs in patterns of either total flexion or extension. They have been studied and described by numerous authorities (Sherrington, 1939; Fay, 1954; Roberts, 1967). They may or may not be elicited in normal infants up to two months of age. The persistence of the infantile, nonintegrated form of some of them beyond two months may be an indication of CNS immaturity or dysmaturity (pathology).

The simple stretch reflex is elicited by stretch of a muscle and serves to regulate the length and the rate of change of the length of the muscle. An example of this elemental reflex or CS is the familiar kick reaction following the sudden stretch of the patellar.

The plantar reflex is characterized by plantar flexion of the toes in response to scratch or stroke stimuli applied to the sole of the foot. In early infancy and later in pathology, Babinski's reflex (dorsiflexion of the great toe and fanning of others) may be observed. (A frog manifests a physiologic Babinski when it (a) descends in water, (b) reflexly reaches with its hind legs to touch the bottom, (c) stimulates the "soles" of its hind legs as it touches, (d) and, in turn, elicits the Babinski and extension reflexes, thus propelling itself back to the surface.)

The flexion reflex, or flexor withdrawal pattern, is characterized by flexion at all joints of a limb, dorsiflexion of the foot, and extension of the toes in response to a stimulus (usually pricking) applied to the sole of the foot. Such flexion reflexes have been observed in the arms of children with cerebral palsy who do not show them in the legs.

The extension reflex is characterized by a sudden extension of a limb or contraction of all extensor muscles and inhibition of the flexor muscles in response to a moving stimulus from the ball of the foot onto the toes.

The cross reflex is characterized by flexion of one limb eliciting, in turn, extension of all joints of the contralateral limb or the extension of all joints of a limb accompanying the flexion reflex in the opposite limb. Prolonged stimulation may result in alternating movements that resemble stepping activities.

The long spinal reflexes are elicited by the application of a noxious stimulus to the foot and the response is characterized by flexion of the stimulated limb and the one diagonally opposite with extension of the other two limbs.

Coitus, shake, and scratch reflexes are also mediated at the spinal cord (extended) level. These are considered elemental reflexes, but of the kind that represent complete but primitive motor acts, rather than as components of a particular motor act. In other words, they are already reflecting more complex reflex patterns emerging from simpler ones.

Other reflexes that appear elemental to crawling patterns and that are found in human infants are the upper limb movement, the Moro reflex, and spontaneous and reinforced crawling.

The infantile upper limb movement was described by Thomas (1960, p. 21) in his discussion of the examination of the newborn. The reflex is elicited by placing the child in prone and extending the upper limbs alongside the trunk. A positive response consists of head turning, flexion of arms and forearms, and a moving forward of the upper limbs (that may be facilitated by tactile stimulation of the hands).

The Moro reflex (Magnus, 1926), when elicited in the typical, supine "examination position," is characterized by an abductor-extensor reaction of various body parts in response to sudden noise, movement of the supporting surface, tapping of the abdomen, blowing on the face, and tipping the child backward. Following the response, the arms may be seen to return to the more usual flexed position. The reflex is strong during the first three months of life and becomes weaker and disappears by about four to six months. When viewed from the more functional prone position, it may be interpreted as a body-stabilizing response to sudden disquieting stimuli. The integrated form of the Moro reflex is the startle reaction (McGraw, 1962, p. 19) observed in older children and adults and marked by an adductor-flexor pattern in response to sudden stimuli.

Spontaneous and reinforced crawling may be observed in the newborn infant (Prechtl and Beintema, 1964, p. 48). The activity is elicited by placing the infant in the prone position and waiting for about half a minute. A positive response (likely after the first three or four days of life) is spontaneous crawling movements. Pressing hands gently on the soles of the feet (reinforcing stimulus) may increase crawling movements and may actually cause some movement of the baby (Bauer's response).

The elemental nature of the flexion, extension, and cross reflexes, and the upper limb and reinforced crawling movements, and the more complex long spinal reflexes elicited in prone to homologous, homolateral, and cross-pattern crawling may be obvious. The reason why this elemental nature is not always discernible is that the flexion, extension, and cross reflexes are routinely stimulated in the supine or typical "examining position." In such a position, they have been and still are viewed by many as isolated withdrawal, protective, or defensive reflexes. Also, the upper limb movement and reinforced crawling movements may be viewed as "prone forms" of the flexion reflex (of the arms instead of the legs) and of the cross reflex.

Tuning Brainstem (Medulla and Pons) Reflexes

Brainstem reflexes may be considered the other half of the amphibiotic-reptilian mode of progression. Brainstem reflexes are considered tuning, tonic, or postural reflexes and effect changes in the distribution of muscle tone throughout the body. They are activated when there is a change in the position of the head and body in space (stimulation of the labyrinths), or when there is a change in the position of the head in relation to the body (stimulation of neck proprioceptors). They were studied in laboratory animals (Sherrington, 1939, 1947; Magnus, 1926) and in human infants (Gesell, 1938). They may or may not be elicited in the normal child within the first four to six months, and reflect a higher level of integration than the spinal reflexes in keeping with the integration-elaboration concept. Persistence of these reflexes in their infantile, nonintegrated forms may be an indication of CNS immaturity or dysmaturity.

The tonic neck reflexes (TNR) are elicited through head rotation (asymmetrical TNR) or neck flexion (symmetrical TNR) and are characterized by postural changes in the limbs that tune the musculature in favor of movement toward the direction of gaze. The asymmetrical TNR is obtained from muscles of the neck and probably from receptors of the ligaments and joints of the cervical spine; the reflex increases extensor tone in the face limbs and increases flexor tone in the skull limbs. The change in tonus is primarily seen in the arms. The symmetrical TNR is also obtained from sense receptors of the neck; head extension increases extensor tone in the arms and flexor tone in the legs and head flexion increases flexor tone in the arms and extensor tone in the legs.

The tonic labyrinthine reflexes (TLR) are elicited through changes of the angle of the head with the horizontal, probably through stimulation of the otoliths of the labyrinths, and are characterized by postural changes of flexion or extension in all four limbs. It is obvious that symmetrical TNRs and TLRs are interacting. The supine position of the head produces maximal extensor tone, while the prone position produces maximal flexor tone. Again, position of the head and moving or preparing to move in the direction of gaze tunes the muscles and facilitates the movement.

Pattern Analysis of Spinal and Brainstem Reflexes

The analysis of reflex patterns of spinal and brainstem reflexes was done early by Fay (1954). He recognized that TNRs and spinal automatisms like the flexion, extension, and cross reflexes when elicited in supine and individually appeared to have no functional significance. However, if combined and organized in prone they form a total pattern movement of an amphibian or reptilian type.

In fact, with appropriate alternation of head flexion and extension in prone one might elicit a symmetrical TNR that may tune the muscles in the direction of gaze such that a homologous crawling pattern is stimulated. In this example, the symmetrical TNR in prone reflects the integration and elaboration of the spinal automatisms into a new whole. So, too, a fully expressed asymmetrical TNR in prone tunes musculature in such a way as to stimulate the homolateral crawling pattern. Finally, head rotation in combination with the long spinal reflexes forms cross-pattern crawling.

Figure 1.1 illustrates the integration of spinal (symbolized by the circle) and brainstem (symbolized by the square) reflexes and their elaboration into various crawling patterns. For many years the author used the "tree" analogy to depict sensorimotor integration of the CNS only to find that Easton (1972) has also used the analogy but in not quite the same way.

Figure 1.2 shows the functional test position for spinal reflexes; Figure 1.3 shows the functional test position for the brainstem reflexes.

Fig. 1.1. Tree of progressive integration and elaboration in bipedal evolution

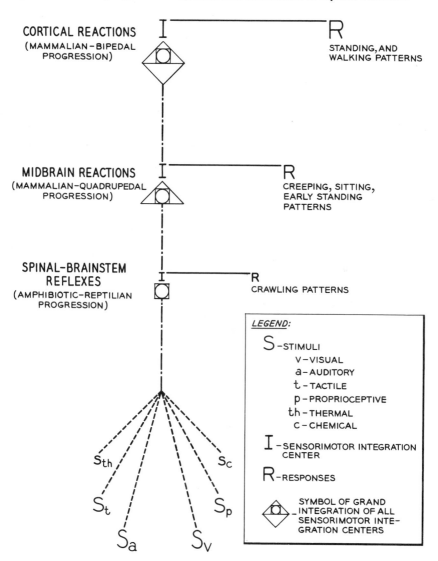

Fig. 1.2. Spinal reflexes elicited in the functional prone position

flexion reflex

(a)

(b)

extension reflex

(a)

(b)

cross reflex

(a)

(b)

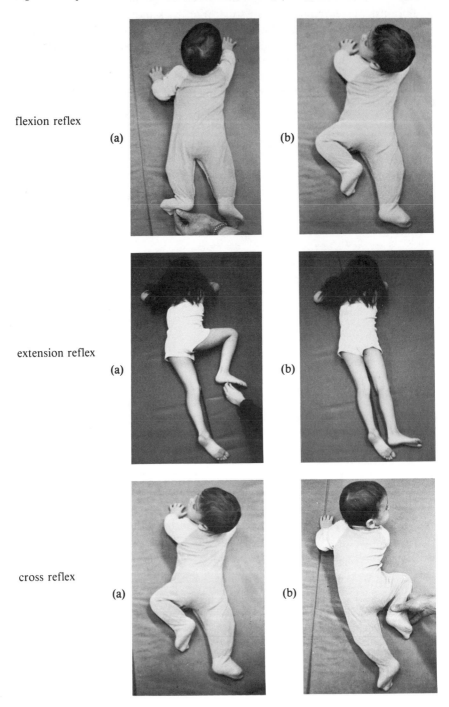

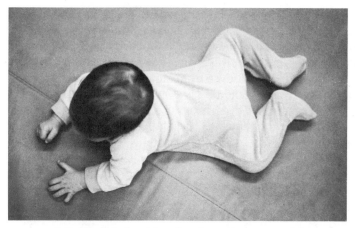

symmetrical tonic neck reflex (homologous crawling)

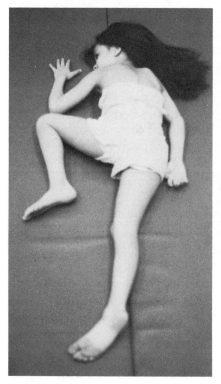

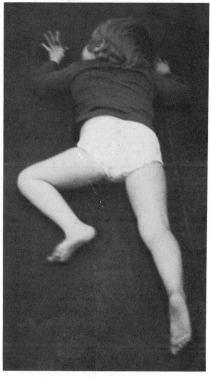

asymmetrical tonic neck reflex
(homolateral crawling)

long spinal reflex
(cross-pattern crawling)

MAMMALIAN-QUADRUPEDAL MODE OF PROGRESSION

The mammalian-quadrupedal mode of progression is characterized by (a) preparatory movements that bring the child into a "four-foot" standing position and (b) reciprocal movements of the four limbs that carry the child forward. More specifically, this integration-elaboration stage is marked by the child's capacity to roll over from supine, to sit up, to stand on hands and knees, and even to stand on two legs with assistance. The actual mode of body progression, however, is on all fours or the creeping position. As with the development of crawling, there are usually various phases in creeping development, which are not always reflected in the creeping development of every child. First, the child may push himself up onto his hands and knees and hold the position without moving. Then, he begins to move without rhythm or pattern similar to his early attempts at crawling. Then, as in crawling, homologous creeping ("bunny walk"), homolateral creeping, and finally, cross-pattern creeping phases follow (four to fifteen months). The phases in creeping reflect the direct integration of the phases in crawling, but with the elaboration of them reflected by the "four-limb standing," anti-gravity position. The associated development of sitting is marked by complete rotation of the child in supine into prone, then on fours, and into side sitting. Partial rotation pattern and symmetrical pattern into long sitting and chair sitting follow. Midbrain reflexes appear as the CSs of these four-foot walking or creeping patterns and sitting patterns.

The analysis of midbrain reactions in terms of elemental and tuning reactions follows. In keeping with the integration-elaboration concept, the change from reflex to reaction here signifies that these responses are less automatic, more complex, and less organized reflexes.

Elemental Righting Reactions

Righting reactions are integrated at the level of the midbrain above the red nucleus, not including the cortex. They interact with each other and combine to establish a normal head and body relationship in space, as well as in relation to each other, and bring the creature to its feet or the child to all fours. Righting reactions develop in a definite sequence from birth onward and their appearance coincides with the recognized milestones of the child's motor development. As cortical influences increase, they are gradually integrated by around the age of three to five years. Early studies of these reactions were reported by Magnus (1926). The Bobaths (1964) also studied these reactions in terms of their application in neurotherapy. Seven of the righting reactions are identified here.

The neck righting reaction is characterized by rotation of the body as a whole in the direction to which the head is rotated. Neck proprioceptors appear to be the essential receptors. The reaction is present at birth, is strong until four months, and diminishes thereafter. A lack of neck righting after one month or the persistence of the infantile, nonintegrated form after six months may be an indication of CNS immaturity or dysmaturity.

The labyrinthine-on-head righting reaction is characterized by head raising in prone between one and three months and head raising in supine between four and six months. For a true evaluation of the reaction the child should be blindfolded, so as to eliminate the influence of the optical-on-head righting reaction. The reaction may be observed in the upright position by holding the child in space in the pelvic area and tipping him to the right and to the left. Tipping should elicit automatic righting reactions of the head maintaining the head in the normal, face vertical-mouth horizontal position. Reactions in prone, supine, and in the upright position may be elicited throughout life. A lack of response in the prone after the second month, in the supine after the sixth month, and in the upright position after the eighth month may be indications of CNS immaturity or dysmaturity.

The optical-on-head righting reaction is characterized by the head following movements of the eyes (and thus the eyes contribute to head orientation). The reaction is of secondary importance at first but gains quickly in influence as the child develops. Testing is similar to that for the labyrinthine-on-head righting reaction minus the blindfold. The child is moved through prone, supine, and right and left upright positions. However, if the labyrinthine-on-head righting reaction is active, it will confound testing for the optical reaction. As with the labyrinthine reaction, optical reactions are elicited throughout life. Accordingly, they should be elicited in prone at about one to two months, in supine at about six months, and in right-left tilting in the upright position at about six to eight months.

The body-on-head righting reaction serves to right the head in response to some part of the body touching a surface; for example, automatic head righting follows when an individual's feet touch the ground or when the side of the body presses against a surface. This reaction interacts closely with the labyrinthine-on-head reaction to maintain the normal position of the head in space. It may be observed at about four to six months and is integrated between one and five years.

The quadrupedal righting reaction is prerequisite to assuming the quadrupedal position from prone lying. Pressure applied with fingers in the pelvic area of both sides of the body or a lifting maneuver on both sides may result in automatic flexion of arms, hips, and knees. Continuation of this flexor pattern brings the child into the quadrupedal position. (When the stimulus is applied to only one side of the pelvis, unilateral flexion is elicited with the child remaining in prone, and this has been called the "amphibian reaction." The unilateral form may be functional for homolateral crawling activities but not for assuming the first stage of homolateral creeping.) The quadrupedal righting reaction may be observed at about six to eight months and remains active throughout life.

The body-on-body righting reaction modifies the neck righting reaction by the addition of a rotation of the trunk between the shoulders and the pelvis. For example, first there is head rotation, then there is pectoral or shoulder girdle rotation, and, finally, pelvic girdle rotation. Neck proprioceptors and the tactile sense organs of the body surface are among the essential sensory receptors stimulated. The reaction appears around the sixth to eighth month and is integrated by about two years.

The sitting righting reaction reflects the progressive integration of the body-on-body righting reaction as follows: (a) The complete rotation pattern from supine is characterized by the child rolling over to his abdomen, getting onto all fours (quadrupedal righting reaction), and then side sitting. (b) The partial rotation pattern from supine is characterized by the child rolling over toward one arm, raising himself onto the forearm, and, finally, pushing up into the long sitting position. (c) The symmetrical sitting pattern from supine reflects the complete integration of body-on-body righting reactions by the child symmetrically flexing the head and hips and bringing the head and trunk into the long sitting position. The complete rotation pattern may be observed from ten to twelve months on, the partial rotation pattern from about two to three years on, and the symmetrical pattern after five years and on throughout life. Depending on fatigue, illness, degree of sobriety, sleepiness, and so on, the adult may use complete rotation or partial rotation patterns to assume sitting.

Other reactions that appear elemental to sitting and creeping patterns and that are found in human infants are the bowing reflex, primary sitting, arm walking, arm-support reactions, hopping reactions, and placing response of upper limb.

The bowing reflex, originally reported by Gamper, was described by Peiper (1963, p. 71). The reflex is characterized by head and neck ventroflexion, followed by ventroflexion of the trunk, and eventual sitting with a curved back in response to pressure applied to lower limbs, or to extension of the thighs at the hip joints with the child in supine. The primitive sitting position is accomplished by frequent sideward turns of the head and trunk (tuning movements). The reflex is occasionally elicited in healthy, premature infants. It may be viewed as a "rehearsal phenomenon" for the eventual symmetrical sitting pattern.

Primary sitting, or infantile passive and spontaneous sitting reactions, were described by Thomas (1960, p. 41). Sitting reactions are elicited by pulling the infant by his hands from supine into sitting. During the first weeks, the posture is accomplished with a head lag. At about three months, the head assumes a more normal position, but the baby still takes no active part in the movement. However, near the end of the first six months, only a slight pull by the hand is needed to elicit the primary sitting pattern.

Arm walking, or "wheelbarrow reaction," may be observed during the second to sixth month and prior to the emergence of spontaneous creeping activity. A tendency toward rhythmic progression of the arms might be observed when the child is held up by the trunk and legs and moved forward. The initial response is usually a forward movement on forearms with clenched fists; eventually, the arms and fingers extend and alternating movements of the arms gradually improve. Arm walking is apparently an early form of dynamic arm-support reactions.

Arm-support reactions are marked by automatic extension of the arms with abduction and extension of the fingers. Depending on how they are elicited, they may serve a protective function or a dynamic one. The protective function may be elicited by lifting a child freely in the air from the prone position by the ankles, and then moving his head suddenly toward the surface. Early studies of such a reaction were reported by Schaltenbrand (1927). Similar reactions have been studied by various individuals and called by different names, for example, the parachute reaction. It has also been referred to as the precipitation reflex (Rademaker, 1935). Under this name, it may be tested by holding the baby upright in space by his trunk and then moving the child downward and sideways toward a surface. A positive response consists of upper limb extension, including fingers, toward the surface in a seeking-for-support pattern. The response appears before actual contact is made by the upper limbs. The limb-supporting activity is strong enough to support the body weight. Also, each limb can be evaluated separately. In sitting, the reactions are first active when the child is tipped forward (around six months), then sideways (around eight months), and then backward (around ten months) (Thomas, Dargassies, and Chesni, 1960, p. 41). In general, the arm-support reactions may be observed from about four to six months, and they remain active throughout life. (They are also observed in the creeping posture, on-knees, and standing positions).

Dynamic arm-support reactions describe those involved in alternating and reciprocal arm-support activity as seen in arm-walking and in various forms of creeping.

Hopping reactions (quadrupedal) are movements that continue to bring the limbs beneath the body so as to maintain its support. For example, if someone attempts to push an on-fours child off balance to the right or left the limbs automatically lift, follow the body, and are replaced in their appropriate supportive positions.

Placing reaction of upper limb (quadrupedal) was described by Thomas (1960, p. 39). The reaction is elicited by holding the infant upright and then applying the back of one of his hands to the edge of a surface like a table. The first stage of the reaction consists of upper limb flexion bringing the hand above the surface; the second stage consists of limb extension in a supporting movement, the supporting reaction of the upper limb taking place first with the use of the fist and later on with the use of an open palm. The reaction may be observed by about the third or fourth month on. It appears elemental to creeping patterns and functions as a response to the child's hand coming in contact with a raised surface, for example, a step, or to the child's hand and arm suddenly dropping as a result of an unexpected depression in the surface like a hole.

Tuning Midbrain Reactions

The Landau and Schaltenbrand reactions, the chain-in-prone reaction, and the ocular reactions may be considered as tuning reactions. As with the tuning brainstem reflexes, tuning midbrain reactions serve to influence musculature so as to facilitate particular volitional movements.

The Landau reaction (Schaltenbrand, 1927; Byers, 1938) represents a combination of tonic and righting reflexes. To elicit the reaction, the child is held in the air in the prone position (support by one hand under the trunk); this stimulates on-head righting reactions causing head raising into the normal vertical position, which, in turn, stimulates tonic extension of the spine and legs. Stimulation of this synreflexic pattern or chain reaction in the upright position results in early or "midbrain standing," or standing that requires the child to hold on or to be assisted. It is standing without balance reactions and thus is not self-maintaining. In this case, it is the on-head righting reactions that tune and facilitate extension of spine and legs, thus allowing primitive standing. The reaction appears at about six months and is integrated by two or three years of age when cortical integration allows true bipedal standing supported by bipedal balance and support reactions.

The Schaltenbrand reaction is the reverse of the Landau. That is, once the synreflexic activity has resulted in the normal head position and spine and leg extension, the head is physically flexed and this is followed by flexion of the spine and legs. In effect, it represents an "untuning" maneuver. Stimulation of the reaction in the upright position results in body flexion or "midbrain sitting."

The chain-in-prone reaction, described by Peiper (1963, pp. 180–91) may very well be an early form of the Landau reaction. "As soon as the infant succeeds in righting his head in space, his whole body tries by means of reflexes to adjust to this position. Chain reflexes starting from the head regulate the position of the neck, trunk, arms, pelvis, and legs down to the tips of the toes in order to maintain equilibrium." The reaction is elicited by placing the child in prone on a table, and moving his head and trunk forward over the edge of the table so that only the pelvis remains supported by the table (examiner holds child in the area of the upper thighs). The response consists of on-head righting reactions, stimulating body-on-body righting reactions causing upward arching of the head and trunk; and tonic neck and tonic labyrinthine reflexes causing tonic extension of the spine and legs and simultaneous raising and sideways stretching and flexing at the elbows of both arms. The reaction gradually appears during the first month of life and is integrated at about two years.

The Landau and chain reactions are good examples of the integration of tuning brainstem reflexes by tuning midbrain reactions.

Eye movement reactions were studied by Easton (1972). Eye movements, at least in the cat, provide data from stretch receptors that appear useful in modifying muscle tone and possibly in modifying labyrinthine reflexes. "The principal effect of stretch of the horizontal eye muscles appears to be a pattern of inhibition tending to foster a turn of the head and neck away from the direction of gaze. The principal effects of stretch of the vertical muscles are on the forelimb muscles, such that downward directed gaze might foster forelimb extension and upward directed gaze forelimb flexion." The tuning of the head to move away from the direction of gaze may be useful in serialized head movements in crawling, visual scanning, and change-of-direction movements.

Pattern Analysis of the Midbrain Reactions

The pattern analysis of midbrain reactions is more straightforward than the analysis of spinal and brainstem reflexes. In general, the midbrain reactions are involved with head righting, aligning the body with the head, and with bringing the child into on-fours, or the creeping position. The role of the neck righting, on-head righting, body-on-body righting, and quadrupedal righting reactions as components or parts of the total pattern of assuming the on-fours position from the supine is obvious. The role of the elements of arm walking, dynamic arm-support reactions, and quadrupedal hopping, and placing reactions to the development of homologous, homolateral, and cross-pattern creeping should also be evident. The bowing reflex and primary sitting are viewed as elemental reflexes of the crude-but-complete motor-act variety. Some of the tuning reflexes on this level appear to be preparing the child for early bipedal standing. The role of eye-movement reactions as tuning reflexes appears tied to the concept that the head leads all motor activities and that eye and head movements are intimately related. Eye movements could facilitate certain muscle patterns directly, or could stimulate particular head movements, which subsequently may bias particular musculature in favor of particular movement patterns.

Figure 1.1 on page 33 illustrates the integration of spinal and brainstem reflexes by midbrain (symbolized by the triangle) reactions and their elaboration into creeping, sitting, and early standing activities.

Figure 1.4 depicts the quadrupedal or on-fours righting reaction elicited from prone; Figure 1.5 shows homologous, homolateral, and cross-pattern creeping; and Figure 1.6 shows three stages of the integration of body-on-body righting reactions resulting in the sitting position.

Fig. 1.4. Quadrupedal righting reaction elicited in functional prone position

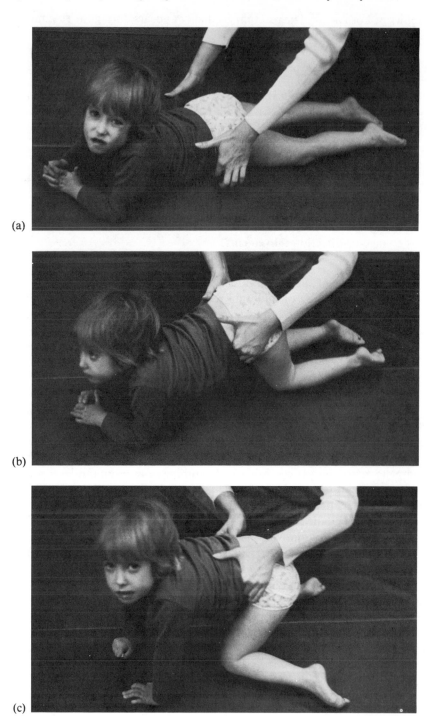

(a)

(b)

(c)

Fig. 1.5. Quadrupedal progression patterns: integration of creeping patterns into cross-pattern creeping

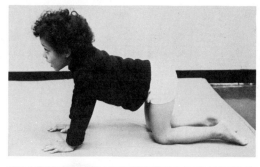

starting position

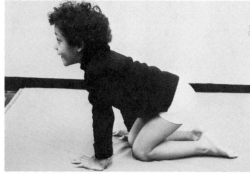

homologous
progression

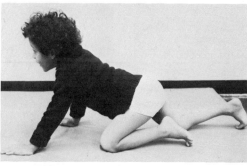

homolateral
progression

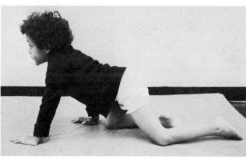

cross-pattern progression

Fig. 1.6. Sitting righting reactions: integration of body-on-body righting
reactions into symmetrical sitting

complete rotation
pattern

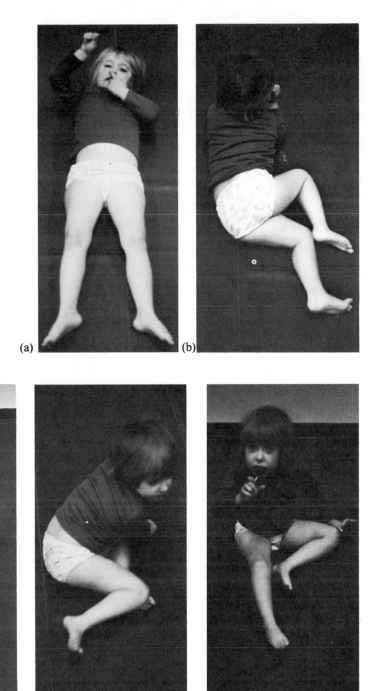

(a)

(b)

(c)

(d)

(e)

partial rotation pattern   symmetrical pattern

(a)   (a)

(b)   (b)

(c)   (c)

MAMMALIAN-BIPEDAL MODE OF PROGRESSION

When the child reaches the mammalian-bipedal mode of progression, she has reached the prerequisite level for the highest form of motor behavior—speech behavior. The child can now assume standing from supine independently, either through a complete rotation pattern (10 to 12 months), partial rotation pattern (2 to 3 years), or a symmetrical pattern (about 5 years).

Again, as with the crawling and creeping stages of progression, bipedal progression also reflects phases in its full development. First, the child assumes kneeling and standing by pulling herself up with someone's assistance or with the aid of some furniture (chair, sofa) or play objects. Erect arm walking follows and is characterized by taking steps and moving sideways along the object; forward walking begins when the child holds on only with one hand. Erect arm walking along furniture and various objects, or side walking, has also been referred to as "cruising" (Doman, Delacato, and Doman, 1960). Erect arm walking is followed by free or patternless forward walking (the "hold-up" position or arms held in a flexor pattern, sometimes above the level of the shoulder as though preparatory for an arm-support or protective reaction in the event the child falls forward). Finally, forward walking in cross-pattern is observed (10 to 25 months). Upright arm walking, or upright creeping (i.e., side walking), may be observed as the early stage of integration of midbrain quadrupedal progression by cortical centers; cross-pattern walking may be viewed as the ultimate stage of integration of quadrupedal progression.

Cortical reactions are involved with planned volitional movements (concatenated or orchestrated basic coordinative structures or reflexes), the full development of equilibrium reactions, as well as with bipedal placing and supporting reactions. The analysis of cortical reactions in terms of elemental and tuning reactions follows.

Elemental Equilibrium Reactions

Equilibrium reactions are mediated by the efficient interaction of the cortex, basal ganglia, and cerebellum. Body proprioceptors are the main receptors; labyrinths are active to a lesser degree. They occur only when muscle tone is normal or near normal and provide for body adaptation in response to a change in the center of gravity of the body. They emerge from about six months on, are active throughout life, and find their full development in human beings. Early studies of these reactions were made by Rademaker (1935), Weisz (1938), and Zador (1938). These reactions have also been studied by the Bobaths (1964), specifically as they apply to their treatment approach.

Equilibrium reactions, or adjustments to changing gravitational and spatial relationships, have at least two components: a balance component and a supportive-protective one. For example, if the trunk of an individual in standing is slowly pushed laterally by the application of pressure on the opposite side of the trunk, and if the individual resists this body displacement, the following sequence of activities may be observed:

1. On-head righting reaction, maintaining the head in the normal position of face vertical, mouth horizontal
2. Shifting muscle tonus in the arm toward which the trunk is being pushed in preparation for the extension and abduction of that limb (supportive-protective activity), and shifting muscle tonus in the opposite arm and leg in preparation for extension and abduction of those limbs (balance activity)
3. With continued trunk displacement, the eventual emergence of an extensor-abductor pattern of the upper limb toward which the weight is being transferred, and the concomitant emergence of abductor-extensor patterns of upper and lower limb opposite to the side of weight transference
4. Continued lateral displacement of the body causing balance failure resulting in hopping reactions of the legs to keep the legs beneath the body, and balance-support movements of the upper limbs to keep the body from falling

The last phase describes equilibrium activities designed to regain equilibrium. If all fails, and there is actual loss of balance, arm-support reactions become functional as the arms reach out and protect the head and upper body as the individual falls to the ground. This example of the dynamics of maintaining, regaining, or losing equilibrium reflects the integration and elaboration by the cortical level of elemental, midbrain arm-support and hopping reactions and various brainstem and midbrain tuning reactions.

Equilibrium reactions are discussed further in terms of their pre-walking and walking functions.

Pre-walking equilibrium reactions are involved with stabilizing various levels of motor development. When a child achieves a new developmental motor level, for example, sitting, it is stabilized only if the child develops the necessary arm-support and balance reactions in the sitting position. (At one level of motor development, such reactions usually indicate that the next higher level is possible.) Following are descriptions of the full range of pre-walking equilibrium reactions beginning from their earliest appearance.

1. Prone and supine equilibrium reactions may be elicited on a tilt board by slowly tipping the child to one side. Arching of the head and body toward the raised side and abduction and extension of the arms and legs in balance movements (limbs on raised side) and support

movements (limbs on lowered side) is the expected response. The reaction may be observed in prone at about four to six months and in supine at about seven to ten months.

2. Side-lying equilibrium reactions are primarily demonstrated by shifting muscle tonus and an arm-support reaction. If a child in the side-lying position is slowly raised by the upper arm, angulation of the head toward the raised side with leg abduction on that side and abduction and extension of the arm on the opposite side is the expected response.

3. On-elbows equilibrium reactions are stimulated with the child in the prone-on-elbows pattern. Gently pushing the child from front-to-back and from side-to-side should result in alternating shift of muscle tonus to support arm-balance movements and arm-support activity. The on-elbows, or on-twos position, may be viewed as preliminary to the on-fours position.

4. On-heels (on-threes) equilibrium reactions are elicited with the child in the heel-sitting position. Again, gently pushing the child from front-to-back and from side-to-side should result in an alternating shift of muscle tonus resulting in arm-support reactions, or extensor-abductor patterns of the limbs toward the side of weight transference (support reactions) and similar patterns on the opposite side (balance reactions). The on-heels position is also preliminary to the on-fours position, and on-heels equilibrium allows for homologous creeping or "bunny-hop progression."

5. On-fours, or quadrupedal, equilibrium reactions are elicited by gently rocking the child in a forward-backward or side-to-side fashion. Alternating muscle tonus representing limb balance and support reactions should be observed. Loss of balance in side-to-side displacement should result in quadrupedal hopping reactions. On-fours equilibrium allows for homolateral and cross-pattern creeping. It appears at about 8 to 10 months.

6. Sitting equilibrium reactions may be elicited in side-sitting, long-sitting, and chair-sitting positions. In chair-sitting, for example, displacing the child's trunk backward results in a forward extension of head, shoulders, arms, and legs in an overall balance reaction to compensate for the backward weight displacement; displacing the child's trunk forward results in flexion of legs, extension of neck and spine, and backward movement of the arms as a balance reaction to compensate for the forward weight displacement. Displacing the trunk toward one side results in an on-head righting reaction and the typical support reaction (extension-abduction of limbs) to the side of weight transference and the typical balance reaction on the opposite side.

Sitting equilibrium reactions should be observed at about 10 to 12 months.

A lack of response in the pre-walking equilibrium reactions at the times specified may be an indication of CNS immaturity or dysmaturity.

Walking equilibrium reactions are concerned with bringing the individual into the bipedal position and finally to bipedal progression. Reactions involved in assuming and stabilizing standing are described first.

1. On-knees equilibrium reactions may be elicited in side-to-side and front-to-back modes. Sideward displacement of the body by applying pressure on one side of the trunk should result in an on-head righting reaction, balance reactions in the arm and leg opposite to the side of weight transference with the knee on that side raising off the support, and arm-support reactions toward the side of weight transference, without the hand on that side touching the ground. Backward displacement of the body results in a forward movement of the head, shoulders, and arms, while forward displacement results in on-head righting with extension of neck and spine and backward movement of the arms. On-knees equilibrium allows for a form of upright creeping. It appears at about 13 to 15 months.

2. Half-kneel equilibrium reactions are observed with the foot of one leg brought forward and set on the ground. Gentle displacement from front-to-back and side-to-side rocking movements should elicit appropriate head and trunk righting and arm balance and support reactions. Half-kneel equilibrium is prerequisite to bipedal standing.

3. Simian stance equilibrium reactions represent those found in a position that links quadrupedal creeping with bipedal walking. With the child on his feet, his body crouched, hands open and touching the floor between abducted knees, appropriate balance and arm-support reactions may be observed in response to side-to-side rocking movements. Pushing forward on the child's back may stimulate semi-upright walking and eventual bipedal standing. The reaction may be observed at about 15 to 18 months.

4. Standing equilibrium reactions may be observed in a number of forms. With the child in standing, hold him by the knees or at the level of the pelvis and gently displace the knees or hips in a front-to-back, side-to-side, and rotatory manner. Head and trunk righting and appropriate arm balance and support reactions should be observed.

   Or the child's weight may be shifted to one side by pressure applied to the side of the trunk or hips resulting in extension and abduction of his weight-free leg (balance reaction) with extension and abduction of the opposite arm (support reaction). Or, hold the child from behind under his shoulder girdle, tip him backwards and observe the forward movement of his head, shoulders and arms, and dorsiflexion of the feet. These reactions may be observed at about 12 to 18 months.

Preparatory reactions for bipedal progression are described next.

1. Step-position equilibrium reactions are stimulated with the child standing with one foot in front of the other. Arm-balance and support reactions are stimulated by gentle forward-backward displacement of the trunk.
2. One-leg equilibrium reactions are stimulated by flexing the knee of one leg from behind and by gently moving the child in various directions over the standing leg. Support may need to be given the child by holding the opposite arm. Head and trunk righting and appropriate arm balance and support reactions should be elicited. Another one-leg equilibrium reaction has been called the seesaw reaction (Weisz, 1938). At the side of the child, the examiner raises the leg on that side into flexion with the dorsiflexed foot held in the palm of the examiner's hand and with the arm on that side held by the examiner's other hand. The examiner then pulls the child gently forward by the arm, which should stimulate strong extension and abduction of the lifted leg plus righting and balance reactions of the head, arms, and thorax. Finally, the examiner lowers the extended leg to the ground in a heel strike manner as in a normal stepping action. This reaction may be observed at about 15 months.
3. Hopping reactions in the bipedal posture represent reactions designed to regain equilibrium. They are stimulated by holding the child from behind under the shoulder girdle and moving him quickly for a certain distance through space in forward, backward, and sideways directions. The response is characterized by the lifting and replacing of the legs beneath the displaced trunk. Such reactions may be observed at about 15 to 18 months.

Other elemental standing or walking reactions are the positive and negative leg-supporting reactions, placing response of the lower limb, and primary and definitive walking.

1. Positive and negative leg-supporting reactions may be viewed as precursor activities to standing and walking. The positive leg-supporting reaction is characterized by simultaneous contraction of flexors and extensors, exerting a synergic action and resulting in fixation of the joints of the legs. Stretching of the intrinsic muscles of the feet by contact of the soles of the feet with the ground or other surface

is the appropriate stimulus for the reaction. Reflex relaxation of the extensors of the proximal joints to allow flexion for reciprocation characterizes the negative leg-supporting reaction. Although lack of a positive leg-supporting reaction may be abnormal after four months, a continuous, positive leg-supporting reaction may be abnormal after eight months. The elements of future standing and bipedal progression are obvious in these reactions.

2. Placing reactions of the lower limb (Prechtl and Beintema, 1964, p. 53) are important for equilibrium when the leg approaches a step or when it suddenly descends into a hole or depression. The reaction may be tested by lightly pressing the dorsum of one foot against the edge of a table or other surface. The first stage of the reaction consists of lower limb flexion bringing the limb above the table; the second stage consists of limb extension upon contact of the sole of the foot with the table. The reaction may be observed as early as after the first 10 days of life and a form of it remains active throughout life.

3. Primary and definitive walking activity may be seen as precursory or "rehearsal phenomena" for later walking. Primary walking activity in the newborn was described by Thomas (1960, p. 31). Walking movements with good coordination and regular rhythm but without balancing or associated movements of the upper limbs may be stimulated by holding the newborn upright with feet on the surface and by gently moving him in a forward direction. The reaction does not occur backwards. It may be observed up to several weeks.

Primary walking activity changes after several weeks. There is increasing use of the toe-tips, and speed, rhythm, and coordination diminish. During the period of transition from primary to definitive walking, or between the second and sixth months, the feet begin to drag, and near the end of the period the infant tends to jump or to beat the floor with the feet in an alternating fashion. At about the sixth or seventh month, the stage of definitive walking emerges and the infant again takes steps if he is lifted and pushed along. These first steps do not show the coordination characteristics of primary walking. The sequence of foot contact with the ground is first by the toes, then by the whole sole, and later the heel touches first.

Related to the phenomena associated with transition from primary to definitive walking and to the concept of progressive integration and elaboration of the CNS are statements by McGraw (1962, p. 23) on neonatal neuromuscular behavior. McGraw indicated that the course of development in each function represents "a period during which the behavior reflects further maturation of subcortical or nuclear mechanisms; a period of diminution in overt expression, which seemingly reflects the onset of cortical inhibition upon the functioning of nuclear centers; the invasion of cortical control over the function, as indicated by the deliberate or voluntary quality of overt activity; and, finally, the integration of the various neural centers involved in a function, as evidenced by a smooth, frictionless type of performance.'' McGraw's statement is specific to the integration-elaboration concept of CNS maturation.

Tuning Cortical Reactions

Forms of the tonic neck, tonic labyrinthine, on-head righting, and eye movement reflexes may be considered as tuning cortical reactions.

Tonic neck reflexes apparently provide a facilitatory influence on volitional efforts related to stylized movements such as in sports, dance, and so on, and to natural work movements such as in lifting loads.

Head and body righting reactions are used to facilitate sitting and standing from supine and prone-lying positions.

Eye movement reactions facilitate head movements that, in turn, facilitate various volitional movements. More direct influence of eye movements may be seen in stylized movements such as in a golf swing where a downward directed gaze may facilitate upper limb extension; or in jumping over a high object where an upward directed gaze may facilitate lower limb flexion.

Changing direction during walking may also be facilitated by eye-head reflexive movements.

Pattern Analysis of Cortical Reactions

A pattern analysis of cortical reactions shows that all patterns necessary for bipedal standing and walking are already present at the midbrain level of maturation. Cortical equilibrium and associated reactions have two major roles: (a) They stabilize all lower-level motor milestones like the prone-on-elbows position and the quadrupedal position and various forms of sitting and (b) they allow for bipedal standing and bipedal progression.

Standing on lower limbs and "upright creeping," so to speak, reflect the ultimate integration by the cortical centers of spinal, brainstem, and midbrain reactions. More specifically, true standing and walking reflect the integration of righting reactions that bring the child into standing; arm-balance and support reactions that stabilize the bipedal posture; and leg support, hopping, and placement reactions that contribute to the bipedal mode of body progression. In short, fully developed cortical reactions allow the child who is capable of cross-pattern creeping to rise on his "hindlegs" and engage in erect cross-pattern creeping or bipedal walking. In erect creeping, the positive support function of the upper limbs is integrated into associated arm-swing movements used for balance and support movements. Bipedal progression waits upon the cooperation of the frontal lobes of the neocortex and is usually concomitant with or heralds speaking activities.

Cortical integration of tuning reflexes and reactions reveals the use of a pattern of head, neck, and eye tuning reflexes and reactions from all levels of CNS maturation to facilitate bipedal standing and walking behavior.

Figure 1.1 on page 33 illustrates the grand integration of spinal, brainstem, and midbrain centers by cortical (symbolized by the diamond) centers and the elaboration of their motor patterns into bipedal standing and walking. Figure 1.7 shows pre-walking equilibrium reactions stabilizing the on-forearms, on-fours, and chair-sitting positions. Figure 1.8 shows walking equilibrium reactions in on-knees, standing, and one-leg positions.

Fig. 1.7. Pre-walking equilibrium reactions

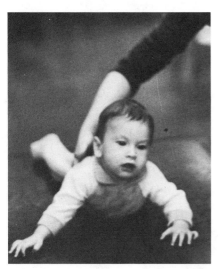

(a) on-forearms balance

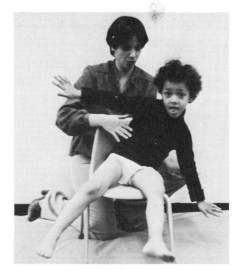

(c) chair-sitting balance

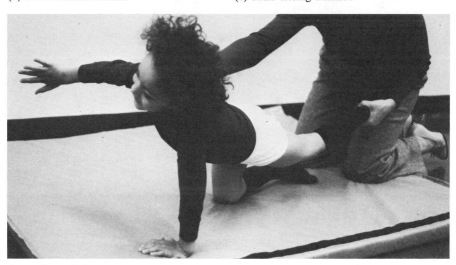

(b) on-fours balance

Fig. 1.8. Walking equilibrium reactions

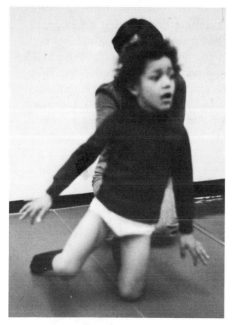

on-knees

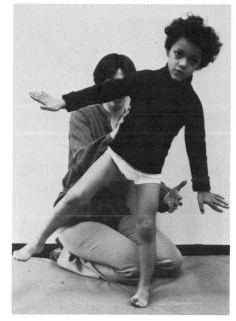

standing

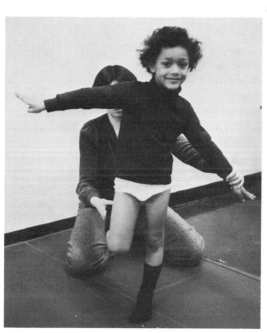

one-leg position

Although the concept is not universally accepted, the author believes the progressive integration-elaboration concept of neuroevolution is well supported by the discussions of Jackson's evolution and dissolution of the nervous system, recapitulation theory, triune brain, reflexization of movement, and the progressive integration and elaboration of modes of human body progression.

Evolution of Expressive Communication

The progressive integration-elaboration concept of CNS maturation is developed further through a discussion that relates the concept more specifically to the speech central nervous system (SCNS), or to the evolution of expressive communication. Discussions of corticalization and speech and the origins of speech are included here.

CORTICALIZATION AND SPEECH

The emergence of speech waits upon a particular type of brain evolution—one characterized by a vertical-lateral integration. Cerebral maturation, the uncommitted cortex, and cerebral dominance are important factors in this vertical-lateral integration of the SCNS. The discussion of corticalization and speech is based on knowledge of the ontogenesis of the SCNS, and its relationship to the phylogenesis of the SCNS is inferred based on recapitulation theory.

Cerebral Maturation

Cerebral maturation is discussed in terms of the maturational control of the emergence of speech and physical data on the maturation of the brain.

Maturational control of the emergence of spoken language appears well established. Lenneberg (1966, p. 219) asked why children regularly begin to speak between 18 and 28 months of life, and after referring to the contributions of training of, need for, and pleasure from speech, he stated, "the most important differences between the prelanguage and postlanguage phases of development originate in the growing individual and not in the external world or in changes in the availability of stimuli." Lenneberg (p. 235) identified four criteria for determining whether the onset of speech may be attributed to a maturational process: regularity in onset, differential use of environmental stimulation with growth, independence from use, and superfluousness of practice.

In response to the criteria, Lenneberg (pp. 221–35) offered the following information:

- The normal interlinking of the sequential development of oral language with the development of functions more easily connected to physical maturation like gait and motor coordination

- The frequent maintenance of the interrelationships between language development and other developments, even when the whole maturational process is slowed because of various types of mental retardation
- The regularity in the emergence of language, for example, approximately 100 percent of children acquire single words by 22 months, and two-word phrases by 36 months
- The existence of no evidence that intensive language stimulation can accelerate language development in a child who is maturationally still a toddling infant.

"Complimentary to the question of how old a child must be before he can use the environment for language acquisition is that of how young he must be before it is too late to acquire speech and language" (p. 235). The concept of age limitation on language acquisition as well as on onset of language acquisition should be of special interest to specialists concerned with the cerebral palsied. Evidence offered by Lenneberg to support the concept of a developmental phase of primary language acquisition, a period that runs from about 2 to 13 years, includes: (a) Symptoms of acquired aphasia tend to become irreversible at about the time cerebral lateralization becomes well established (about puberty). (b) Language-learning appears to cease after puberty in Down's syndrome. (c) Profoundly deaf children have a better chance of developing adequate speech if amplification and training begin as close to the age of two as possible.

Physical data on brain maturation around the period of primary language acquisition have also been collected. Anatomical, histological, biochemical, and electrophysiological data on the maturation of the brain have been collected before, during, and after the period of primary language acquisition. Findings revealed that, in all those aspects of brain maturation studied, about 60 percent of the mature values are reached before the onset of speech (about two years of age), then the maturation rate slows down and the brain reaches its mature state by the close of the period of primary language acquisition (Lenneberg, 1967, pp. 158–79).

Vertical Integration

The concept of vertical integration of the speech brain was touched on in a previous work (Mysak, 1976, pp. 14–29) and is specifically related to the larger concept of the progressive integration and elaboration of the CNS. The SCNS is also viewed from the standpoint of levels of sensorimotor integration that are progressively integrated and elaborated upon. The concept of vertical integration of the SCNS may be developed on the basis of progressive motor elaboration or progressive language elaboration. Vertical integration of motor speech is more appropriately discussed in the last section of the chapter; the vertical integration of oral language is discussed here in terms of the triune model of the brain.

As previously described, the triune brain includes a foundation for the three brains called the neural chassis (spinal cord, medulla, pons, midbrain) and three drivers or brains: the R-complex (including olfactostriatum, corpus striatum, globus pallidus), the limbic system (including olfactory cortex, thalamus, hypothalamus, amygdala, pituitary gland, hippocampus), and the neocortex (including frontal, parietal, temporal, occipital lobes). The neural chassis is responsible for directly activating the most simple as well as more complex reflex units of the motor speech program, that is, reflexive respiration and vocalization, and even nonverbal, faciovocal expression (laughter, crying).

"R-complex speech" represents ritual-type speech, such as memorized speech and social-gesture speech. Specific examples include memorized recitation, repetition of prayers, chants, nursery rhymes, and so on. Regressed adults and very young children might be expected to use such speech excessively because of loss of integration or incomplete integration of this center by cortical centers.

"Limbic speech" represents emotional speech including love, hate, and fear forms. Examples of such talking include emotional appeals from politicians, sermons, love proposals, and so on. Again, children's speech is replete with such talk as a function of incomplete vertical integration of this level.

"Cortical speech" represents reasoning or logical speech. Cortical speech is the only true speech. Theoretically, the other two brains cannot "talk" without the cortex. Examples of logical talk include conversation, description, narration, and persuasion forms.

The progressive integration and elaboration of the lower levels of language by the cortical level may be demonstrated in cortical speech used in a proposal of marriage, for example. A true cortical speech proposal begins with a logical argument why the individual should agree to marry. If that doesn't appear to be going well, the cortex may engage in limbic speech, or romantic love talk; if that doesn't work, the cortex may use not only cortical and limbic speech, but also resort to R-complex talk composed of repetitive and chant-like "why don't you want to?," "ya gotta," "Oh, please," and so on.

Lateral Integration

The discussion of lateral integration includes the evolution of the speech cortex and the development of a major speech cortex, or the integration of the right cortex by the left cortex.

Uncommitted cortex is a concept discussed by Penfield (1966). "Man's brain is remarkable among mammals because of the greatly increased volume of cerebral cortex that covers it with deeply folded convolutions. . . . Unlike the cortex of the rat, which is completely motor or sensory except for a small undefined area, most of the human cortex is neither sensory in function nor motor.'' Successively greater increases in the proportion of uncommitted cortex are found in the brains of the ground shrew, tree shrew, tarsius, chimpanzee, and, finally, man. ''The temporal and parietal lobes have made their appearance in man as an outbudding from the thalamus which seems to push the visual sensory cortex back and away from the somatic sensory and the auditory sensory.''

Motor and sensory areas of man's cortex are committed to function, but this is not so with the new cortex between the auditory and visual areas. Organizational and functional connections of the new cortex are established during the first decade of life. The new cortex is responsible for speech in the major hemisphere (usually left) and to perception in the minor hemisphere.

Support for Penfield's concept is based on data he collected from conscious patients undergoing surgery for relief of focal epilepsy. When electrical current was applied to particular parts of the cortex in the major hemisphere, an immediate aphasic-like interference with speech was observed; however, no such speech interference was observed when similar stimulation was applied to the corresponding area in the minor hemisphere. Instead, stimulation of the minor hemisphere resulted in two types of phenomena: (a) The patient reported that ''what he sees and hears seems suddenly familiar, or strange, or frightening, or coming closer, or going away, etc.'' (p. 221). (b) The patient suddenly experiences ''awareness of some previous experience,'' or a sudden ''flashback.'' Similar ''psychical responses'' were elicited with stimulation ''of the temporal cortex that lies farther forward on the nondominant side and on the dominant side as well. Thus, except for the speech area and the audiosensory area, the cortex that covers the superior and lateral surfaces of the temporal lobe on both sides may be taken as a functional unit'' (p. 221). The interpretive cortex was the name given to this area by Penfield.

Penfield believed that the speech cortex of the uncommitted cortex is composed of a major speech area (Wernicke's area) and two minor speech areas (Broca's and the supplementary motor area of Penfield). He believed further that destruction of the major speech area results in loss of speech, but that if the damage occurs before the age of ten or twelve, the homologous area on the nondominant side may develop into a speech area within the period of a year or more. Damage to this homologous area in the nondominant hemisphere of the adult causes problems in body scheme awareness and of spatial relationships.

Speech cortex, or the cortex of the dominant hemisphere, has also been discussed by Roberts (1966) and Geschwind (Roberts, 1966, pp. 26–40). Roberts commented on the concept of "brainedness" and discussed further the various speech cortices in the major speech brain or dominant hemisphere, and Geschwind (1979) has considered anatomical differences in the two hemispheres and the role of the limbic system in speech.

1. On the concept of brainedness, Roberts stated that, "Handedness is a form of behavior in a particular individual. It may be influenced by psychological abnormalities, heredity, environment, brain damage, and perhaps other factors" (p. 18). Regardless of handedness, however, Roberts believes that the left hemisphere is usually dominant for speech purposes except in those cases where individuals have suffered damage to the left cerebral hemisphere at an early age. A left hemisphere dominant for speech is the most important thing that man inherits. Roberts believes "that right-handedness may have developed secondarily to speech dominance." Conversely, if in fact the right hemisphere is dominant for speech, the chances are the individual will be left-handed. It is this belief by Roberts that gives rise to the idea of "brainedness."

   The concept of lateral integration in the SCNS is directly supported by the concept of brainedness for speech function. Roberts' findings on the effects of lesions in, and of electrical stimulation of, various areas of the cortex on speech and language also contributes to the concept of intrahemispheral integration and elaboration of the SCNS.

   The location and effects of lesions on speech and language function are:
   a. Bilateral lesions in the region of the inferior Rolandic fissure cause symptoms of pseudobulbar palsy and anarthria or dysarthria.
   b. Lesions in the supplementary motor area of Penfield result in aphasia and difficulty in producing rapidly alternating movements, especially in the opposite foot—similar difficulty may be experienced in oral activities. However, the entire supplementary motor area may be excised without permanent aphasia.
   c. Lesions in the region of the posterior part of the second frontal convolution cause aphasia associated with writing difficulties, but this is transient.
   d. Lesions in the region of the posterior part of the third frontal convolution, or Broca's area, causes an aphasia that will resolve itself.
   e. Roberts (1966, p. 21) says that "the most pronounced and prolonged disturbances in speech occur with lesions of the posterior speech area—the posterior temporal, inferior parietal, and anterior

occipital region. The more anterior the lesion, the more the auditory aspects are involved, and the more posterior the lesion, the more the visual aspects are affected."

2. On the question of anatomical differences in the two hemispheres, Geschwind reported findings that tend to show differences in Heschl's gyri in the temporal lobes of both hemispheres. In contrast, Heschl's gyri in monkeys are similar bilaterally and appear in pattern like those usually found in the right hemisphere of man. If these differences actually exist, Geschwind believes that Wernicke's area has developed to the point where it has pushed the auditory cortex forward. The posterior inferior parietal region also appears more developed in man.

Geschwind also discussed the anatomical background of learning in the monkey and in man and the significance of the limbic system.* In teaching a monkey to select a certain visual form, the monkey receives a piece of food only if he selects the form desired by the experimenter. When successful, the monkey has formed an association between a visual stimulus and a food stimulus, or monkey-learning in this instance is the result of a visual-limbic association. Such a task is usually easy for a monkey and, in fact, the monkey's brain appears anatomically designed for such activity since the largest number of connections of the visual system are with the limbic system. Monkeys also form tactile-limbic and auditory-limbic associations. What is difficult for the monkey is to form associations between two nonlimbic stimuli.

Nonlimbic associations are relatively easy for man, and this is usually attributed to the fact that man uses "verbal mediation." Man "learns in the visual experiment to choose the object named 'circle'; when the tactile experiment is done he again chooses the object named 'circle.' " Geschwind believes that "What is important is not that we need language in order to have cross-modal associations: it is rather that in order to develop language we must be able to form non-limbic cross-modal associations" (p. 30). Man learns to name objects by associating the sight or feel of it with a particular auditory stimulus, its name; it is just this kind of nonlimbic, crossmodal association that is a problem for the monkey to make. Language acquisition in children would be expected when the child develops the capacity to form nonlimbic, crossmodal associations, of which language is considered a special kind.

---

*Geschwind defined the limbic system as "that portion of the brain which connects with regions in which are represented both the subjective and objective manifestations of behavior related to the survival of the individual or the species—the motor aspects of rage, flight and sexual behavior, the feelings of hunger or thirst with the corresponding feelings of satiation, and other similar behaviors and emotions."

The development of the angular gyrus region in man is considered the basis for forming nonlimbic, intermodal associations, according to Geschwind. The angular gyrus region is situated at the junction of the visual, auditory, and somesthetic association regions, and appears well suited to function as an association area of association areas, and may be considered the anatomical substrate for man's ability to make nonlimbic, intermodal transfers.

From the standpoint of language acquisition then, serious damage or destruction of the angular gyri region should be considered among the most serious in man.

ORIGINS OF SPEECH

The phylo-ontogenesis of expressive human communication reveals the progressive integration and elaboration of earlier modes of communication by later ones. Again, this integration is marked by higher modes assuming a directive and regulatory control over lower modes, which continue to serve their basic functions. General theories on the origins of speech and the integration-selection theory and support for the theory are presented here.

General Theories

The beginnings of speech must be inferred rather than objectively studied. There is "no evidence in the form of archeological remains of early stages of language evolution, though we must assume that language like other aspects of culture underwent a period of evolutionary development" (Hoijer, 1966, p. 232). Similarly, Simon (1957, pp. 8–23) stated that "speech, practically alone of all man's activities, has left no record of its origin and development" (p. 8).

According to Simon, information on the beginnings of speech must be inferred from the structure of primitive people and from the records of the kinds of lives they lived:

1. Primitive people probably gestured and used calls and yells much before they began to use speech sounds. "The transition from the merely representative use of preverbal sounds to the arbitrary symbols of speech may well have been most gradual" (p. 10).
2. About 30 to 40 million years ago, one division of primate slowly developed toward terrestrial living patterns and evolved into human beings. Over the next millions of years came the bipedal posture and the development of manual dexterity and hence freedom of the mouth from grasping and manipulative activities. Such bipedal-manual development also meant corresponding changes in the sensorimotor areas of the cortex. Freedom of the mouth allowed oral and throat

structures to evolve slowly into the various organs needed to support the speech process. The brain also underwent a progressive increase in size and complexity.

3. The archeological remains of Java man and Peking man, thought to be contemporaneous about a million years ago, indicate "usable speech structures and probably just adequate brains" to justify the inference that these primitive people used a human type of oral communication.

4. Improvement in speech equipment was shown by Heidelberg man (around 500,000 years ago). Greatly improved equipment for speech was shown by Neanderthal man (100,000 to 150,000 years ago) and Cro-Magnon man (about 50,000 years ago), who was similar to modern man in appearance and showed through his cultural remains "considerable use of his fully developed speech mechanism."

Throughout human history numerous explanations have been offered for how speech began; some of these theories are identified here.

Natural theories are those that posit that some type of natural and inherent relationship exists between oral symbols and the things, acts, and so on that they represent.

Onomatopoeic theories are those that view the source of many words as oral imitations of the sounds made by the things they represent.

Vocal emotion theories are those that indicate the source of words as the reflexive utterances made during various kinds of emotional experiences.

Common effort theories are those that indicate words emerged from the vocalizations made by people engaged in group physical effort in order to synchronize their physical efforts.

Social pressure-control theories are those that indicate people joined groups for purposes of safety and economy of effort and also they desired group control, so the need for oral symbols grew.

Body language theories are those that view words as oral gestures emerging out of bodily gestures.

Vocal play or babble-luck theories are those that suggest certain involuntary utterances or play vocalizations become associated with various acts.

Cortical emergence theories are those that indicate oral symbols are the product of the development of the cerebrum which, in turn, is responsible for the meaningful linking and associating of neuromotor patterns responsible for already present reflexive sounds.

Combination theories are those that indicate more than one source for the origin of oral symbols. Since speech has different functions, it may be reasonable to assume that different types of words have different sources. Along these lines, Van Riper (1963, pp. 2–11) discussed the roles of speech in (a) the formulation of thought, (b) communication or in the transmission of information, (c) social control or its use as a way of manipulating others or controlling the environment, (d) emotional expression or as a way of informing others how speakers feel about themselves or about others, and (e) self-identification or self-expression or as a way of exhibiting the self or calling attention to the self.

Integration-Selection Theory

The author's integration-selection theory of the origins of speech is based on the assumption that there were multiple sources for meaningful human vocalization; that speech behavior, like other sensorimotor behaviors, proceeded from more generalized, relatively undifferentiated behaviors to specific, more highly differentiated behaviors; that natural selection processes resulted in the emergence of those speech behaviors that were most efficient; and, finally, that speech evolution was marked by the progressive integration of all major steps of speech evolution and that the highest forms assume a directive and regulatory control over lower forms that continue to serve their basic functions. Four major evolutionary steps in the phylogenesis of speech are identified, and, in accordance with the recapitulation theory, may be observed in the ontogenesis of speech in the infant.

Body talk was characterized first by relatively unorganized bodily, hands, head, face, and mouth movements in association with relatively unorganized vocalizations—or, in short, generalized, undifferentiated bodily and vocal responses. Such responses may have been observed in prespeech people when they were moved by pain, emotion, or strong needs, for example.

In time, general bodily and head movements became more expressive, but hands, face, and mouth movements and associated vocalization remained relatively unorganized. A small step toward integration, selection, and differentiation of body talk was made. Now prespeech people might have assumed certain prefight stances, for example, and be observed to use associated yells, screams, and growl-like sounds. In terms of ontogenesis, this period is recapitulated around the first six months of life.

Hands talk was characterized by the emergence of expressive bilateral and unilateral hand movements superimposed on the general body talk. Associated vocalizations were more organized and might be differentiated according to sounds of frustration, anger, pain, and pleasure, for example. Prespeech people may have used their hands to communicate "come here," "go-away," "that's mine," "that's good," "that's bad," and so on. In terms of ontogenesis, this period is recapitulated during the second six months of life and characterized by hands talk signifying "pick-me-up," "give me," "I want," "I'm excited," and so on.

Face talk was characterized by the emergence of a repertoire of facial expressions used for communication. Associated vocalization now included articulatory patterns to imitate animal sounds and other environmental sounds. The face-talk repertoire of prespeech people might have included the following dichotomies of basic facial expressions: happy-sad, excitement-boredom, security-fear, and love-hate. In terms of ontogenesis, this period is recapitulated during approximately 12 to 18 months and characterized by similar facial expressions, but with a continuum of expressions within each dichotomy of facial expression.

Mouth talk was characterized by the emergence of the use of an arbitrary code of utterances superimposed on appropriate face, hands, and body talk. In terms of ontogenesis, this period is recapitulated during approximately 18 to 24 months; however, true speech in infants appears earlier in many instances.

Reflections of the Theory

The integration-selection theory of the origins of speech gains support from the concepts of integration-elaboration of CNS development, phyletic traces of early vocalization, and tuning influences of early forms of communication.

The integration-elaboration concept of CNS development is reflected in the integration-selection of emerging speech. The emergence of mouth talk reflects the integration of face, hands, and body talk, that is, during a conversation mouth talk is the figure language while face, hands, and body languages are the ground languages continuing to serve their basic functions.

Phyletic traces of early vocalization and communication may also be observed today under certain communication situations. For example, during heated argument, individuals may be observed to accompany their mouth talk with gross body movements, exaggerated bilateral and unilateral hand movements, and with extremes of facial expression. Further, under such conditions, loss of fine control of vocalization, articulation, and even of choice of words may be observed.

Primitive or vestigial communicative sounds may also be observed under particular conditions. Primitive signal sounds are still heard in the yells, screams, and cries of infants, children, and adults during terror, sorrow, and life-threatening situations. Other categories of primitive vocalization might include: the "a-ha group" uttered during moments of insight or discovery; the "h-rr group," uttered during moments of anger or hostility; the "m-mm group," uttered during moments of pleasure or contentment; the "ow group," uttered during moments of pain; and the "ee group," uttered during moments of excitement.

The concept of vestigial utterances is hypothetical and unprovable, but it is supportable in terms of the recapitulation theory and the models of the triune brain and reflexization of movement.

Tuning influences of body, hands, and face talk are apparent in many speaking situations. For example, one may observe the use of mouth talk at its highest level when an excellent lawyer is presenting a logical argument on behalf of a client. Early in the presentation, the lawyer may be quite composed and almost entirely "oral symbolic." In time, and with pressure from his opposing counselor, however, he may be required to verbalize more quickly or may need to verbalize about unexpected points. Pressures for rapid and novel verbal exchanges may trigger tuning or facilitating forms of "old language." Early on there may be an increase in speech-associated facial expressions, then an increase in arm-hand gestures, and, finally, an increase in overall bodily movements such as pacing and assuming different stances. Verbal tuners are indispensable to individuals who frequently encounter unusual verbal demands such as lawyers, teachers, politicians, salespeople, and those involved in arguments.

Implications for Cerebral Palsy

The concept that speech neuroevolution is best understood in phylo-ontogenetic terms and that cerebral palsy may best be understood in terms of delayed, retarded, or arrested neuroevolution invests this chapter with great importance for specialists concerned with the understanding and care of children with cerebral palsy.

The developments that appear pertinent to the phylogenesis of speech are apparently recapitulated in the ontogenesis of speech: bipedal-manual development, hand-mouth rather than rooting-feeding development, and associated differences in the stimulation of certain cortical areas of the brain.

A thorough evaluation of cerebral palsy speech problems, therefore, should include an assessment of the child's level of bipedal evolution, and of his level of expressive communication. Correspondingly, both these factors must be considered in the speech management plan.

REFERENCES

Bobath, K., and Bobath, B. The facilitation of normal postural reactions and movements in the treatment of cerebral palsy. *Physiotherapy,* August, 3–19 (1964).

Byers, R. K. Tonic neck reflexes in children. *Am. J. Dis. Child.,* 55, 696–742 (1938).

Denny-Brown, D. Disintegration of motor function resulting from cerebral lesions. *J. Nerv. Ment. Dis.,* 112, 1–45 (1950).

Doman, G. J., Delacato, C. H., and Doman, R. J. The Doman-Delacato Developmental Mobility Scale. Philadelphia: The Rehabilitation Center (1960).

Easton, T. On the normal use of reflexes. *American Scientist,* 60, 591–599 (1972).

Fay, T. The use of pathological and unlocking reflexes in the rehabilitation of spastics. *Am. J. Phys. Med.,* 33, 347–352 (1954).

Fukuda, T. Studies on human dynamic postures from the viewpoint of postural reflexes. *Acta Oto-Laryngologica,* Suppl. 161 (1961).

Geschwind, N. Specializations of the human brain. *Scientific American,* 241, 180–199 (1979).

Gesell, A. The tonic neck reflex in the human infant. *J. Pediat.,* 13, 155 (1938).

Greene, P. H. Cybernetic problems of sensorimotor structure. *Univ. of Chicago Inst. for Comp. Res. Quart. Reports* (1969).

Hellebrandt, F. A., Schale, M., and Carnes, M. L. Methods of evoking the tonic neck reflexes in normal human subjects. *Am. J. Phys. Med.,* 41, 90–139 (1962).

Hoijer, H. The problem of primitive languages. In E. C. Carterette (Ed.), *Brain function: speech, language, and communication.* Berkeley and Los Angeles: University of California Press (1966).

Jackson, J. H. Evolution and dissolution of the nervous system. In J. Taylor (Ed.), *Selected writings of John Hughlings Jackson,* Vol. 2. New York: Basic Books (1958).

Lenneberg, E. H. *Biological foundations of language.* New York: John Wiley and Sons, Inc. (1967).

———. The natural history of language. In F. S. Smith and G. A. Miller (Eds.), *The genesis of language.* Cambridge: The M.I.T. Press (1966).

MacLean, P. D. *A triune concept of the brain and behavior.* Toronto: University of Toronto Press (1973).

Magnus, R. Some results of studies in the physiology of posture. *Lancet,* 2, 531–535 (1926).

McGraw, M. B. *The neuromuscular maturation of the human infant.* New York: Hafner Publishing Co. (1962).

Mysak, E. D. *Neuroevolutional approach to cerebral palsy and speech.* New York: Teachers College Press, Teachers College, Columbia University (1968).

———. *Pathologies of speech systems.* Baltimore: Williams and Wilkins (1976).

Peiper, A. *Cerebral function in infancy and childhood.* New York: Consultants Bureau (1963).

Penfield, W. Speech, perception, and the uncommitted cortex. In J. C. Eccles (Ed.), *Brain and conscious experience.* New York: Springer-Verlag (1966).

Prechtl, H., and Beintema, D. *The neurological examination of the full term newborn infant.* London: William Heinemann Medical Books Ltd. (1964).

Rademaker, G. *Reactions labyrinthiques et equilibre.* Paris: Masson et Cie (1935).

Roberts, L. Central brain mechanisms in speech. In E. C. Carterette (Ed.), *Brain function: Speech, language, and communication.* Berkeley and Los Angeles: University of California Press (1966).

Roberts, T. D. M. *Neurophysiology of postural mechanisms.* London: Butterworths (1967).

Sagan, C. *The dragons of eden.* New York: Balantine Books (1977).

Schaltenbrand, G. The development of human motility and motor disturbances. *Arch. Neur. and Psych.,* 20, 720–730 (1927).

Sherrington, C. S. *Selected writings,* ed. D. Denny-Brown. London: Hamish Hamilton Medical Books (1939).

Sherrington, C. S. *The integrative action of the nervous system.* London: Cambridge University Press (1947).

Simon, C. T. The development of speech. In L. E. Travis (Ed.), *Handbook of speech pathology*. New York: Appleton-Century-Crofts (1957).

Swineyard, C. A. Developmental aspects of neurological structure relevant to cerebral palsy. *Develop. Med. Child Neurol.*, 9, 216–221 (1967).

Thomas, A. Dargassies, S., and Chesni, Y. *The neurological examination of the infant*. London: National Spastics Soc. (1960).

Travis, L. E. *Speech pathology*. New York: Appleton Century (1931).

Twitchell, T. E. On motor deficit in congenital bilateral athetosis. *J. Nerv. Ment. Dis.*, 129, 105–132 (1959).

Van Riper, C. *Speech correction*. Englewood Cliffs: Prentice Hall (1963).

Weisz, S. Studies in equilibrium reaction. *J. Nerv. Ment. Dis.*, 88, 150–162 (1938).

Zador, J. *Les reactions d'equilibre chez l'homme*. Paris: Masson et Cie (1938).

2

Neuro-ontogenesis
of Speech

THE NEUROGENESIS OF speech is best understood from both phylogenetic and ontogenetic standpoints. Chapter 1 emphasizes the neurophylogenesis of speech, and this chapter emphasizes its neuro-ontogenesis.

Topics included in this chapter are the evolution of listening, speech
postures, hands talk, basic speech movements, skilled speech movements,
and the communisphere. Also, since the focus of the book is on neuroevolution of, and neurospeech therapy for, skilled speech movements, no specific
discussion of language development, as it is more commonly understood, is
presented here.

Evolution of Listening

Though it may appear somewhat inappropriate in a chapter devoted to
the neuro-ontogenesis of movements involved in speech, information on the
evolution of listening is presented for a number of reasons. First, the hearing mechanisms are contained within the head and hence efficient hearing
for speech requires trunk and head balance and localizing ability; in short,
posture and movement are involved in listening. Second, primary talking

and early true talking are, of course, dependent on hearing. Third, listening, or hearing for speech, like other speech functions, unfolds through a progressive integration and elaboration of auditory reflexive centers by cortical centers.

BASIC LISTENING POSTURES

Corresponding to basic speech postures are basic listening postures. As a minimum, adequate hearing for speech requires head, neck, and trunk balance and the ability to localize easily the source of speech signals. Hence, basic hearing postures include the back, elbow, and sitting patterns described in the next section on basic speech postures.

In terms of neurointegration, such basic hearing postures require the integration of spinal and brainstem reflexes by on-head righting and body-on-body righting reactions, the Landau reaction, and the various arm-support reactions. Basic hearing postures are stabilized by the full emergence of sitting equilibrium reactions by about 10 to 12 months.

BASIC LISTENING RESPONSES

Basic listening responses are observed through various kinds of bodily movements as well as through changes in autonomic activities. For the most part, they appear to be protective responses. Auditory reflexive behavior may be observed in fetuses as well as in young infants.

Auditory Reflexive Behavior in Fetuses

Fetal auditory reactions have been observed by the seventh month and appear strongest by the ninth month. Murphy (1964) reported that the auditory mechanism is stimulable by the 20th to 25th week of pregnancy. Loud sounds produced near the position of the fetal head have elicited "kick" and restlessness reactions in fetuses (Peiper, 1963, pp. 83-92). Fetal heart rate has also shown temporary increases in response to sound stimuli.

Auditory Reflexive Behavior in Infants

Peiper described various kinds of auditory reflexive behavior in infants. Among the reactions observed are: cochleopalpebral reflex, fright reaction, respiratory changes, restlessness, grimacing, cessation of crying and suckling, eye opening, forehead wrinkling, mouth opening, crying, smiling, suckling, tongue protrusion, and arm extension and finger spreading (probably elements of the auditory Moro reflex).

More specifically, various studies have shown: (a) changes in respiratory traces in response to auditory stimuli in infants during the first hour of life; (b) eye blink in reaction to noisemakers and high-pitched tuning forks in newborns and premature infants; (c) conditioned suckling in newborns in response to sound stimuli on the 27th day of life; and (d) suckling and smiling in response to human voice during the third week and second month, respectively.

Pattern Analysis of Basic Listening Responses

Auditory reflexive behavior may also be analyzed in terms of elemental and tuning reflexes. The palpebral reflex, restlessness, eye opening, forehead wrinkling, mouth opening, crying, arm extension and finger spreading may be viewed as elemental auditory-protective movements, while cessation of crying and suckling and smiling may be viewed as early elemental listening reactions.

Tuning listening reflexes are considered those which serve to sensitize or maximize the efficiency of the auditory system and which orient it to sound sources. Changes in respiration and heart rate in response to sound may be indicating autonomic conditioning that may facilitate or sensitize auditory processing, while some of the more general bodily reactions toward the sound source are precursory to orienting movements.

SKILLED LISTENING RESPONSES

Integration and elaboration of basic listening responses by cortical levels is manifested by various behaviors, such as selective inhibition of startle, localizing behavior, and early speech perception.

Selective Inhibition of Startle

Inhibition of startle, or more accurately, the integration of the auditory Moro reflex, is the "first sign of cortical function in relation to auditory stimuli" (Murphy, 1964). The infant may ignore familiar sounds, while less familiar, and even softer sounds, may cause startle. "Rudimentary cortical function precedes selective inhibition and at this stage hearing can be distinguished from auditory reflex."

Localizing Behavior

Auditory localizing may take at least two forms: the orientation of the head toward the sound source or the orientation of the head and eyes, or just the eyes, toward the sound source. Initial head and eye orientation to sounds, with eye orientation being somewhat slower, has been observed by about the third month. Details on the development of head-eye orientation to sound was provided by Murphy (1964).

Normally, the 8-to-10-week old infant in supine orients his head, or shows head-roll toward a 50dB sound source, a response that may be preceded by "stilling" and often accompanied by a "batting" of the hand or a "kicking" of the leg of the stimulated side. Eye turn, often accompanied by head roll, may be observed at 9 to 12 weeks. From the age of 12 weeks on, head control in the normal infant may be sufficient to allow for testing in the seated position. Localization downward occurs before localization upward and, in the majority of cases, localization toward the right precedes localization toward the left. Consistent turning to one side irrespective of the source of the sound may indicate monaural problems, while consistent turning toward only one source of sound with no reaction toward the other may be a function of maturation.

Speech Perception

Developing auditory perception for speech may be estimated by observing the infant's reaction to the speech of others as well as through intrapersonal and interpersonal echolalia.

Listening responses to the speech of others may be observed even during the first weeks of life when whimpering may cease in response to human voice. Later observations reveal: stare or smile in response to mother's voice at about three months; immediate localization of, and differential response to the tone of the mother's voice at about six months; meaningful reactions to the calling of the infant's name, appropriate responses to "no" and "bye-bye" at about nine months; and quick recognition of name, and some responses to "give me" requests by about 12 months.

Echolalia behavior, or the repetition of self-produced sounds, a crucial step in speech development, may be observed after six months, and echolalia on an interpersonal basis, or attempts at imitating sounds made by others, may be observed after about nine months.

Pattern Analysis of Skilled Listening Responses

Cortical integration of lower-level, auditory-movement reflexes is reflected by the full development of tuning orienting reflexes. The gradual emergence of the tuning orienting reflexes appears to follow the sequence of first auditory "startle" (body excitation) to sound, then auditory "stilling" (body immobilization), then auditory "searching" (head-scanning movements), and, finally, definitive auditory localizing.

The emergence of listening appears to be characterized by first smile or recognition of mother's voice, then differential response to tonal aspects of mother's voice, and finally, appropriate responses to symbolic speech.

Evolution of Basic Speech Postures

Basic speech postures are those that provide appropriate background muscle tonus and appropriate background stability for the speech effectors, that is, for the respiratory-phonatory-resonatory-articulatory complex. In that sense, speech postures are facilitatory or have a tuning influence on speech movements. At least four basic speech postures may be recognized: back, elbow, sitting, and standing.

BACK PATTERNS

Speech postures in supine, the earliest type, represent various forms of symmetrical supine or semireclining "back patterns."

Infant Form

The young infant may be observed with the head in normal alignment with the body, with the lower limbs gently flexed and abducted, and with hands brought together and to the mouth. In this posture, she may explore her hands and mouth and may be observed to engage in reflexive vocalization.

Older Forms

Older children and adults may also be observed to speak from various "chaise lounge" or back-pattern positions, such as occiput-in-hands, hands-on-crown, and hands-on-knees positions. Hands-on-one-knee and chin-in-hand positions represent somewhat asymmetrical versions of this back-pattern speech posture.

Level of Neurointegration

The infant should be able to roll over into this position from prone and be able to engage in symmetrical flexor activities. The posture reflects the integration of spinal automatisms and tonic neck and tonic labyrinthine reflexes by neck righting, on-head righting, and body righting reactions. The posture is stabilized through the emergence of upper limb and lower limb support and balance reactions in supine at about seven to ten months. Back-pattern speech postures are used throughout life.

ELBOW PATTERNS

Symmetrical and asymmetrical forms of the on-elbows speech posture may be observed. These are the "elbow-pattern" speech postures.

Infant Form

This posture shows the child in prone and is characterized by extension of the neck and trunk, with lower limbs extended, abducted, and outwardly rotated. The child displays excellent head balance and supports the upper part of the body with the upper limbs and hands. The pattern allows for an expansion of the child's visual and auditory perceptual fields, and for exploratory activities with one hand when the child shifts to weight-bearing on only one upper extremity. Primary talking in the form of babbling and some auto-echolalia may be observed.

Older Forms

Various forms of the on-elbows speech posture are observed in children and adults; for example, the head-in-hands-cradle position. Various on-upper-arm forms may also be seen including face-in-hand cradle, occiput-in-hand cradle, and chin-in-three-finger cradle positions.

Level of Neurointegration

The child should be able to assume the prone-lying position by rolling over from supine and be able to raise the upper part of the body and support it on elbows. Assumption of the elbow-pattern speech posture reflects the integration of tonic neck and tonic labyrinthine reflexes and neck righting reflexes by body-on-body and on-head righting reactions, as well as by the chain-in-prone reaction, the Landau reaction, and the arm-support reaction in the forward position. Elbow patterns are stabilized by the emergence of arm-support and balance reactions at about six to eight months. Elbow-pattern speech postures are used throughout life.

SIT PATTERNS

A number of speech postures in sitting may be observed including floor-sit, chair-sit, and squat-sit patterns. And they may be referred to as "sit patterns."

Infant Form

Primary sitting reactions have been reported even during the first weeks of life. Pulling the infant by his hands from supine elicits a sitting movement characterized by head lag. At about three months, the head assumes a more normal position, but the infant continues not to take an active role in the sitting movement. Primary sitting is elicited with only a slight pull of the hands by about six months and is characterized by erect sitting with extended spine, flexed hips, and extended knees; however, since the child does not enjoy trunk balance and fully formed arm-support reactions, she can sit unsupported for only short periods. Because of the lack of full stability in sitting, these early forms are considered precursors to sit-pattern speech postures.

The first true sit-pattern speech posture emerges when the child is able to roll over from supine into prone, raise her body off the ground and move into side-sitting or long-sitting positions. Arm-support reactions in sitting may be observed at 6 months when the child is tipped forward, at 8 months when tipped sideways, and at 10 months when tipped backward. Tailor-sitting and heel-sitting are other infant forms of sit-pattern speech postures. Sitting allows for further expansion of the child's visual and auditory perceptual fields and for exploring objects with the hands. Primary talking may be marked by true echolalia.

Older Forms

Various chair-sit forms of speech postures may be seen in older children and adults; for example, chin-in-hands cradle, and chin-on-fist cradle positions. In-front-of-table postures include forearms-on-table and chin-in-hands cradle positions.

Level of Neurointegration

The child should be able to assume independently a floor-sit position from supine. This reflects the integration of spinal and brainstem reflexes by on-head righting, and body-on-body righting reactions, the Landau reaction, and arm-support reactions toward the front, side, and back. Sit patterns are stabilized by the full emergence of sitting equilibrium reactions by about 10 to 12 months. Sit-pattern speech postures are used throughout life.

STAND PATTERNS

Speech postures in standing include standing with one hand holding on to something, free standing, and dynamic standing or walking.

Infant Form

The first stand-pattern speech posture is observed when the child is able to move from supine into a quadrupedal position and then pull himself into kneeling, half-kneeling, and, finally, into standing while holding on to some form of support. Standing and walking allows for the ultimate expansion of visual and auditory perceptual fields and for exploring the environment. It is at this time that true speech may be heard.

Older Forms

Various forms of standing speech postures may be observed in older children and adults. Among them are hands-to-mouth, hands-on-hips, hands-in-back, hands-in-pockets, and clasped hands positions.

Level of Neurointegration

The child must be able to assume independently the standing position from prone or supine-lying positions. This reflects the grand integration of spinal, brainstem, and midbrain reactions. Standing and walking are stabilized by the full emergence of balance and support reactions in standing by about 12 to 18 months. Stand-pattern speech postures are used throughout life.

Figures 2.1, 2, 3, and 4 illustrate some of the back, elbow, sit, and stand-pattern speech postures.

Fig. 2.1. Basic speech postures: back patterns

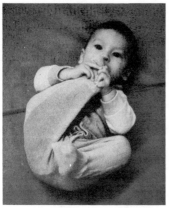
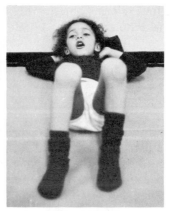
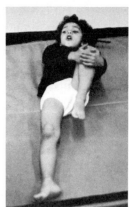

symmetrical supine   occiput-in-hands   hands-on-knee

Fig. 2.2. Basic speech postures: elbow patterns

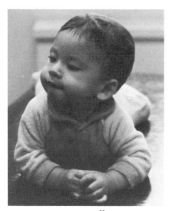
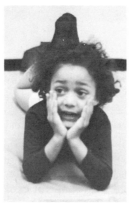
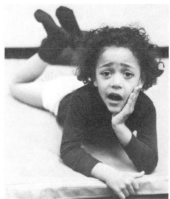

prone-on-elbows   head-in-hands cradle   face-in-hand cradle

Fig. 2.3. Basic speech postures: sit patterns

long
sitting

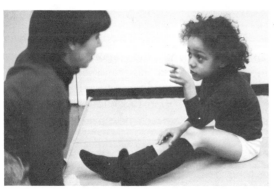
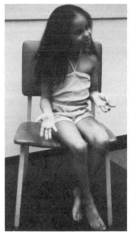

chair
sitting

Fig. 2.4. Basic speech postures: stand patterns

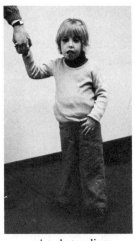 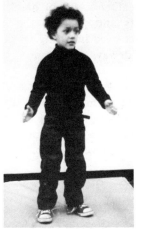 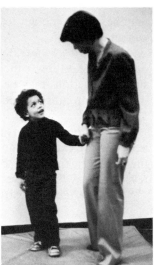

    assisted standing   free standing   walking

Evolution of Basic Hands Talk

Chapter 1 described hands talk as a stage in the integration-selection theory of the origins of speech. The hypothesis was that this stage in the origins of speech may be recapitulated in the infant during the second six months of life and reflected in infant hands talk requesting such things as "pick me up," "I don't want . . . ," "give me," and so on.

Hands talk emerges from reflexive hand movements and serves the infant first as symbolic communication in the form of pointing, for example, "I want" gestures, or pushing away, or "I don't want" gestures; and then serves as adjunctive communication to true speech in the form of speech-associated hand gestures. The discussion of the emergence of hands-talk movements is divided, therefore, into reflexive hand movements and expressive hand movements.

REFLEXIVE HAND MOVEMENTS

Reflexive hand movements are divided into three categories: protective, progression, and vegetative.

Protective Reflexes

Reflexive holding, stabilizing, and protection against falling are forms of hand-protective reflexes.

The grasp reflex is one of the earliest forms of hand-protective reflexes. Pressure applied to the palms of the newborn elicits the grasp reflex that may be strong enough to allow the child to be lifted free in the air (Darwinian reflex).

Arm-support reflexes are other forms of hand protective reflexes. The on-elbows position supports and protects the head and trunk. Arm-support reactions may be observed in sitting when the child is tipped forward at 6 months, tipped sideways at 8 months, and tipped backward at 10 months.

Arm-balance reactions may also be viewed as protective. They are characterized by extension and abduction of arms and hands in response to the displacement of the center of gravity of the body. Such arm-balance reactions may be observed from six months on.

Scratch reflexes may also be viewed as a form of hand-protective reflex.

Progression Reflexes

Reflexive hand movements involved in push-pull activity or moving the body forward as in crawling or creeping are considered hand-progression reflexes. Infantile upper-limb movement and hand-pulling reflexes may be observed during the crawling phase of body progression. Arm walking, placing reaction of the upper limb, and hopping reactions of the upper limbs are arm reactions important to the creeping phase of body progression. Arm-balance reactions are also indispensable to successful body progression movements.

Vegetative Reflexes

Reflexive hand movements involved with feeding may be referred to as hand-vegetative reflexes. Two such hand-mouth reflexes have been identified—the palmar-mental and the palmar-mandibular reflexes—and are discussed in the next section of the chapter.

EXPRESSIVE HAND MOVEMENTS

Hands talk takes two forms: symbolic gestural and adjunctive gestural.

Symbolic Gestural

From about six months on, the infant may use hand movements in a voluntary fashion to indicate he wants something or wants to be taken somewhere (points), he wants to be picked up (reaches out), he doesn't want something (pushes away), or something tastes good (rubs tummy). He may also wave bye-bye, wave come here, and so on. Symbolic gesturing remains active throughout life.

Adjunctive Gestural

As the child learns to speak, he continues to use symbolic hand movements, but, in addition, adjunctive gestural behavior may also be observed.

For example, the child may use scolding language to a doll and simultaneously uses general supportive hand gestures. Or, the child in attempting to describe something big, fat, or far away may lose a key word and supportive hand gestures may become exaggerated and evolve into facilitatory hand gestures as the child struggles to find the word.

PATTERN ANALYSIS OF REFLEXIVE AND EXPRESSIVE HAND MOVEMENTS

The integration and elaboration of reflexive hand movements by cortical centers results in the emergence of various skilled hand movements and in speech-facilitating hand movements.

Skilled Hand Movements

The integration and elaboration of protective, progression, and vegetative hand reflexes by cortical centers results in the child being able to do the following: bring his hands together and to the mouth by about two or three months; hold objects with both hands (grasp the bottle with whole hand, for example) by about four or five months; reach, grasp, and hand-mouth feed with one hand by about six months; scissor grasp by about eight or nine months; pincer grasp and release by about 10 months; and supinate by about 11 or 12 months.

Expressive Hand Movements

The integration and elaboration of symbolic gestural movements by cortical centers is manifested by the emergence of adjunctive gestural movements accompanying speech. Adjunctive gestural movements in their fully developed form serve at least two purposes: (a) they may be used in an exaggerated fashion to facilitate word-finding during certain difficult speaking situations, and (b) they serve as general tuning reactions for the speech system. Supination ability is considered a key expressive hand movement.

Figures 2.5, 6, and 7 illustrate some protective, progression, and vegetative hand reflexes, and Figure 2.8 some expressive hand movements.

Evolution of Basic Speech Movements

Basic speech movements represent the coordinative structures or reflexes of which skilled speech movements are composed. In accord with the concept of reflexization of voluntary movement, they are the reflexes that form the basic language of the motor speech program. These reflexes are basic to feeding movements, later preverbal speech movements, and, finally, to skilled speech movements. For the sake of exposition, they are divided into protective, emotional, and vegetative reflexes and reflexive vocalization.

Fig. 2.5.   Reflexive hand movements: protective reflexes

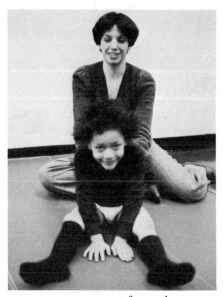
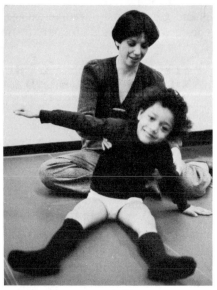

arms-support-forward   arm-support sideways

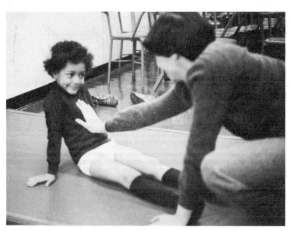

arm-support-backward

    Many of the reflexes and reactions discussed under the headings of protective, vegetative, and emotional responses vary in terms of ease, place, and time of elicitation. Time of integration of these infantile reflexes also varies from child to child. In general, those reflexes that are associated with infantile feeding behavior are integrated before, or by approximately, one year. Reaction is distinguished from reflex on the basis of increased complexity and decreased consistency of response pattern.

Fig. 2.6. Reflexive hand movements: progression reflexes

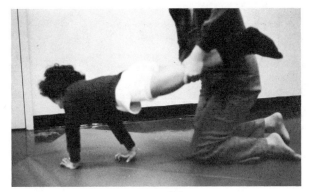

arm walking

upper limb placing

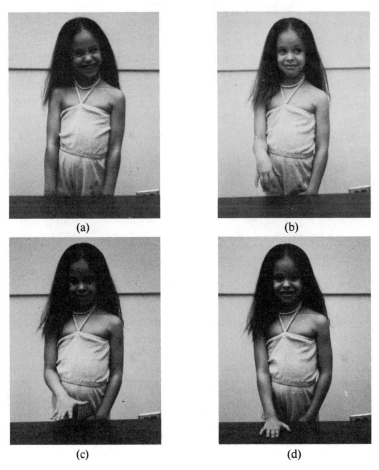

(a)

(b)

(c)

(d)

Fig. 2.7. Reflexive hand movements: vegetative reflex

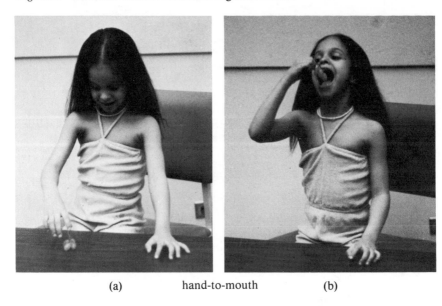

(a)   hand-to-mouth   (b)

Fig. 2.8. Expressive hand movements

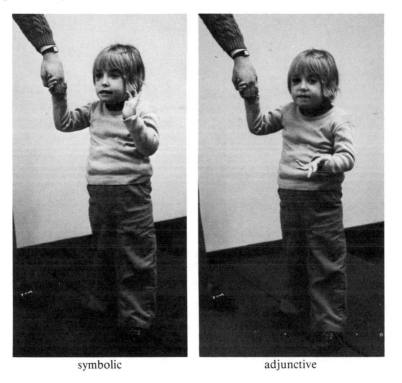

symbolic   adjunctive

PROTECTIVE REFLEXES

Two categories of protective reflexes may be recognized: head and neck-mouth-face reflexes.

Head Reflexes

Irregular movements of the head in infants may be elicited by stimulation of the face. Auriculocephalic and nasocephalic reflexes may be elicited by rubbing the lobe of the ear or tickling the nostril, respectively. Head rotation toward the opposite side is the expected response. These reflexes have been observed during the neonatal period (Thomas, Chesni, and Dargassies, 1960, p. 5). They may be regarded as reflexes that ensure unobstructed breathing.

Neck-Mouth-Face Reflexes

A number of protective reflexes are found in the larynx, pharynx, tongue, lips, jaw, and face.

Laryngeal reflexes include the glottic closing and opening and cough reflexes. Laryngeal-closing activity is even present during aquatic fetal life. Schwartz (1961) cited excessive rehearsal of this reflex as a possible cause of infantile voice difficulty, or congenital laryngeal stridor. Laryngeal closing during swallowing is an important reflex for air-breathing organisms, and Schwartz believed that prenatal practice of this pattern contributes to its establishment. Adults may also experience the glottic-closing reflex during a sudden descent, as in the sudden drop of an elevator or plane, when suddenly splashed with cold water, or when first entering cold water for a swim. Schwartz says the reflex suggests "the glottis reacting as if it recalled menacing stimuli of an earlier period (immersion reflex)." Reflexive glottic closing also occurs during the lifting of heavy objects and other activities requiring the buildup of intrathoracic air pressure.

Reflexive glottic opening is elicited whenever there is a threat to breathing as with various forms of nasal or oral obstructions.

Cough reflexes are also regarded as laryngeal protective responses. Both glottic closing and cough reflexes remain active throughout life and protect the individual against aspiration of foreign objects into the lungs and from choking.

Pharyngeal and palatal reflexes marked by reflex constriction of the pharynx and elevation of the velum are protective against foreign objects entering the throat. Both reflexes remain active throughout life.

Tongue reflexes characterized by reflexive tongue protrusion, or the lingual counteracting response, may be observed if the tongue is steadily forced back into the throat, as in tongue swallowing. The response represents another protection against choking.

Lip reflexes, characterized by reflexive puckering, or the lip counteracting response, may be observed in response to the corners of the lips being steadily spread apart. This reflex protects the lips against damage by placing limits on mouth opening.

Jaw and jaw-jerk reflexes are characterized by reflexive contraction of jaw flexors in response to steady or sudden stretch of the mandibular extensors. These reflexes protect the jaw against damage by limiting the extension of the jaw.

Face reflexes, characterized by reflexive eye closure and grimacing, are observed in response to sudden air pressure like blowing in the face or to an object suddenly approaching the face.

Pattern Analysis of the Protective Reflexes

The protective reflexes may be seen as elemental reflexes of the primitive-but-complete-pattern variety, or as primitive but complete motor acts, rather than as component parts of a larger pattern.

Integration of protective head reflexes and neck and mouth reflexes by speech centers could result in their use as speech-associated head movements, and as movements contributing to the production of voicing, pressure sounds, and lingual, labial, and mandibular speech sounds.

EMOTIONAL REFLEXES

A number of emotional reflexes associated with fear, pain, or pleasure may be identified or observed in the infant. All are displayed primarily in the face.

Spreading Reflex

Peiper (1963) described a reflexive spreading or retracting of facial muscles and reflexive eye opening in response to fright or fear.

Cry Reflex

A companion reflex to the spreading reflex is the cry reflex. It may be seen and heard in response to fright, pain, frustration, or discomfort. Mouth opening and facial grimacing and tearing characterize the response. Sobbing and sighing are considered as elements of the cry reflex. As any new parent will attest, the cry reflex is present at birth and continues throughout life.

Because of the potential importance of cry breathing to the development of speech breathing, a series of studies on the development and relationships of cry, vegetative, and vocalization breathing are discussed here. The studies were conducted at the Speech Research Laboratory of Teachers College, Columbia University (Wilder and Baken, 1974; Langlois, Wilder, and Baken, 1975; Langlois and Baken, 1976; and Wilder and Baken, 1978). Respiratory patterns in normal infants from birth until about 13 months of age were explored.

Cry breathing showed a 50 percent decrease in mean bpm (breaths per minute) based on a steady increase in the mean duration of respiratory cycles over the first eight months of life. Approximate figures are as follows: 1 month—50 bpm; 2 months—40 bpm; 3 months—37 bpm; 4 months—35 bpm; 5 months—34 bpm; 6 months—31 bpm; 7 months—29 bpm; and 8 months—23 bpm. The steady decrease in bpm was based on the increased duration of the expiratory phase that more than doubled during the period. A steady decrease in the I-fraction (ratio of inspiratory duration to the total duration of the respiratory cycle) during crying over the first eight months of life was also observed. Approximate figures are as follows: 1 month—19 percent; 2 months—18 percent; 3 months—16 percent; 4 months—15 percent; 5 months—15 percent; 6 months—14 percent; 7 months—12 percent; 8 months—11 percent. (Wilder and Baken, 1978).

Bpm continued to decrease over the entire 13-month-age-range studied. Cry bpm at 13 months (19 bpm) fell within the bpm range reported for adult speech. I-fraction remained relatively stable over the first six months but showed more variability as infants began to develop the upright position. By about seven months, the infant is apparently able to negotiate a short inspiration and a prolonged voiced expiration; by about 13 months, expiratory duration and I-fraction values during crying closely resembled those found for adult speech.

Vegetative and vocalization breathing also showed interesting developmental trends. During the first year of life, vegetative breathing showed slight irregular increases in breathing cycle duration with a reciprocal decrease in rate and an I-fraction that remained stable. Whereas cry respiration and vegetative respiration showed developmental changes during the first year of life, respiration during noncrying vocalization did not (Langlois, Wilder, and Baken, 1975). A possible explanation offered for this finding was the small number of syllables uttered by the infants (mean length of syllable utterance never exceeded 1.84). Therefore, the relatively similar respiratory rates and high I-fraction could be attributed to the absence of multisyllabic babbling.

The relationship of thoracic-abdominal activity in the various types of infant respirations studied during the first year is also pertinent to the purposes of this chapter. Vegetative breathing was characterized predominantly by abdominal movements. Cry respiration and respiration during noncrying vocalization showed a developmental increase in thoracic participation. Also, abdominal contraction usually led the expiratory phase and this "physiologic asynchrony" was reminiscent of the asynchronisms observed during adult speech. Fitting well with the larger concept of the neuro-ontogenesis of speech was the finding that increased thoracic participation and improved thoracic movement organization corresponded with advances in developmental level from simple prone, through aided sitting, independent sitting, standing, and walking.

Smile Reflex

Reflexive smiling in response to the maternal voice may be demonstrated at about four to six weeks (Illingworth, 1962, p. 25). The smile reflex may also be elicited by auditory, visual, or movement stimuli.

Laugh Reflex

Tickling may elicit uncontrollable laughter in infants. Laughing behavior may be observed in infants at about 16 weeks (Illingworth, 1962, p. 24).

Pattern Analysis of Emotional Reflexes

Infantile emotional reflexes are considered to be primitive but complete motor acts.

Integration of these reflexes results in their use as speech-tuning reflexes. For example, such reflexes may be used to influence vocal color, speech rate and rhythm to project better the verbal expression of happiness, sadness, fear, and so on. Integration of crying respiration would appear to make an important contribution to the development of speech breathing.

VEGETATIVE REFLEXES

Vegetative reflexes include those involved with breathing, or oxygen nourishment, and those involved with feeding, or food nourishment.

Breathing Reflexes

Basic breathing is observed during approximately the first six months of life. It may be described in terms of type of lung expansion, either diaphragmatic or abdominal; cycles, depth, or breaths per minute; mode of inspiration, either nasal or oral; and level of control, either medullary or cortical.

Inspiratory reflexes in the infant include the essential primal breath, or the fundamental inspiratory reflex. Ongoing inspiratory reflexes are activated and regulated in accordance with changes in CO_2 levels in the blood. Deep, involuntary inspiration with the mouth open, or the yawn reflex, is another form of inspiratory reflex. In the young infant abdominal or diaphragmatic breathing predominates (phylogenetically older), while thoracic breathing is minimal. Breathing is shallow, with essentially symmetrical inspiratory-expiratory phases, and breaths per minute is high. The usual mode of inspiration is nasal, and the level of control is the pneumotaxic center of the medulla.

Peiper (1963, p. 311) reviewed studies of vegetative breaths per minute during the first six months of life. For the first month of life, a range from about 22 to 72 bpm (mean of about 35 bpm) was reported; and for the first through six months a range from about 21 to 58 bpm (mean of about 33 bpm) was reported.

Inspiratory reflexes for feeding vs. voicing are different. The oral mode of inspiration serves the crying and screaming function, while the nasal mode of inspiration is essential for breast and bottle feeding. Nasal inspiration also characterizes at-rest breathing at all ages.

Feeding Reflexes

A number of reflexes associated with infantile feeding, or rooting-feeding, have been studied. They usually are described in elemental reflex fashion. In actuality, they form a pattern or a chain of reflexes devoted to orienting toward, obtaining, and ingesting food.

Hand-mouth reflexes are of two types: the palmar-mental reflex and the palmar-mandibular reflex (Peiper, 1963, p. 116, pp. 416–17). They are found in the newborn and have been explained on a phyletic basis. The palmar-mental reflex is elicited by scratching the thenar eminence. Simultaneous contraction of the chin muscles that lifts the chin up constitutes the response pattern. The reflex has been observed in newborns, infants up to the last months of the first year, and occasionally in children between six and twelve years of age.

The palmar-mandibular reflex, or Babkin's reflex, is elicited by applying pressure to the palms of both hands. Mouth opening, closing of the eyes, and head ventroflexion constitutes the response pattern. The response weakens during the first month and usually "disappears" by the third month.

The phyletic heritage of these patterns relates to manner of food intake. Rooting-feeding, or food intake by direct mouth seizure and oral manipulation, may be seen in fish, amphibians, and reptiles, and in the human infant during the first months of life. Hand-mouth feeding, which represents an integration and elaboration of rooting-feeding, is characterized by grasping of the food first with the forelimbs and then bringing it to the mouth. Such feeding may be observed in squirrels, raccoons, monkeys, apes, and in the infant at about six months of age. Hand-mouth reflexes are apparently basic to the voluntary hand-mouth movements used in later eating behavior.

Rooting reflexes are those that orient the infant's head and mouth toward the source of nourishment: the breast or bottle. Prechtl (1958) described two phases of rooting, a side-to-side phase and a directed head-turning phase. The side-to-side phase lasts from birth to about three weeks and is characterized by side-to-side head turning that decreases in extent as the head is gradually directed toward the stimulus. After about three weeks, a single well-guided movement of the head, which brings it in contact with the touch stimulus, or the directed head-turning reflex, emerges. Gentle tapping or stroking of the cheek, perioral skin, or lips constitutes the adequate stimulus. Time of integration of the directed head-turning reflex varies, but it is not unusual to observe it at the age of one year. Testing techniques for eliciting the rooting reflex were discussed by Thomas (1960, p. 15). Lightly stroking outward at the angle of the mouth causes the lowering of the respective half of the lower lip; if the tester's finger is moved away but kept in contact with the cheek, the tongue moves toward the stimulus and the head follows. Stimulating the middle of the upper and lower lips causes lip and tongue elevation and lip and tongue depression, respectively; if the tester's finger continues to move upward or downward toward the chin, the head extends, or the head flexes and the mouth opens, respectively.

Lip reflex is characterized by involuntary movements of the lips in addition to eventual lip closure and pouting activity. It may be seen in preparation for, and during, suckling (Thomson, 1903). Time of integration of the reflex varies, and it has been elicited in some normal children in a drowsy or sleepy state up to twelve years of age.

Mouth-opening reflex allows the infant to bring the source of nourishment into the mouth for processing. A visual stimulus alone, such as a breast, bottle, or finger, may elicit reflexive mouth opening (Mysak, 1959).

Biting reflex is characterized by mouth-closure and holding behavior in response to a stimulus object placed between the gums. It could be viewed as a reflex that secures the nipple in the mouth. Integration of this reflex may occur by approximately four months (Mysak, 1959).

Tongue reflex is characterized by take-in, push-out, and lateralizing movements. Take-in movements are associated with pleasant stimuli, push-out movements with noxious ones. Lateral movement in the direction of a touch stimulus applied to the lateral margin of the tongue was reported in neonates (Weiffenbach, 1972).

Suckling reflex allows the infant to obtain the nourishment after orienting toward its source, the nipple, taking it into the mouth, and stabilizing it there. Suckling involves a forward, upward, and backward movement of the tongue, and may be differentiated from what is commonly called sucking, which is basically a holding of the stimulus object between the lips while creating negative pressure within the mouth. Suckling may be elicited by placing a finger or nipple in contact with the lips, tongue tip and blade, gums, or hard palate. The reflex may be facilitated by gentle movement of the stimulus. Integration of the reflex may be observed during the period from about four months up to the first year (Mysak, 1959); however, it has been elicited in drowsy, older children by gentle stroking of the lips.

Chewing reflex, or reflexive flexion and extension movements of the jaw, may be elicited by stimulating the gum or teeth with a finger or biscuit at about seven months (Illingworth, 1962, p. 25).

Swallow reflex, or the reflex responsible for the actual ingestion of food, follows suckling activity. Anticipatory swallowing may also be observed prior to suckling activity. Coughing, sneezing, and hiccoughing may also elicit swallowing. Stimulation of the palate, fauces, posterior pharyngeal wall, or back of the tongue may cause swallowing activity (Miller and Sherrington, 1915).

In the neonatal period, the swallowing reflex is usually preceded by mouth-opening and lingual protrusion-retrusion, or the suckling reflex. This synreflexia may be regarded as only a part of the chain of feeding reflexes. At about 12 weeks, the suckle reflex part of the chain may be integrated; however, in many normal infants, and children even up to the age of 10 or 12 years, the tongue protrusion pattern may remain unintegrated for as yet undetermined reasons in many cases. It is possible that some varieties of forward-tongue-movement swallow patterns are physiologic, especially those that do not disturb dentition.

Palatal and pharyngeal reflexes already discussed under the protective reflexes section also participate in vegetative motor patterns.

Studies of feeding reflexes that relate to the purpose of this section of the chapter were done by Hooker (1952), Sheppard (1979), and Belfiore-Cohen (1974).

Hooker (1952) found infantile cranio-oropharyngeal patterns similar to the rooting, lip, mouth-opening, biting, suckling, and head reflexes described here in human fetuses between 7.5 and 26 weeks menstrual age (number of weeks since onset of last menstrual period before conception). The patterns were described as reflexive, appearing in an orderly progression with fetal development and resulting from stimulation of the trigeminal nerve. This indicates that these reflexes are already available for use in the fetal stage even before they are functional.

Sheppard (1979) conducted a videotaped, longitudinal study of oral reflexes and evolving skill movements of chewing and social vocal behavior. The focus was on two infants during their first eight months of life. At least a part of this study may be considered an extension of Hooker's work. Perioral, labial, gingival, and palmar reflexogenous sites were studied. These reflex sites are commonly associated with rooting, lip, lateral tongue, mouth-opening, biting, and Babkin reflexes. Responses related to these sites were found throughout the eight-month period. A trend toward diminishing reflex complexity as a function of age was found in all but lip and lateral tongue reflexes. Also, in keeping with the concept of integration and elaboration of basic reflexes into skilled movements, similarities in gestures were found between the reflexes and the emerging chewing and vocal skills.

In a cross-sectional study of oroneuromotor development in normal children aged three, five, and seven, Belfiore-Cohen (1974) studied, among other factors, the status of feeding reflexes. An unexpected finding was that some of these reflexes could still be elicited in some form throughout this age range, especially the suckling reflex. The suckling reflex was present significantly more often in three and five year olds than in seven year olds. Apparently, complete integration of all these basic reflexes by higher speech centers may not be necessary for adequate speech sound maturation.

Pattern Analysis of Vegetative Reflexes

A separate analysis is made of the breathing and feeding reflexes.

Breathing reflexes are elemental reflexes of the primitive-but-complete pattern variety. The early integration of basic breathing reflexes is observed in the shift from nasal to oral inspiration as a function of when the infant is feeding or crying, for example. Cry respiration patterns in infancy appear remarkably similar to speech respiration patterns: between 8 and 13 months, waveforms are similar; I-fractions are almost identical; at 13 months bpms fall within the speech range; and a similar asynchrony of thorax and abdomen during the expiration phase may be observed. The developmental patterns "seen throughout the first year in the decrease of breathing rate and the increase of thoracic participation indicate that some essential characteristics of adult speech are rehearsed and refined in crying" (Langlois and Baken, 1976). Cry talking, or the ability to speak while crying, may be observed throughout life. The ultimate integration of breathing reflexes is reflected in the automatic shift from "medullary vegetative breathing" to "cortical speech breathing" when the at-rest, speaking child begins to talk.

Feeding reflexes are also elemental reflexes, but, in this instance, they are component parts of a more complex reflexive pattern. It could be considered unphysiologic to study these reflexes as separate phenonema, as they have been. Rooting, mouth-opening, biting, lip, suckle, and swallow reflexes are all parts of a reflexive feeding pattern, and it would be more informative if they could be studied as a pattern. Meader (1940) spoke of articulatory movements as modified vegetative reflexes and recommended the buildup of vegetative reflexes such as swallowing, sucking, and chewing reflexes in therapy for certain speech problems. Chew talking, or the ability to speak while chewing, may be observed throughout life.

An analysis of the integration and elaboration of these reflexes by midbrain and cortical centers results in the following possible patterns:

1. Preverbal symbiotic communication and auditory conditioning may arise from the special head or rooting reflex. The primary purpose of the head reflex is to orient the infant to the source of food nourishment, but simultaneously the child receives "verbal nourishment" through maternal face and mouth talk. Future automatic head orienting toward the maternal voice is very likely a manifestation of this early positive conditioning. Early "face reading" or preverbal symbiotic communication also begins with the head reflex toward nourishment. This early face-to-face behavior also serves as a base for later speaker-listener attitudes.

2. Mandibular speech movements may arise from hand-mouth and mouth-opening reflexes. Such movements are responsible for vowels and consonant sounds requiring wide or narrow mouth openings, or varying degrees of mandibular extension, as well as labiodental sounds.

3. Labial speech sounds may arise from movements associated with the lip reflex such as pucker, spread, and close movements. Movements required for lip-round and lip-spread vowels and bilabial nasals, plosives, and glides, and labiodental sounds are included here.
4. Linguadental, lingua-alveolar, linguapalatal, and linguavelar speech sounds may arise from movements associated with the biting, suckle, chewing, and swallow reflexes.
5. Pressure sounds, or those requiring movements associated with adequate velopharyngeal closure, may arise from movements associated with suckle, swallow, pharyngeal, palatal, and yawn reflexes.

REFLEXIVE VOCALIZATION

Just as all the coordinative structures needed for crawling, creeping, sitting, standing, and walking may be observed in the newborn and early infant period, so, too, all the speech reflexive units required for speech may be observed in the infant during the first 12 months or so.

Basic speech movements are revealed during cries and screams associated with pain, discomfort, and hunger. Some are observed concomitant with feeding, and some during hand-mouth play activities. Reflexive-movement vocalization, hand-mouth vocalization, and imitative vocalization are among the categories of reflexive vocalization that may be identified.

Movement Vocalization

During the first months of life, automatic movements of the arms and legs, on-head righting movements, turning over, and reaching movements may be accompanied by automatic vocalization. Such reflexive-movement vocalization may be explained on the basis of reflexive glottic closing required to build up intrathoracic pressure needed to facilitate various movements. Movement-associated vocalization may be observed throughout life in activities like karate, dancing, lifting, elimination, infant delivery, and so on.

Hand-to-Mouth Vocalization

Reflexive vocalization may also be observed during hand-to-mouth play, during feeding, and during teething. Hand-to-mouth play may stimulate increased vocalization because it causes "interesting" variations in sound production, or because it focuses and increases touch, pressure, and movement feedback from the articulators. Teething vocalization results from a combination of pain-eliciting vocalization and vocalization resulting from a focus on touch, pressure, and movement feedback from the gingival area. Vocalization during feeding may emanate from a combination of pleasure-induced laryngeal activity and voicing in conjunction with lip-holding movements around the nipple giving rise to various bilabial sounds; tongue-stroking movements during suckling or chewing giving rise to various lingua-alveolar and linguapalatal sounds; and tongue-back-elevation movements during swallow giving rise to linguavelar sounds.

Forms of Vocalization

This introductory section to imitative vocalization, which defines forms of preverbal vocalization, should contribute to the understanding of the section on imitative vocalization.

Crying, cooing, babbling, lalling, and echoing are terms that describe forms of preverbal vocalization. Sounds referred to below are based on Irwin and Chen (1943) and Irwin (1947, 1951).

Crying denotes the crying and screaming behavior that appears to predominate during the early months of life. Such reflexive behavior is usually in response to hunger, fear, pain, discomfort, and frustration and remains active throughout life.

Cooing (gurgling, snorting, grunting, laughing, chuckling) denotes the reflexive sounds heard in response to "pleasant feelings" and may be observed in its early form during at least the first four months of life. Sounds heard during this period are primarily vocalic with an increasing amount of gutteral sounds: [i, ɪ, ɛ, u, ʊ, h, k, ʔ]. Forms of "cooing" persist throughout life.

Babbling denotes sounds made not only because of good feelings but also as "vocal play." This stage marks a shift to the use of more labial sounds. Part of vocal play includes self-echoing of spontaneous sounds, sometimes called lalling. Babbling-lalling may be observed during the middle months of the first year, or from four to eight months (Ingram, 1976, p. 15). Single syllables may be heard at this time [gʊ, mʌ, bæ, kɑ], and various other sounds [e, æ, oʊ, g, ɑ, ɔ, ə, j, m, p, b, w]. Babbling is not observed after speech has developed except in cases of regression related to neuropathology or psychopathology.

Echoing denotes sounds made in imitation of others as well as self-echoing or lalling. This stage is a continuation of the important vocal play stage begun in the babbling period. This behavior may be observed during the 8- to 12-month period. Sounds heard during this period include: [t, d, n, l, ʃ, s, z, tʃ].

Various analyses of preverbal vocalization have been made that have pertinence to the discussion. For example:

1. The infant's earliest noncrying sounds are vowels.
2. The infant at about six months can produce most of the vowels and about half the consonants.
3. The infant at 12 months can produce more consonants than vowels.
4. Vowel development proceeds from front to back.
5. Consonants develop from back to front. The sequence in preverbal vowel and consonant development has been explained in terms of

motor development: since the infant is usually in supine during the first six months, gravity pulls the velum and tongue backward, thus favoring the production of front vowels and back consonants.

6. The infant's phonemic vocabulary changes when the infant assumes the sitting position "because of the relational shifts in position of the resonatory and articulatory organs" (Berry, 1969, p. 164). Babbling and a marked increase in labial and dental consonants occur. Sitting is also related to development of the thorax, descent of the ribs to an oblique position, and consequent deeper breathing. The beginning of dentition, and spoon and cup feeding also co-occur with sitting.

Imitative Vocalization

The importance of self-echoing and true echoing to later speech development requires further discussion of the phenomena. Ingram (1976, p. 16) discussed Piaget's (1962) belief in the importance of imitation in the development of language. Preverbal imitative ability during Piaget's sensorimotor stages are as follows:

1. From 0 to one month of age, the infant cries when he hears others crying.
2. From one to four months, the infant vocalizes when the adult does, but this "vocal contagion" or mutual imitation depends on the adult making sounds similar to the child's. In other words, the child's cooing may be extended by the adult reflecting it. It is basically auto-echolalia.
3. From about four to eight months, the infant may imitate specific sounds of the adult when those sounds are similar to those made spontaneously by the child. Such extended or provoked babbling may be viewed as a form of auto-echolalia as well.
4. From about 8 to 12 months, there may be initial attempts by the infant at imitating sounds not yet made by him. This marks the beginning of true echolalia.
5. From about 12 to 16 months, the infant shows initial attempts at reproducing true words—a more advanced form of true echolalia.
6. From about 16 to 18 months, the infant exhibits an important step in imitative ability when the infant shows deferred imitation of words heard earlier or delayed echolalia.

Pattern Analysis of Reflexive Vocalization

Babble talk may be viewed as elemental reflexive voicing that is integrated and elaborated upon by higher speech centers into first words. Findings of a preliminary study have suggested that in certain children speech patterns appeared similar to their babble-talk patterns (Oller et al., 1974).

Also, first words appear to emerge from a background of automatic sound-making and echoic behavior. More specifically, speech arises from a bank of automatic sounds and sound combinations that are progressively shaped into arbitrary symbols through the following sequence of imitative behavior: auto-echolalia, or externally sustained cooing or babbling; true echolalia, or the imitation of new sound combinations and words; and finally, delayed echolalia or deferred imitation. Echolalia could be considered primary talking.

Evolution of Skilled Speech Movements

Skilled speech movements emerge from basic speech postures and speech-associated arm-hand movements and basic speech movements. They represent the integration and elaboration of all subcortical and nuclear mechanisms involved in speech function.

Pertinent to this concept of speech neuro-ontogenesis are McCarthy's (1954, p. 513) criteria for the emergence of first words somewhere after the tenth month: (a) establishment of adequate respiration, (b) development of the erect position, (c) cessation of nursing, (d) use of solid food, and (e) eruption of frontal incisors. "As control of the tongue and lips proceeds and dentition provides the frontal wall of the oral cavity, cortical control of speech sounds begins and the infant voluntarily imitates the speech of others and imitates his own speech sounds."

A manifestation of the evolution of skilled speech movements is the emergence of speech breathing and effector coordination.

SPEECH BREATHING

Heralds of emerging speech breathing are (a) deeper-breathing babbling associated with the development of sitting, the thorax, and the descent of the ribs to an oblique position and (b) multisyllabic babbling indicating development of regulation of air pressure for speech purposes at about seven or eight months.

More specifically, the progressive integration of reflexive breathing by speech breathing is seen through changing (a) thoracic-abdominal relationships during crying and noncrying vocalization, (b) I-fraction, and (c) mode of inspiration.

Thoracic-Abdominal Relationships

The progressive increase in thoracic participation and movement organization during crying and noncrying vocalization during the first year appears related to developing speech respiration. Also, abdominal-thoracic asynchrony where abdominal movements precede thoracic movements at the start of the expiratory phase "may reflect the infant's increasing ability to control the elastic recoil forces of expiration" (Langlois, Wilder, and Baken, 1975). The phenomenon is also important to developing speech breathing.

I-fraction

Another indicator of readiness for speech breathing is shifting I-fraction. The capacity of the 10-month-old infant to shift from an I-fraction of about 40 percent during vegetative breathing to one of about 15 percent during crying serves as such an indicator.

Mode of Inspiration

Speech breathing is also marked by a shift from primarily nasal to primarily oral inspiration. Cortical integration of reflexive breathing is also reflected by the ability to voluntarily cease breathing, change inspiratory mode, or alter bpm.

Manifestations of cortical integration of reflexive breathing for speech purposes, therefore, are oral inspiration, thoracic-abdominal asynchrony, and a small I-fraction.

EFFECTOR COORDINATION

As echolalia or primary talking is progressively integrated and elaborated by cortical centers into true talking, the speech effector system, composed of the respiratory effector, resonatory effector, and articulatory effector shows increasing degrees of intra- and intersystem coordination. Required accuracy, speed, and rhythm of speech effector function are reflected through measures of differentiation, praxis, and diadochokinesia.

Effector Differentiation

Speech effectors are contained within the trunk, neck, and head. A prerequisite of speech effector coordination is the emergent specificity of movement or differentiation of movement of the trunk, neck, and head, already discussed under basic speech postures. Following this is laryngeal and articulator differentiation from the head, and finally, articulator differentiation from other articulators.

Laryngeal differentiation from the head describes the growing development of the child to phonate with a minimum of associated head movements. A part of Sheppard's study (1979) on transient oral reflexes and emerging oral motor skills in infants involved gesture patterns that characterize emerging social vocal behavior. She found a high percentage of head dorsiflexion immediately preceding the onset of vocalization—the head posture was usually maintained throughout or during part of the vocalization event. Phonation-associated head movements continue to be seen in young children and in adults during emotional talking such as during arguments or "sad talking."

Articulator differentiation from the head describes the emerging capacity within the child to extend and flex the mandible, pucker or spread the lips, or protrude and retrude the tongue with a minimum of associated head movements.

Articulator differentiation from other articulators describes the developing capacity within the child to extend and flex the mandible in isolation from the lips and tongue, to spread and pucker the lips in isolation from the mandible and tongue, and to protrude-retrude and elevate and depress the tongue in isolation from the mandible and lips.

As part of a larger study of oroneuromotor development in normal children, Belfiore-Cohen (1974) studied articulator differentiation. She was concerned with establishing preliminary data on articulator differentiation in boys and girls aged three, five, and seven years. As expected, articulatory differentiation increased significantly from three to five and from five to seven years. Measured was the ability for various isolated movements of the mandible, lips, and tongue.

Effector Praxis

Praxis as used here is defined as the ability to perform coordinated actions or movements. Such ability at the level of the larynx may be called laryngopraxis, or at the level of the articulators, articulopraxis.

Laryngopraxis describes the developing ability in the child to produce a series of discrete on-off vowel phonations—the speed of production is not a factor in laryngopraxis. Regression in this ability is sometimes an early sign of neuropathology.

Articulopraxis describes the developing ability within the child to show good intra-articulatory coordination during the production of various combinations and increasing numbers of syllables. Syllabic forms, in front-to-back and in physiologic terms, include bilabial, labiodental, linguadental, lingua-alveolar, and linguavelar forms.

As a function of development, children show increasing capacity to produce with good coordination various two-syllable combinations: for example, bilabial-labiodental /bʌ-vʌ/, bilabial-linguadental, bilabial-lingua-alveolar, bilabial-linguapalatal, and bilabial-linguavelar combinations. Using a receding, neurodevelopmental pattern, the labiodental syllable may then serve as the base syllable /vʌ-bʌ/ combined with preceding syllables and then receding ones to form a new, two-syllable set. Eventually all syllables may serve as base syllables in combination with all other syllables.

Similarly, three-syllable and four-syllable combinations are produced well and in coordinated fashion by developing children. Again, initiatory norms on articulopraxis were offered by Belfiore-Cohen (1974).

Children aged three, five, and seven were asked to reproduce various two-syllable, three-syllable, and four-syllable sound combinations. The sound combinations constructed were samples of front-to-middle (mʌ-nʌ), front-to-back (mʌ-kʌ), middle-to-front (nʌ-mʌ), middle-to-back (nʌ-kʌ), back-to-middle (kʌ-nʌ), and back-to-front (kʌ-mʌ) combinations. All subjects were able to do the two-syllable series; seven- and most five-year-olds were able to complete the three-syllable series, but the majority of three-year-olds could not; and most seven-year-olds and the majority of five-year-olds were able to complete the four-syllable series; and, again, the majority of three-year-olds could not.

Effector Diadochokinesia

Effector diadochokinesia is the ability to engage in serial, repetitive movements of the various speech effectors. Rates of diadochokinesia increase as a function of age. In assessing diadochokinesia, not only the rate is considered, that is, syllables per second, but also the duration (at least 10 seconds) and rhythmicity of performance.

Respirodiadochokinesia is measured by having the child "pant" as quickly as possible. Care should be taken against the possibility of hyperventilation. Estimates of respirodiadochokinesia can be made on the basis of a five-second performance.

Laryngodiadochokinesia is measured by having the child produce a series of discrete, on-off vowel phonations as quickly as possible.

Velodiadochokinesia is measured by having the child produce, in alternating fashion, and as quickly as possible /mʌ-bʌ/, or /nʌ-dʌ/, or /ŋ-gʌ/.

Articulodiadochokinesia may be measured by having the child repeat as quickly as possible various syllables, for example, /pʌ/, /tʌ/, /kʌ/, or syllable combinations, for example, /pʌtʌ/ or /pʌ, tʌ, kʌ/.

Data on articulodiadochokinesia have been collected by numerous investigators over the years. Rates of "articulodiado" are clearly age-related. Belfiore-Cohen (1974) found a steady increase in rates of /pʌ/, /tʌ/, and /kʌ/ for three-, five-, and seven-year-olds. For all syllables, three-year-olds scored significantly lower than five-year-olds and seven-year-olds, and five-year-olds scored significantly lower than seven-year-olds. Table 2.1 displays the means and ranges of the rates.

TABLE 2.1 *Articulodiadochokinesia Rates**

		pʌ		tʌ		kʌ	
Age		Males	Females	Males	Females	Males	Females
3	Mean	2.5	2.6	2.5	2.8	2.5	2.5
	Range	1.7–3.1	1.7–3.6	1.7–3.0	1.7–3.6	1.6–3.5	2.1–3.2
5	Mean	3.6	3.7	3.5	3.6	3.1	3.3
	Range	2.3–5.0	2.0–5.5	2.2–5.1	2.5–5.5	1.8–4.0	1.6–4.7
7	Mean	4.3	4.2	4.2	4.0	3.7	3.6
	Range	3.4–5.5	2.6–5.0	3.4–5.4	3.0–5.0	2.3–5.2	2.8–4.8

*Average number of repetitions per second based on a 10-second sample. The table is from Belfiore-Cohen (1974).

VOICE AND SPEECH PRODUCTION

Adequate speech breathing and effector differentiation, praxis, and dia-dochokinesia are the major indicators of adequate voicing for speech, as well as of accurate, coordinated, and rhythmical speech articulation. Voluntary differentiation, praxis, and diadochokinetic movements are manifestations of cortical integration and elaboration of the basic speech movements found in certain protective, emotional, and vegetative reflexes and reflexive vocalization.

Communisphere

Among the various factors contributing to the emergence of spoken symbols among early people was the decreasing "space" among and between them. As man's biosphere became more crowded through the increase in population and community living, a concomitant need arose for communication; and thus began the gradual integration and elaboration of man's basic biosphere into a more complex communisphere.

In terms of speech neuro-ontogenesis, at least four ranges of communisphere may be recognized: the intimate, personal, family, and public ranges.

The intimate communisphere represents the infant's first communisphere—the one that develops when mother holds the baby closely during nursing or feeding. During this time, mother and child gaze at each other's face and into each other's eyes. The mother is inclined to talk to her baby during these special communicative moments. The intimate communisphere may be considered as setting the foundation for all future face-to-face communicative encounters; and, therefore, how this communisphere is established and developed may be considered significant to future speech development.

The intimate communisphere is maintained throughout life during kissing and caressing behavior and while dancing, as examples.

The personal communisphere, or the communisphere delineated by approximately the arms-length range, is the person-to-person communisphere. Mother or father and child create such a communisphere when the infant is in back, elbow, sit, and stand speech postures.

It is through positive experiences in the intimate and personal communispheres that the child learns to talk.

The family communisphere, or the communisphere delineated by approximately the six- to 12-foot range, is the person-to-small group communisphere. Child and parents or a family create such a communisphere while around a dinner table or during play activities. It is through good experiences in the family communisphere that personal communication expands into sociocommunication.

The public communisphere, or the communisphere delineated by distances that extend beyond approximately the 12-foot range, is the person-to-larger group communisphere. Children enter the public communisphere when first reciting at a larger family gathering, or to a group of classmates. The public communisphere represents an extension of the sociocommunication emerging in the family communisphere.

The comparative importance of intimate, personal, and family communispheres for overall speech development, or the best proportion of time spent in the various communispheres for overall speech development, are unanswered issues at this point in time.

Implications for Cerebral Palsy

As with the chapter in neurophylogenesis of speech, this chapter contains many implications for the understanding and care of cerebral palsy speech problems.

Again, if cerebral palsy is best understood in terms of delayed, retarded, or arrested neuroevolution, then a proper evaluation of the speech problem in cerebral palsy must include an exploration of the child's listening behavior and basic speech postures, his speech-associated hand movements, his basic speech movements, and the development of communispheres, as well as his skilled speech movements.

Correspondingly, such an evaluation invites the incorporation of all these factors into the overall plan of neurospeech therapy for any particular child with cerebral palsy.

REFERENCES

Belfiore-Cohen, A. Oroneuromotor development in normal children. Unpublished doctoral dissertation, Teachers College, Columbia University (1974).

Berry, M. F. *Language disorders of children.* New York: Appleton-Century-Crofts (1969).

Hooker, D. *The prenatal origin of behavior.* Lawrence, Kansas: University of Kansas Press (1952).

Illingworth, R. S. *An introduction to developmental assessment in the first year.* London: National Spastics Society (1962).

Ingram, D. *Phonological disability in children.* New York: Elsevier (1976).

Irwin, O. C., and Chen, H. P. Speech sound elements during the first year of life: A review of the literature. *J. Speech Dis.,* 8, 109–121 (1943).

――――. Infant speech: Consonantal sounds according to place of articulation. *J. Speech Hearing Dis.,* 12, 397–401 (1947).

――――. Infant speech: Consonantal position. *J. Speech Hearing Dis.,* 16, 154–161 (1951).

Langlois, A., and Baken, R. J. Development of respiratory time-factors in infant cry. *Devel. Med. Child Neurol.,* 732–737 (1976).

――――, Wilder, C. N., and Baken, R. J. Pre-speech respiratory patterns in the infant. Paper presented at the annual meeting of the American Speech and Hearing Association, Washington, D.C. (1975).

McCarthy, D. Language development in children. In L. Carmichael (Ed.), *Manual of child psychology,* 2nd ed. New York: John Wiley and Sons, Inc. (1954).

Meader, M. H. The effect of disturbances in the developmental processes upon emergent specificity of function. *J. Speech Dis.,* 5, 211–219 (1940).

Miller, F. R., and Sherrington, C. S. Some observations on the buccopharyngeal stage of reflex deglutition. *Quart. J. Exp. Physiol.,* 9, 147–186 (1915).

Murphy, K. Development of articulation and hearing. In *Learning Problems of the Cerebral Palsied.* London: The Spastic Society (1964).

Mysak, E. D. Dysarthria and oropharyngeal reflexology: a review, *J. Speech Hearing Dis.,* 28, 252–260 (1963).

———. Significance of neurophysiological orientation to cerebral palsy habilitation. *J. Speech Hearing Dis.,* 24, 221–230 (1959).

Oller, D. K., Wieman, L. A., Doyle, W. J. and Ross, C. Child speech, babbling, and phonological universals. *PRCLD,* 8, 33–41 (1974).

Peiper, A. *Cerebral function in infancy and childhood.* New York: Consultants Bureau (1963).

Perlstein, M., and McDonald, E. Nature, recognition, and management of neuromuscular disabilities in children. *Pediatrics,* 11, 166–173 (1953).

Piaget, J. *Play, dreams, and imitation in childhood.* New York: Norton (1962).

Prechtl, H. F. R. The directed head-turning response and allied movements of the human baby. *Behavior,* 13, 212–242 (1958).

Schwartz, A. B. Congenital laryngeal stridor—speculations regarding its origin. *Pediatrics,* 27, 477–479 (1961).

Sheppard, J. Transient oral reflexes and emerging oral motor skill in infants. Unpublished doctoral dissertation, Teachers College, Columbia University (1979).

Thomas, A. Chesni, Y., and Dargassies, S. *The neurological examination of the infant.* London: National Spastics Society (1960).

Thomson, J. On the lip-reflex (mouth phenomenon) of newborn children. *Rev. Neurol. Psychiat.,* 1, 145–148 (1903).

Wilder, C. N., and Baken, R. J. Respiratory patterns in infant cry. *Human Communic.,* 3, 18–34 (1974).

———. Some developmental aspects of infant cry. *J. Genet. Psychol.,* 132, 225–230 (1978).

Weiffenbach, J. M. Discrete elicited motions of the newborn's tongue. In J. M. Bosma (Ed.), *Oral sensation and perception,* Springfield, Ill.: Charles C Thomas (1972).

3

Neurospeech Disorders

NEUROSPEECH DISORDERS IN cerebral palsy are based on the concept of the neurophylo-ontogenesis of speech and, therefore, are more inclusive than traditional descriptions of cerebral palsy speech disorder. Neurospeech disorders include problems in basic listening movements, speech postures, basic hand movements, basic speech movements, and skilled listening responses, skilled speech movements, and expressive communication.

Estimates of the incidence of communicative problems among cerebral palsied children vary for a number of reasons, among them are definition of disorder and severity and types of children included. Some estimates found in the literature include: 70 percent (Wolfe, 1950), 75 percent (Hopkins, Bice, and Colton, 1954), 79 percent (Lorenze, 1962), and 86 percent (Achilles, 1955).

Theories on Symptoms in Neuropathology

A discussion of theories of symptoms in neuropathology and the significance of these theories to the neuropathology of cerebral palsy is necessary prior to beginning the central discussion of this chapter.

DISSOLUTION THEORY

As discussed in Chapter 1, Jackson (1958, p. 46), with respect to adult neuropathology, developed the concept of dissolution of the CNS. The concept defines dissolution as a reverse of evolution, meaning that with progression of the disease there is a progressive dissolution in behaviors from behaviors that are least organized, most complex, and least automatic to behaviors that are most organized, most simple, and most automatic. Dissolution could also be uniform or local; by uniform dissolution Jackson meant a relatively even reversal of the evolution of the entire CNS; by local dissolution, he meant a more local reversal of evolution resulting from disease of a part of the CNS. The concept of dissolution also refers to depth of involvement by which Jackson meant that, depending on the amount of injury, the highest centers being least organized suffer first and most; the middle centers being more organized resist longer; and the lowest centers being most organized suffer the last and the least. Finally, dissolution also means duplex symptomatology: that is, negative symptoms, or loss or defect-of-function symptoms; and positive symptoms, or release-of-involuntary-activities symptoms.

DYSINTEGRATION THEORY

The dissolution theory of symptoms of neuropathology formed the basis for the author's dysintegration theory of symptoms in developmental cerebral palsy. The concept of dysintegration of the CNS also includes level, form, and depth of dysintegration and types of symptomatology.

Level of Dysintegration

Dysintegration in cerebral palsy may be reflected by a delay in the integration and elaboration of basic reflexes. In such cases, spinal automatisms like the flexion, extension, and cross reflexes, and brain-stem reflexes like the tonic neck and tonic labyrinthine reflexes may persist and remain unregulated and undirected by higher brain centers. This, in turn, implies problems in developing back, elbow, and sit speech postures, for example.

Retardation of integration implies a slower-than-expected integration of lower sensorimotor integration centers by higher ones. For example, a child of three or four may only be developing elbow and sit speech postures, and just beginning to develop expressive hand movements and imitative reflexive vocalization.

Arrestment of integration means that the child's integration-elaboration processes reach a certain level and appear to remain fixed at that level.

Form of Dysintegration

As in dissolution, dysintegration in cerebral palsy may be uniform or more local in form. Uniform dysintegration may be reflected by relatively even dysintegration of (a) various functions at a particular integration level; (b) sensory and motor aspects, (c) sides of the body, and (d) speech, intellectual, and social activities.

Local dysintegration may be manifested by local delays, retardation, or arrestment of function at various sensorimotor integration levels: sensory features may be more involved, or the upper limbs more than the lower limbs, or vice versa. There may be uneven developments of general motor, speech, or cognitive functions.

Depth of Dysintegration

Depth of dissolution refers to the observation that, in neuropathology, functions related to the highest CNS centers are involved first, then middle-center functions, and finally, lowest-center functions.

In developmental cerebral palsy, depth of dysintegration refers to the observation that the lowest sensorimotor integration centers, being most organized, dominate sensorimotor integration; middle centers, being less organized, contribute less to sensorimotor integration; and the highest centers, being the least organized, contribute least to sensorimotor integration. Such dominance by lower centers over CNS function occurs even though higher centers may be capable of better functioning. This discrepancy or unused neurophysiological potential is one of the bases for neurospeech therapy.

Triplex Symptomatology

Instead of the duplex symptomatology that characterizes the dissolution theory of symptoms in neuropathology, the dysintegration theory of symptoms in developmental cerebral palsy is characterized by triplex symptomatology. The triplex symptomatology is manifested by three sets of three symptoms: (a) the concept of delay, retardation, and arrestment of neurointegration, (b) the observation of tone, posture, and movement symptoms, and (c) the concept of atrophic, hypertrophic, and dystrophic symptoms.

Delay, retardation, or arrestment symptoms have already been discussed under level of dysintegration. Here the concept relates to the possibility that in any one child with cerebral palsy some functions may be delayed in appearance, some may be retarded or slowed in development, and others may be arrested in development.

Tone, posture, and movement symptoms represent the set of symptoms found in most cases of developmental cerebral palsy. Muscle tone may be low or hypotonic as in cases of ataxic cerebral palsy, or high or hypertonic as in cases of spasticity and rigidity, or fluctuating as in cases of athetotic cerebral palsy. Abnormal postures are associated with dysintegration and with irregular tone. And since normal movement is dependent on normal tone and posture, and since tone and posture are usually irregular in cerebral palsy, movement is irregular as well. Movement is also irregular because of dysintegration. Tone, posture, and movement symptoms form a triad of symptoms; that is, they are closely related if not inseparable.

Atrophic, hypertrophic, and dystrophic symptoms refer, respectively, to the absence of the appearance of coordinative structures or reflexes, the overdevelopment of these basic movements, and the incomplete integration of these reflexive units.

For example, atrophic symptoms describe the absence of (a) elemental righting reactions or stabilizing equilibrium reactions, (b) reflexive hand movements, or (c) feeding reflexes.

Dystrophic symptoms refer to the partial integration of basic movements by higher, sensorimotor integration centers. For example, a child's walking pattern may include only partially integrated spinal automatisms and tonic neck reflexes, or a child involved with eye-hand activity may exhibit only partially integrated grasp-release reflexes and tonic neck reflexes. Also, when speaking, a child's mouth may extend in an unregulated manner while articulating an open-mouth sound, indicating only partial integration of the mouth-opening reflex; or the child's tongue may protrude or lateralize in an unregulated manner while articulating tongue-tip sounds, indicating only partial integration of the suckle and lateral tongue reflexes.

Hypertrophic symptoms refer to the "overgrowth" of basic movements, or the nonintegration of them. This nonintegration of the basic units of movement leads to their exaggeration.

The concept of hypertrophic symptoms was discussed by Twitchell (1965): "In a sense, the patient with cerebral palsy represents a still more profound physiological defect in sensory-motor maturation or integration with a hypertrophy of various infantile reflexes." According to Twitchell, the defect in voluntary movement and in reflex mechanisms in cerebral palsy have a common basis which "is a defect in sensory-motor integration with conflict between hypertrophied infantile reflexes."

Examples of symptoms of hypertrophy include: problems in roll over from supine because of exaggerated asymmetrical tonic neck reflexes stimulated by head lateralization in preparation for roll over; problems in reaching out in sitting because of exaggerated symmetrical tonic neck reflexes stimulated by the child's head, which may be held in a ventroflexed position; and problems in initiating voice because of unregulated glottic-closing or glottic-opening reflexes.

Dysintegration of Basic Listening Movements

Basic listening movements include the assumption of head and trunk positions that facilitate listening for speech (corresponding to basic speech postures) and the emergence of elemental protective and listening reflex movements and tuning reflex responses.

PROTECTIVE REFLEXES

The auditory Moro and eye-opening and eye-closing reflexes, restlessness, mouth-opening, and crying responses to sound are viewed as auditory protective responses. Atrophy, hypertrophy, or dystrophy of these responses may interfere with auditory processing of speech signals to various degrees.

LISTENING REFLEXES

Cessation of crying, suckling, or stilling in response to speech stimuli are considered early reflexive listening responses. Atrophy, hypertrophy, or dystrophy of these responses may also have negative implications for auditory processing of speech.

TUNING REFLEXES

Changes in heart rate, respiration, and hormonal flow in response to speech sounds are viewed as positive autonomic conditioning for auditory processing. Such positive auditory conditioning responses may be considered as auditory tuning reflexes. Atrophy, hypertrophy, or dystrophy of these responses may also interfere with auditory speech processing in various and subtle ways.

Dysintegration of Basic Speech Postures

The law of developmental direction in humans is well known, that is, behavior organization is cephalocaudal, or head to feet. First comes control of eye movements, then face movements (e.g., smiling), and then head movements (e.g., turning and lifting). Then, after six months or so, motor control of the arms and upper trunk region is observed with grasping and sitting. Finally, after 10 or 12 months, motor control proceeds to the legs, allowing for standing and early walking activities. An important feature of the progression in motor control is that postural control of a part of the body always precedes movement control of that part. In other words, coordinated movements in any given posture are dependent on adequate maintenance of that posture.

The concept of the importance of postural control to movement control has not been well developed in the field of speech pathology. The importance of trunk balance to speech breathing and neck and head balance to voicing and articulation should be obvious. Stated differently, coordinated movements of the speech effectors (respiratory, phonatory, resonatory, and articulatory) are dependent to a substantial degree on postural control of the trunk, neck, and head; therefore, difficulty in developing and maintaining basic speech postures should be viewed as an integral part of the speech problem in cerebral palsy.

BACK PATTERNS

Back-pattern speech postures are the earliest to develop and remain operative throughout life. They become functional when the infant can roll over into supine from the prone position, assume a normal head position in relation to the body, and be able to bring his hands together and to the mouth.

Dysintegration of back patterns may be based on atrophic, hypertrophic, and dystrophic symptoms. Atrophic symptoms include the nonappearance or delayed appearance of basic spinal and brainstem reflexes, and later the delayed or nonappearance of neck, and on-head righting reactions, and stabilizing equilibrium reactions in prone and supine. Hypertrophic symptoms may include exaggerated tonic neck and tonic labyrinthine reflexes resulting from nonintegration of brainstem centers. Dystrophic symptoms may include the partial integration of spinal and brainstem reflexes and hence the incomplete emergence of neck righting, on-head righting, and supine equilibrium reactions.

Dysintegration of back patterns may have negative effects on breathing reflexes and on emerging speech breathing patterns; feeding reflexes; hand-to-mouth vocalization, cooing, and babbling; and auditory localization movements.

ELBOW PATTERNS

Elbow-pattern speech postures become functional when the child can roll over from supine, fully extend his head, neck, and trunk, and extend, abduct, and outwardly rotate his lower limbs. The child must show good head balance and good support of the upper trunk with upper limbs and hands. Various forms of elbow patterns remain functional throughout life.

Dysintegration of elbow patterns may be manifested by atrophic features such as the delay or nonappearance of the elemental on-head righting, body-on-body righting, and arm-support-forward reactions; the tuning midbrain reactions—the Landau and the chain-in-prone reactions; and the stabilizing equilibrium reactions in prone, side lying, and on-forearms. Dystrophic features or the incomplete emergence of the elemental and tuning midbrain reactions and stabilizing equilibrium reactions may also be observed. Hypertrophic symptoms include exaggerated spinal and brainstem reflexes and accompanying abnormalities of tone and movement.

Dysintegration of elbow patterns has negative implications for the normally expanding auditory and visual perceptual fields, for hand exploratory activities, and for early auto-echolalia behavior.

SIT PATTERNS

Sit patterns become functional when the child is able to roll over from supine, assume the quadrupedal posture, then side sit, long sit, heel sit, or tailor sit. Various sit postures remain functional throughout life.

Dysintegration of sitting is characterized by the atrophic features of delay or nonappearance in the elemental righting reactions of complete rotation and quadrupedal righting and hopping, and in stabilizing equilibrium reactions in the on-fours and in-sitting positions. Hypertrophic and dystrophic symptoms may also be contributory to dysintegration of sitting.

Dysintegration of sit patterns has negative implications for the expanding auditory and perceptual fields associated with sitting and for early true echolalia behavior.

STAND PATTERNS

Stand patterns become functional when the child is able to roll over from supine, assume the quadrupedal position, push up into the simian position (or move into the half-kneeling position), and finally, into the standing position.

Dysintegration of standing is manifested by the atrophic features of delay or absence of elemental righting reactions; of elemental and stabilizing equilibrium reactions in the on-knees, half-kneel, and standing positions; and of tuning cortical reactions including head-lead and eye-movement reactions. As in back, elbow, and sit pattern dysintegrations, hypertrophic and dystrophic features may also accompany dysintegration of stand patterns.

Dysintegration of stand patterns has negative implications for development of critical auditory and visual perceptual fields in standing and for the onset of true talking.

Dysintegration of Basic Hand Movements

Basic hand movements are viewed as those reflexive movements that give rise to various "hands talk" movements. Included as basic hand movements are particular protective, progression, and vegetative reflexes.

Dysintegration of reflexive hand movements is indicated by the atrophic features of delay or absence of arm-support and arm-balance reactions, of various hand progression movements such as upper limb movement, arm walking, and upper-limb placing and hopping reactions, and hand-to-mouth feeding movements. Dystrophic symptoms are reflected by partial emergence of these movements. Hypertrophic symptoms are manifested by exaggerated upper limb flexion patterns associated with nonintegrated long spinal reflexes, and exaggerated symmetrical and asymmetrical arm postures associated with nonintegrated tonic neck and tonic labyrinthine reflexes.

Dysintegration of basic hand movements has negative implications for the development of hand movements that serve symbolic gestural and adjunctive gestural roles. More is said about these roles in the section of this chapter devoted to expressive communication. Hands talk, so important to normal children, is infrequently available to cerebral palsied children.

Dysintegration of Basic Speech Movements

Basic speech movements are defined as the underlying reflexes of which skilled speech movements are composed. Stated in another way, skilled speech movements are a manifestation of the integration and elaboration of these reflexes by higher speech centers. Included as basic speech reflexes are certain protective, emotional, and vegetative reflexes, and particular forms of reflexive vocalization. Atrophy, dystrophy, or hypertrophy of these basic movements may influence substantially the development of skilled speech movements.

PROTECTIVE REFLEXES

Basic glottic closing-opening, cough, pharyngeal, and palatal, and jaw, lip, and tongue protective reflexes serve to protect the organism against invasion from foreign bodies and also protect certain organs per se.

Dysintegration of protective reflexes is characterized by atrophic features of delay or absence of laryngeal closing-opening and palatal reflexes, the jaw-jerk reflex, and lip and tongue protective reflexes. Hypertrophic features, or the exaggerated and unregulated manifestations of the glottic closing-opening or jaw jerk reflexes, may also be observed. Partial integration of glottic closing-opening, palatal, and jaw-jerk reflexes is also observed.

Dysintegration of protective reflexes may have negative implications for the development of voicing, pressure sounds, and labial and lingual sounds.

EMOTIONAL REFLEXES

Basic cry, smile, and laugh reflexes serve at least two purposes: (a) they are behaviors that signal pain, fear, discomfort, or contentment and happiness and (b) they serve as precursors to "speech color," or sounds used to accompany later "happy talk," "sad talk," "excited talk," and so on, and to speech respiration.

Dysintegration of emotional reflexes may also be characterized by atrophic, hypertrophic, or dystrophic features. Delay or absence of smile and laugh reflexes, which may be regarded as speech tuning reflexes, has negative implications for the development of speech color—just as their exaggeration may interfere with later speech messages. Reduced or weak crying carries negative implications for the important development of crying respiration which, in turn, may have repercussions on the development of speech respiration.

VEGETATIVE REFLEXES

Breathing vegetative reflexes and feeding vegetative reflexes are necessary to sustain life and to serve as coordinative structures for various skilled speech movements.

Breathing Reflexes

Dysintegration of basic breathing movements is manifested by at least atrophic and dystrophic symptoms. Atrophic features are characterized by delay or absence of participation of the thorax in breathing, of a decreasing bpm, and of an increasing depth of breathing cycle; dystrophic features imply the partial emergence of these characteristics. Such atrophic and dystrophic features hold significance for future development of speech breathing.

Feeding Reflexes

Feeding reflexes are primarily designed for orienting the infant toward a food source, allowing him to obtain the food, and finally, ingesting it. Two levels of feeding activities may be recognized—rooting feeding and hand-to-mouth feeding. Rooting feeding is primal feeding, and involves the ingestion of liquids and soft foods via direct oral intake. Hand-to-mouth feeding represents an integration of the rooting-feeding movements and involves the ingestion of solid foods via hand transport of the food to the mouth, the chewing of it, and, finally, the swallowing of it. Hand-to-mouth processing of solid foods begins during the second half of the first year. The chain of reflexes of which rooting feeding and hand-to-mouth feeding are composed contain movement patterns many of which are believed to be integrated by speech centers and used for speech purposes. Symptoms of dysintegration of these reflexes are characterized by atrophic, hypertrophic, and dystrophic features.

Rooting reflex delay or nonappearance may have repercussions on early stimulation of listening and face communication. It might also negatively affect the development of future attitudes toward speaker-listener interactions. Also, hypertrophy of the mandibular portion of this head reflex may result in jaw lateralization during attempts at /s/ production and consequent lateralization of sibilants.

Mouth-opening reflex hypertrophy may interfere with articulation in at least two ways: (a) vowels requiring an open-mouth position like /a/ may elicit an exaggerated mouth-opening reflex and result in the distortion of the vowel and (b) exaggeration of the reflex may interfere with control of the production of sounds requiring narrow mouth opening like /i/ and /s/. An exaggerated mouth-opening reflex may also interfere with running speech, if it is unexpectedly elicited by something passing through the visual field, for example.

Tongue reflex hypertrophy or dystrophy may interfere with articulation through the lateralization of the speech airstream. Stimulation of the lateral margins of the tongue during production of lingual sounds may elicit the lateral tongue reflex and result in lateralized sibilants.

Biting, chewing reflex atrophy may contribute to "habitual open-mouth posture" and have negative implications for the development of sounds requiring narrow mouth positions.

Lip reflex hypertrophy or dystrophy may interfere with /r/ and /l/ development. Attempts at producing these sounds may stimulate concomitant lip movements resulting in "bilabialized" forms of these sounds. Attempts at labiodental sound production may also stimulate exaggerated lip reflexes and cause problems in formation of /f/ and /v/.

Suckle reflex hypertrophy or dystrophy may also interfere with the production of tongue-tip sounds. Attempts to produce /t/, /d/, /n/, /s/, /z/ may excite the suckle movement and result in dentalized and interdental forms of these sounds.

Swallow, palatal, pharyngeal reflex atrophy contributes to drooling, which interferes with articulatory efforts in general. Such atrophy may also interfere with the development of velopharyngeal closure movements required for normal speech resonation. Hypertrophy of palatal and pharyngeal reflexes may result in unregulated closing of the velopharyngeal complex during running speech and periodic hyponasality.

Biting, suckle, chewing, swallow reflex atrophy or dystrophy may in-

terfere with the development of skilled movements required for normal production of linguadental, lingua-alveolar, linguapalatal, and linguavelar
sounds. Manifestations of this interference may include protrusive or
retrusive lingual contacts for /θ, t, d, n, l/ sounds, "diffused" /ʃ, dʒ, tʃ/
sounds, and absent /g, k/ sounds.

Suckle, palatal, pharyngeal, swallow reflex atrophy or dystrophy may interfere with the development of the velopharyngeal closure mechanism and,
consequently, affect the production of all pressure sounds, such as plosives,
fricatives, and affricates.

A number of reports appear in the literature that support the association
of delayed, retarded, or arrested integration of feeding reflexes in children
with speech symptoms, or the reemergence of these reflexes in adults with
speech difficulty.

Avoiding response and grasp reflex as described and as manifested in the
speech mechanisms of athetotic and spastic children (Clement and Twitchell, 1959) could be viewed as dysintegrated rooting and lip reflexes. Sheppard
(1964) found that, in her cerebral palsied subjects, an inverse relationship
existed between the number of infantile reflexes elicited and speech and
feeding proficiency, progress in speech therapy, and age. In a study of
children with the Sjögren-Larsson syndrome, not only were speech and
language problems found but also the persistence of vigorous sucking and
rooting reflexes at age five (Witkop and Henry, 1963). Also, forms of
visceral swallowing might be regarded as suckle-swallow activity, and such
swallow patterns have been associated with various speech sound substitu-
tions (Ward et al., 1961). Finally, in a study of speech problems among
cerebral palsied children (Kamalashile, 1975), it was reported that those
with normal articulation rarely showed vegetative disturbances.

Reemergence of some of these reflexes were reported in various adult
neuropathologies, as well. The reappearance of the suckle reflex has been
reported in severe cerebral degeneration (Brain, 1955, pp. 42–43) and
in cases with vascular, toxic, infectious, and psychotic backgrounds
(Schneider, 1938). The tendency for speech behavior in a case of post-
encephalitic parkinsonian dysarthria to be accompanied with yawning,
biting, and snout movements of the lips and mouth was also reported
(Grewel, 1957). Finally, Morrison et al. (1970) also reported on released
oral reflex phenomena and parkinsonian speech disorder.

Figure 3.1 shows a cerebral palsied individual who has not developed
elbow, sit, or stand speech postures. Figure 3.2 depicts her arm and hand
movements remaining as parts of primitive spinal and brainstem reflexes
and hence not being integrated for use in symbolic or adjunctive gestural
patterns. Figure 3.3a shows her not enjoying full display of reflexive smile,
and Figures 3.3b, c, d, e, and f show her with hypertrophied mouth-
opening, biting, rooting, suckle, and lip reflexes.

Fig. 3.1.
Dysintegration of
basic speech postures

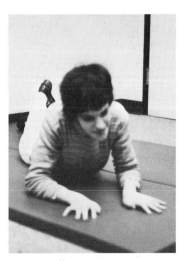

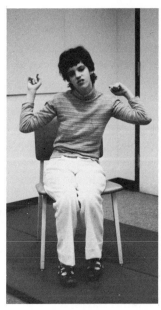

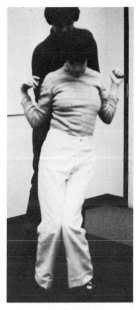

elbow pattern   sit pattern   stand pattern

Fig. 3.2. Dysintegration of
basic hand movements

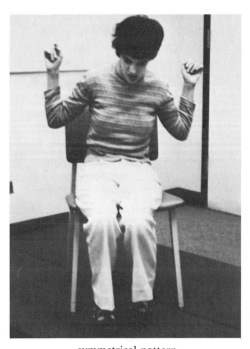

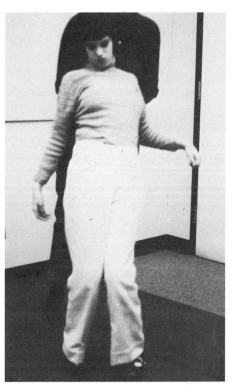

symmetrical pattern   asymmetrical pattern

Fig. 3.3.   Dysintegration of basic emotional and vegetative movements

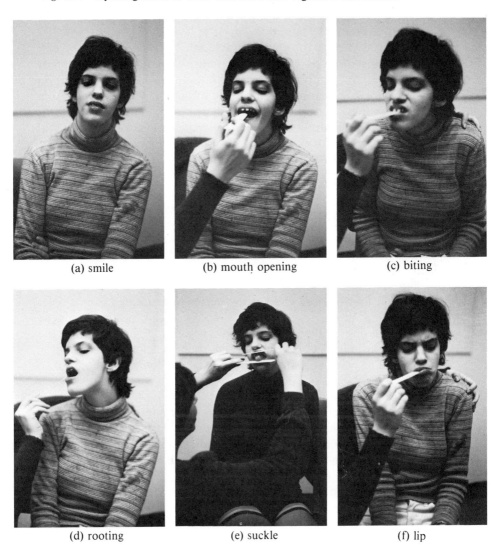

| (a) smile | (b) mouth opening | (c) biting |
| (d) rooting | (e) suckle | (f) lip |

REFLEXIVE VOCALIZATION

Reflexive vocalization appears to have at least three functions: (a) It signals discomfort, pain, frustration, or hunger; (b) it serves as accompaniment to motor activities such as moving and eating, and (c) it serves as preverbal sound material for true speech. Movements associated with preverbal sound production may be considered an early integration of movements associated with protective, emotional, and vegetative reflexes.

Involvement of reflexive vocalization movements may also be characterized by atrophic, hypertrophic, and dystrophic features.

Movement-Associated Vocalization

Atrophy or dystrophy of movement-associated vocalization has at least two implications: (a) It may indicate a problem in automatic adduction of the vocal folds for purposes of creating intrathoracic breath pressure in preparation for large motor activities, like lifting one's upper trunk from the prone position, and hence, has speech posture implications and (b) it may have negative implications for the development of automatic vocal fold presetting in preparation for speech vocalization. Hypertrophy of movement-associated vocalization in a speaking child may be reflected by uncontrolled adductor activity during speaking and consequent voicing anomalies.

Hand-to-Mouth Vocalization

Atrophy of hand-to-mouth play activity results in reduced vocalization, in a reduction in the repertoire of early reflexive vocalization, and in a reduced focus on touch, pressure, and movement feedback from the articulators.

Atrophy or dystrophy of vocalization during lip-grasping of the nipple, tongue-stroking during suckling and chewing, and posterior tongue movements during swallowing may have negative implications for the development of bilabial and labiodental sounds; linguadental, lingua-alveolar, and linguapalatal sounds; and linguavelar sounds.

Happy-Play Vocalization

Atrophy or dystrophy of happy or pleasant-sensations vocalization (cooing) and play vocalization (babbling) would result in delay or disturbance in the use of reflexive vocalic and syllabic sounds. Also affected would be the important association of "talking" and good feelings, and "talking" just for the fun of it.

This ends the section of the chapter describing symptoms of dysintegration of basic movements. The forthcoming section on dysintegration of skilled movements includes further discussion of the role of dysintegration of basic movements in the dysintegration of skilled movements, as well as discussion on other causes of problems in skilled speech movements among the cerebral palsied.

Dysintegration of Skilled Listening Responses

Skilled listening responses include functions of selective inhibition of startle, localizing, and early speech perception.

DYSINTEGRATION OF SELECTIVE INHIBITION OF STARTLE

Atrophy or dystrophy of the capacity for selective inhibition of startle has important implications for auditory processing of speech. Persisting startle is reflective of a lack of cortical participation in auditory processing and also leads to negative responses to auditory stimuli.

DYSINTEGRATION OF LISTENING MOVEMENTS

The development of listening movements in response to speech stimuli progresses from (a) the cessation of whimpering or other "fussing sounds" in response to human voice during the first weeks of life, to (b) the emergence of stare or smile in response to the maternal voice at about three months, to (c) the immediate localization of, and differential response to, the tone of the maternal voice at about six months, to (d) the recognizable response in the child to the calling of his name at about nine months.

Dysintegration of listening movements in the cerebral palsied child may be characterized by atrophic or dystrophic features. A complication of assessing listening movements is that the child's auditory system may be functioning adequately, but stilling, smiling, and localizing movements may not be manifested because of problems in movement in general. Or, the listening movements may be possible, but problems in auditory processing preclude the listening movements from occurring.

HEARING DISORDERS

Because of the fact that, if there are problems with hearing for speech per se, listening movements may not develop, a discussion of hearing disorders among the cerebral palsied is in order.

Incidence of Hearing Loss

Among the cerebral palsied incidence of hearing loss, as reported in various studies, ranges widely. Estimates range from 6 to 41 percent (Nober, 1976, p. 223). Reasons for the variations reported include definition of hearing loss, age of subjects, use of different methods and types of tests, and actual differences in hearing among types of cerebral palsy. High incidence figures are supportable in light of the fact that out of 22 possible causes of cerebral palsy, all may cause central auditory disorders while 73 percent may also cause peripheral disorders (Nober, 1976, p. 223).

Incidence figures according to type of cerebral palsy have been reported but inconsistencies are found. For example, Hopkins, Bice, and Colton (1954) reported (listed here in whole percentages) 22 percent for athetotics,

18 percent for ataxics, 13 percent for rigidities, and 7 percent for spastics; while Nakano (1966) reported 33 percent for athetotics, 38 percent for spastics, and 16 percent for spastic-athetotics. Nober (1976, p. 224) believes that, in general, the incidence of hearing loss among children with cerebral palsy is about 20 percent. Errors or delays in diagnosis of cerebral palsy and deafness also confound incidence figures as well as interfere with prompt initiation of appropriate management (Cunningham and Holt, 1977).

Forms of Hearing Loss

Almost all varieties of loss of hearing are included: conductive, sensorineural, and central forms. Pathology has been found in the external, middle, and inner ears and in the central auditory tracts and cortices.

Middle-ear susceptibility to disease was reported in cerebral palsy, especially among spastics. Also, most unilateral losses were attributed to middle ear involvement (Lassman, 1951).

Inner-ear problems in cerebral palsy were also reported or speculated upon. Possible sources of such involvements are hereditary deafness, kernicterus, viral infections, toxemia, and temporal bone fracture (Nober, 1976, pp. 242–44). Evidence of cochlear damage in the Rh-athetotic child was reported by Blakely (1959). A number of investigators reported on the relationship of hearing loss and kernicterus (Hardy, 1953; Crothers and Paine, 1959, p. 148; Perlstein, 1950; Gerrard, 1952).

Central auditory-tract involvement in cerebral palsy has also been cited. Kernicteric-athetotics have been suspected of showing central deafness (McDonald and Chance, 1964, p. 46). On a particular test of central auditory functioning (Staggered Spondaic Word Test), a group of cerebral palsied children scored more poorly than normals (Katz, Myrick, and Winn, 1966).

Finally, Fisch's (1964) concept of pathology of listening is especially pertinent to children with cerebral palsy. According to Fisch, listening is characterized by three physiological processes: the neuromuscular process, or the adoption of a listening attitude; the neurosensory process, or the ability to inhibit selectively other incoming stimuli and thereby enhance auditory input; and the automatic involuntary process whereby listening is enhanced by, for example, automatic changes in respiration, heartbeat, and adrenalin production. Given the type of pathologies and sensorimotor limitations found in cerebral palsy, such children could suffer problems with all three processes.

Significance of Hearing Loss

Hearing loss has also been studied with respect to speech and its development. Hearing loss considered sufficient to interfere with speech development and language acquisition has been reported (Fisch and Beck, 1961; Byers, Paine, and Crothers, 1955).

Dysintegration of Imitative Vocalization

The sequential development of auto-echolalia and true echolalia—or primary talking—is considered essential to the development of true speech.

Delay in the tendency for the child's automatic cooing to be extended via a speaker's imitation of that cooing (auto-echolalia, I) may interfere with the emergence of the child's imitation of a speaker's sounds when those sounds are similar to those babbled spontaneously by the child (auto-echolalia, II). Problems with these forms of self-imitative vocalization may interfere with the child imitating sounds not yet made by him (true echolalia, I), which, in turn, interferes with the child imitating true words (true echolalia, II). Atrophy, dystrophy, or hypertrophy of any of the aforementioned forms of intrapersonal and interpersonal imitative vocalization ultimately interferes with the child's ability to imitate words heard earlier or his ability for deferred echolalia (true echolalia, III).

Dysintegration of Skilled Speech Movements

Skilled speech movements describes the good production of spoken symbols by a coordinated effector system. Skilled respiratory-phonatory-resonatory-articulatory movements result from the progressive integration and elaboration of basic listening movements, speech postures, and basic speech movements. Dysintegration of these basic speech and listening activities is manifested in dysintegrated skilled speech movements. Such dysintegration may also be characterized by atrophic, hypertrophic, and dystrophic features.

Reflecting the range of dysintegration of skilled speech movements in cerebral palsy are the following comments from various authorities:

No other clinical population will show such a variety of conditions that can delay the use of oral language (Westlake and Rutherford, 1961). There is no speech and language disorder that is uniquely characteristic of the cerebral palsied (Lencione, 1966, p. 221). A very high proportion of children with cerebral palsy and defective speech fall into the category of mixed cases (Ingram and Barn, 1961). And the speech output of the cerebral palsied may range from complete lack to slight or no differences from the normal (Mecham, 1966, p. 24).

For the sake of exposition, the discussion of dysintegration of skilled speech movements is divided into sections on breathing, voicing, articulation, and rhythm. In reality, respiratory, phonatory, resonatory, and articulatory movements are component movements of speech effector output. Put another way, efficient effector output is the result of the coordinated functioning of the respiratory, phonatory, resonatory, and articulatory effectors. Disturb one effector and the entire effector system is changed; or stimulate the integration of one effector and you contribute to the integration of the entire system.

BREATHING

The integration of basic vegetative breathing into skilled speech breathing is manifested by the automatic shift from a medullary, nasal-symmetrical pattern during vegetative breathing to a cortical, oral-asymmetrical pattern during speech breathing. Integrated speech breathing is characterized by a rapid oral inspiration and a prolonged expiration, with an I-fraction of about 15 percent. Such automatic shifting of vegetative to speech breathing requires intact central mechanisms for respiratory regulation and these are frequently involved in cerebral palsy.

Frequency of breathing anomalies among the different types of cerebral palsy has been reported as follows: 80 percent (Wolfe, 1950) or 40 percent (Achilles, 1955) among ataxics and 70 percent among athetotics and 60 percent among spastics (Achilles, 1955). Whatever the actual incidence figures are, it is clear they are high.

Dysintegration of Breathing

Investigators and clinicians have described all sorts of breathing differences among the cerebral palsied. Most of the differences appear related to dysintegration of centers involved with neuroregulation of breathing.

Vegetative to speech breathing transition may be delayed or may not be possible (atrophic or dystrophic features). Symptoms of this difficulty may include delay in voluntary phonation, the ability to produce only one or two syllables per speech expiration, and a generally slow and irregular rate. The sometimes obvious nasal, rather than oral inspiratory, pattern that accompanies speech breathing may also be visually distracting.

Breaths per minute may remain high or decrease more slowly (atrophic or dystrophic features). High and irregular bpm have been reported by numerous investigators (Berry and Eisenson, 1956, pp. 364–65; Westlake, 1952; Achilles, 1955; and Palmer, 1952). Symptoms of this type of dysintegration may include reduction in vocalization (McDonald and Chance, 1964, p. 89) and irregular rate and rhythm.

Abdominal to thoracic breathing shift during transition from vegetative to speech breathing may also be delayed or slow in developing. Such predominance of diaphragmatic-abdominal breathing has been reported (Achilles, 1955). Depending on the depth of cycle, such a pattern may not have speech significance.

Depth of breathing cycle may remain shallow (Achilles, 1955; Blumberg, 1955; Palmer, 1952). Weak or asthenic voice has been associated with shallow breathing patterns.

Abdominal-thoracic asynchrony, or the physiologic asynchrony characterized by abdominal contraction preceding thoracic during speech expiration, may show various forms of immaturity. Observation of simultaneous inspiratory and expiratory movements or so-called reverse or oppositional breathing have been reported (Morley, 1965, pp. 208–9; McDonald and Chance, 1964, p. 89; Achilles, 1955; Westlake, 1952; Perlstein and Shere, 1946; Hull, 1940). Symptoms associated with dysintegrated asynchronies include asthenic voice, inspiratory voice, difficulty in sustaining voice, and interruption of vocalization.

Paralysis of Breathing

Breathing differences among cerebral palsied children include types that cannot readily be attributed to dysintegration of neuroregulatory centers for breathing, but rather appear related to a lack of, or to irregular innervation of muscles directly or indirectly involved with, respiration. For example: airstream obstruction due to irregular movements of the vocal folds, posterior tongue, or oropharynx (Berry and Eisenson, 1956, pp. 364–65); irregular airflow due to trunk dystonia (Crothers and Paine, 1959, p. 45); respiration accompanied by retracted abdominal muscles and little movement of the diaphragm (Morley, 1965, pp. 208–9).

Symptoms associated with such problems include uncontrolled loudness and involuntary respiratory movements (McDonald and Chance, 1964, p. 89) and "forced" voice and fixation of respiratory muscles during speech (Morley, 1965, pp. 208–9).

VOICING

Voicing and resonating for speech purposes implies the integration by speech centers of the basic laryngeal movements associated with the glottic-closing and opening reflexes, basic velopharyngeal movements associated with velar opening and closing reflexes, cry and laugh reflexes, and the various forms of reflexive vocalization, that is, movement, hand-to-mouth, and imitative vocalization. A discussion of voicing dysintegration is complicated by the fact that efficient voicing is the result of the coordination of inspiratory and expiratory movements with laryngeal and velopharyngeal movements. Further complication arises from the frequently found paralytic components in addition to the dysintegration components.

Dysintegration of Voicing

Dysintegration of voicing may be discussed from the standpoints of laryngeal, pharyngeal, emotional-laryngeal, and respiratory-laryngeal dysintegrations.

Laryngeal dysintegration, or the hypertrophy or dystrophy of glottic-closing or glottic-opening reflexes, may result in voicing problems associated with involuntary open-close or over-close activities of the glottis. Symptoms of unregulated open-close activity include inspiratory voice, sudden loss of voice, or intermittent voice. Relatedly, difficulty in initiation of voice, or with interruption of voice, have been associated with adductor or abductor laryngeal spasms (McDonald and Chance, 1964, pp. 990–91). The phenomenon referred to as prevocalization (Farmer and Lencione, 1977), or the intrusion of extraneous vocal behavior before production of initial stops, may also be accounted for on the basis of unregulated open-close activity. Symptoms of over-close activity include forced voicing and uncontrolled loudness of voicing.

Pharyngeal dysintegration, or the atrophy, hypertrophy, or dystrophy of velar opening and closing reflexes, results in unregulated open-close activity of the velopharyngeal closure mechanism. Symptoms of such dysintegration include hyponasality, hypernasality, and mixed and intermittent imbalance in speech resonance. Problems in velopharyngeal closure among the cerebral palsied have been reported (Hardy, 1961; Netzell, 1969).

The five patterns of velopharyngeal dysfunction in cerebral palsied children described by Netzell may be related to dysintegrated open-close activity. A gradual opening pattern was observed with repeated production of/tʌ/; a gradual closing pattern was observed with a speeded production of the syllable; an anticipatory opening pattern was observed during repeated production of /ʌtʌnʌ/; a retentive opening pattern was observed during repeated production of /ʌnʌtʌ/; and a premature opening pattern was observed during repetition of /ʌdʌtʌ/.

Emotional-laryngeal dysintegration refers to the intrusion of reflexive cry and laugh prior to or during speech vocalization.

Respiratory-laryngeal dysintegration refers to the vocal repercussions of various problems associated with previously discussed respiratory dysintegration. Among these vocal repercussions are: delay in initiating voice due to slowness in the vegetative to speech breathing shift; restricted duration of voicing due to use of a vegetative I-fraction pattern; reduced amount of voicing due to a high bpm; and weak phonation due to shallow breathing cycles.

Paralysis of Voicing

Certain laryngeal anomalies have been reported that are not easily related to dysintegration of basic laryngeal movements, but they appear more likely related to problems in direct innervation of laryngeal muscles. For example, aspirate and breathy voices have been attributed to flaccid paralysis of the cords; also, voice problems have been related to spasms of intrinsic and extrinsic laryngeal muscles and of the ventricular folds, and to irregular and arrhythmic laryngeal activity (Mecham, Berko, and Berko, 1966, pp. 38–40).

Cerebral Palsy Type and Dysphonia

Attempts have been made to relate patterns of voice disorder with the major classifications of cerebral palsy.

Athetotic voice has been described as low in pitch, weak and forced in loudness, throaty and forced in quality, and broken and wavering in duration (Clement and Twitchell, 1959); as whispered, hoarse, or ventricular in nature (Berry and Eisenson, 1959, p. 358); as fluctuating in pitch and as weak or irregularly loud (Mecham, Berko, and Berko, 1966, pp. 38–40); and as reflecting inspiratory or intermittent voicing (Ingram and Barn, 1961).

Spastic voice has been described as generally high in pitch, weak and forced in loudness, breathy and hypernasal in quality, and broken and with short vowels in duration (Clement and Twitchell, 1959); as uncontrolled in loudness and as gutteral or breathy in quality (Berry and Eisenson, 1956, pp. 356–60); and as displaying marked or moderate nasal escape (Ingram and Barn, 1961).

Ataxic voice has been described as monotonal or as varying spasmodically in pitch, loudness, and quality (Berry and Eisenson, 1956, p. 360); and as showing pitch rise during speech acceleration and pitch fall during speech deceleration, excessive nasal escape, and abnormalities of intonation and stress (Ingram and Barn, 1961).

Much overlap may be observed in the reports. Also, symptoms of both dysintegration and of paralysis are evident.

ARTICULATION

Speech articulation requires the integration by speech centers of various protective reflexes, feeding reflexes, and hand-to-mouth and imitative vocalization movements. The dysarthria of cerebral palsy not only involves dysintegration of these basic movements but also paralysis of the mandible, lips, and tongue.

On the matter of variability of developmental dysarthrias, Morley (1965, p. 179) observed near normal articulation in the severely handicapped child, severe dysarthria in children with minimal brain symptoms, and dysarthria in the absence of any other neurological symptoms or isolated dysarthria. Incidence figures on dysarthria have been reported as follows: 31 to 59 percent of cerebral palsied cases showed some degree of dysarthria (Wolfe, 1950); 43 percent had poor articulation, 45 percent had fair articulation, and 12 percent had adequate articulation (Achilles, 1955); and 70 to 80 percent of the cerebral palsied had some type of articulation problem ranging from adequate to no ability (Mecham, Berko, and Berko, 1966).

Dysintegration of Articulation
Dysintegration of articulation is related to feeding reflex, protective reflex, and imitative vocalization dysintegrations.

Feeding reflex dysintegration and its potential effects on speech articulation were already mentioned in the section on basic speech movements.

Briefly, hypertrophy or dystrophy of the rooting reflex may contribute to lateralization of sibilants; of the lip reflex to bilabialized /r/ and /l/ and deficits in vowel and /f/ and /v/ production; of the mouth-opening reflex to problems in vowels and sounds requiring narrow mouth postures; of the lateral tongue reflex to lateralization of tongue-tip sounds; of biting and chewing reflexes to sounds requiring narrow mouth postures; of the suckle reflex to lingua-alveolar sounds; and of biting, suckle, chewing, swallow reflexes to problems with linguadental, lingua-alveolar, linguapalatal, and linguavelar sounds.

Grasping-avoiding response dysintegration, or dysintegration of particular protective oral reflexes, may also interfere with articulatory maturation. An attempt was made to differentiate between spastic and athetotic dysarthria on the basis of disequilibrium between grasping and avoiding responses (Clement and Twitchell, 1959).

Different cortical regions are believed to subserve positive exploratory reactions and negative withdrawal reactions. Normally, positive and negative reactions are in equilibrium; however, a lesion abolishing one type of reaction releases the opposite. Lip pursing, tongue protrusion, and velar elevation are viewed as positive or grasping responses, while lip parting, tongue retraction, and velar depression are viewed as negative or avoiding responses.

In spastic dysarthria, the primary problem is considered to be a depression of grasping responses and exaggeration of avoiding responses rather than spasticity of the speech musculature. In athetotic dysarthria, the primary problem is overactive avoiding responses plus periodic alternation with grasping responses rather than involuntary movements of the speech musculature; grasping responses are not depressed in athetosis, but they are in unstable equilibrium with avoiding responses.

Hypertrophy or dystrophy of grasping and avoiding reflexes may disturb production of mandibular, labial, and lingual sounds and nasal and nonnasal sound distinctions.

Imitative vocalization dysintegration, or the atrophy, hypertrophy, or dystrophy of auto- and true echolalia, holds important implications for articulation development. The primary talking period is basic to the child's orienting toward speech sounds; scanning, or "studying" them; tracking, or attempting to reproduce them; comparing, or determining how close his versions of sounds heard are to actual sounds heard; and approximating, or shaping his version of sounds heard until they match the actual sounds heard. This sequence of activities represents the heart of the speech-sound learning process, and atrophy or dystrophy of the processes must be considered a significant factor in inadequate speech-sound acquisition.

Paralysis of Articulation

Articulation disorders among the cerebral palsied are complicated by the presence of various forms of paralytic involvement of the articulators. It is not easy to determine in reports of these involvements the role of dysintegration in the articulation disorder described. The discussion here includes classification of cerebral palsy and dysarthria and characteristics of types of dysarthria.

Classification of cerebral palsy and dysarthria was studied by Ingram and Barn (1961), who related speech data of 258 cerebral palsied children with types of cerebral palsy.

Dysarthria among those with hemiplegia is uncommon as an isolated problem and is more often associated with speech retardation or with dysrhythmia; it was characterized by a slowing of rate and misarticulation, most frequently of the plosives, labiodentals, and interdentals; and does not commonly show an associated hypernasality due to palatal involvement. In another study of 110 children with cerebral palsy, all cases with right hemiplegia had speech problems, while 75 percent with left hemiplegia had speech problems (Kamalashile, 1975).

Dysarthria among those with bilateral hemiplegia (involvement of four limbs, upper limbs more affected) was almost inevitable since the bulbar musculature is involved. These children usually acquire no more than a few single words and rudimentary phrases and show gross dysarticulation and usually marked nasal escape. Since most are severely mentally defective with associated speech retardation, determination of the extent of articulatory organ paresis is difficult. Dysintegration of articulation is definitely a factor in the dysarticulation since most of these children are reported to have more or less severe feeding difficulties in infancy that may involve both suckling and swallowing, or swallowing only, and associated drooling.

Dysarthria among those with diplegia (lower limbs more involved than upper limbs) was usually accompanied by impairment of voluntary movements of the lips, tongue, or palate. The characteristic dysarthria was marked by slowing of utterance and intonation, unchanging and monotonous stress patterns, frequent slight or moderate nasal escape, and labored production of speech sounds with better production of vowels than of consonants. Dysintegration of articulatory movements is a factor in the dysarticulation, because a high proportion of those with severe dysarthria or no speech presented histories of feeding difficulty in infancy or drooling and many showed a positive suckling reflex.

Dysarthria among those with ataxic diplegia (lower limbs more involved than upper limbs and ataxia of cerebellar type) and ataxia (incoordination of movements and impaired balance) showed a slowness and ataxia of movements that caused articulatory problems that were similar to those resulting from the slowness and weakness of movements in children with extensive diplegia, but that in ataxic disorders the articulatory differences tend to be less consistent. It was also not unusual to observe excessive nasal escape during conversational patterns, even though palatal movements appeared intact upon examination. This nasal escape symptom may be reflecting dysintegration of the velar protective reflex, or avoiding response, manifested by unregulated velar-opening movements. A characteristic type of dysrhythmia was also found among these children. Also, most of these children showed speech retardation usually proportional to the degree of mental impairment, and this speech retardation might occur alone but more frequently was associated with dysarthria.

Dysarthria among those with dyskinesia (involuntary movement disorder of the choreoid, athetoid, tremulous, or dystonic varieties) was characterized by involuntary movements of the face, tongue, palate, and often other parts of the body whenever the child attempted to move his articulators; the defective sounds varied widely but /θ, r, l, ʃ, p/ appeared to be particularly difficult. Again, many of these "involuntary movement" symptoms could include hypertrophic or dystrophic dysintegration of lip, mouth-opening, lateral tongue, and suckling reflexes. Also, it was reported that only a small proportion of these children spoke normally (70 percent showed dysarthria) and that a majority of them have complex speech problems.

Characteristics of types of dysarthria reported in the literature are not easily differentiated in terms of dysintegration and paralytic symptoms.

Spastic dysarthria has been characterized as difficulty with linguadental, lingua-alveolar, and fricative sounds (Clement and Twitchell, 1959); as "problems which reflect the inability to secure graded, synchronous movements of the tongue, lips, and jaw" (Berry and Eisenson, 1956, p. 357); and as slow, clumsy articulation with special difficulty in producing sounds that require fine movements of the intrinsic muscles of the tongue (West, et al., 1957, p. 122). Also, the speech mechanism may show hypertonicity, pathologic stretch reflex, and flaccidity (Mecham, 1966, pp. 30–33).

Athetotic dysarthria has been described as "articulatory problems varying from the extremes of complete mutism or extreme dysarthria to a slight awkwardness in lingual movement" (Berry and Eisenson, 1956, p. 358). And as dysarticulation involving all sounds "except at those rare moments when the patient is quiet, and is free from surges of convulsion that sweep over his neuromuscular system, from the labial muscles of articulation to the abdominal muscles of exhalation. In such moments the articulation of the purely athetotic patient is startlingly normal" (West et al., 1968, p. 199). Many of those "convulsions" or unregulated and undirected movements could include various hypertrophic or dystrophic feeding reflexes.

Ataxic dysarthria is "characterized by slurring of articulation which lapses into unintelligibility if speech is continued beyond phrases or short sentences" (Berry and Eisenson, 1956, p. 360). A lack of consistency in incoordinations is another characteristic of ataxic dysarthria. "Ataxic clumsiness alone may be thought of as a sensory, or afferent, deficiency; . . . labored scansion . . . should be regarded as an associative failure'' (West et al., 1968, p. 199). Disordered feedback mechanisms for positional and directional orientations may be found among ataxics and should be viewed as a primary disorder (Mecham, Berko, and Berko, 1966, pp. 30–33).

Apraxic dysarthria may be characterized by both motor programming and/or sensory feedback deficiencies—that is, by kinetic and audio-kinesthetic features. There are those ''who apparently have no difficulty in moving the tongue, lips, or palate for spontaneous movements but have difficulty in directing them for voluntary imitation of movements or for reproduction of the correct articulatory sounds when hearing is normal'' (Morley, 1965, p. 175). Affected children may acquire only a limited number of consonant sounds and usually have insufficient audiokinesthetic control to reproduce such sounds when they appear in conversational patterns. Apraxic dysarthria may appear in cerebral palsied children in isolation or in association with dysarthria or dysphasia. Such apraxia may be complicated further by the development of abnormal, sensory model patterns for articulation as a consequence of the speech system experiencing abnormal, dysarthria-associated movements (p. 182).

Are there primary forms of kinetic (motor programming) and kinesthetic (sensory feedback) dyspraxia?; and eventually are there always secondary kinesthetic features in kinetic dyspraxia? These are questions that continue to demand research attention. Regarding sensory feedback, the tactile sensibility and kinesthetic function of cerebral palsied children, primarily of the tongue, were found to be inferior to normals in most of the tasks (McCall, 1964). Also, measurable breakdown in sensory feedback was reported among certain children with cerebral palsy who had reasonably adequate motor functioning, but yet did not respond to usual therapeutic techniques (Wilson, 1965, p. 56).

In a succinct analysis of the major dysarthrias (Rutherford, 1944), athetotics were viewed as generally being able to make movements for speech but few of these movements are under constant control; spastics as being limited in the direction and extent of movement but control is consistent; and ataxics as not knowing whether appropriate movements have been made or certain whether movements have occurred. Also, investigators reported that, in general, spastics were better than athetotics in speech sound production (Byrne, 1959; Lencione, 1966).

Other Causes of Dysarticulation

Dysarticulation among the cerebral palsied may be attributed to other than dysintegration and/or paralytic involvement of the articulatory organs.

The inability to produce sufficient intraoral breath pressure for speech sound production was cited as a possible background for speech problems (Hardy, 1961). Insufficient breath pressure may be related to malfunctions of the muscles of the palate, respiratory mechanism, and articulators. Malocclusion, related to abnormal orofacial muscle activity, including persistence of infantile suckle-swallow patterns, may also interfere with speech sound maturation (Lyons, 1956). Simple retardation of speech development, usually associated with mental retardation, or hearing loss also contributes to dysarticulation (Ingram and Barn, 1961).

RHYTHM

Dysrhythmia of speech among the cerebral palsied has been reported by many investigators (e.g., Rutherford, 1944; Palmer, 1949; Ingram and Barn, 1961). More specifically, "the proportion of children who stammer or hesitate because of organic disease of the nervous system is small, but it includes a relatively high proportion of the children whose speech disorder is due to cerebral palsy." (Ingram and Barn, 1961).

Speech rhythm requires the integration by speech centers of various protective, emotional, and vegetative reflexes. Cerebral palsy dysrhythmia may be characterized by dysintegration of these basic units as well as by direct involvement of the central neural mechanisms for speech rhythm control.

Dysintegration of Speech Rhythm

Hypertrophy or dystrophy of certain protective, emotional, and vegetative reflexes may be involved in symptoms of speech rhythm dysintegration.

Protective reflex dysintegration may manifest itself in various ways in cerebral palsy dysrhythmia. Hypertrophy or dystrophy of protective head reactions may contribute to unregulated ventroflexion, dorsiflexion, or lateralization of the head preceding or during the moment of speech block; hypertrophy or dystrophy of laryngeal open-close reflexes may contribute to unregulated laryngeal abduction and adduction during speech; and hypertrophy or dystrophy of protective tongue, lip, and jaw reflexes may contribute to unregulated tongue protrusion, lip puckering, and jaw extension preceding and during speech attempts.

Emotional reflex dysintegration may disturb speech flow in various ways. Hypertrophy or dystrophy of fear, sob, and sigh reflexes may contribute to disturbances in speech rhythm indirectly through the negative effects on nerves and muscles of unregulated fear reactions before and during speech efforts, and more directly through unregulated sob and sigh reflexes during speech attempts.

Vegetative reflex dysintegration may affect speech rhythm through hypertrophy and dystrophy of certain breathing and feeding reflexes. The voicing aspect of flow may be interrupted or disturbed by unregulated inspiratory reflexes causing unexpected vocal fold abduction or nasal ("nasal gasp") rather than oral inspiration preceding and during speech production.

Hypertrophy or dystrophy of feeding reflexes may also interfere with speech flow. Preceding or during speech attempts irregular head, jaw, and tongue lateralization may be related to unregulated rooting reflexes; irregular mandibular extension to an unregulated mouth-opening reflex; irregular lip-puckering and pouting movements to an unregulated lip reflex; irregular mandibular flexion to an unregulated biting reflex; and irregular tongue protrusion and lateralization to unregulated suckle and lateral tongue reflexes.

Dysintegration of protective, emotional, and vegetative reflexes have negative implications for the development of effector differentiation, praxis, and diadochokinesia—all of which contribute significantly to normal speech rhythm.

Many years ago Travis (1931, p. 95) made a statement about stuttering that relates to the concept of speech rhythm dysintegration. He said, "The stutterer . . . reflects a certain lack of maturation of the central nervous system which either does not afford integration of the highest neurophysiological levels involved in speech or predisposes these levels to disintegration by various types of exogenous or endogenous stimuli."

Paralysis of Speech Rhythm

Cerebral palsy speech dysrhythmia may, in addition to dysintegration symptoms, include more direct involvement of the central neural mechanisms for speech rhythm control. Because the concept of dysintegration vs. paralytic symptoms of dysrhythmia is still relatively novel, it is difficult to analyze reports regarding neurological dysrhythmia in terms of types of symptoms.

Neurological dysrhythmia in general has been discussed in different ways. West's (1958, Ch. 4) hypothesesis was that the fundamental disorder of stuttering may be related to pyknolepsy and hence may be described as speech epilepsy. Similarities between disorders due to lesions in the striopalidum or mesencephalon and stuttering was reported (Zentay, 1937). Palilalia, or the repetition of a phrase that is reiterated with increasing rapidity, is most frequently found as a symptom of postencephalitic parkinsonism and in pseudobulbar palsy due to vascular lesions (Brain, 1961, p. 106). Stuttering as a manifestation of phonatory ataxia, or temporal dysfunction of voluntary and/or reflex mechanisms regulating the tone of phonatory musculature, was another hypothesis (Wyke, 1970). Also, neurological dysrhythmia marked by articulatory "freezing," palilalia, and episodic silent blocks were reported in parkinsonism (Canter, 1971).

The concept of central neural mechanisms for speech rhythm control and neurological dysrhythmia is also supported by reports of the effects of electrical stimulation of certain parts of the brain on the speech of patients undergoing brain surgery. Hesitation, slurring, distortion, and repetition of words resulting from electrical stimulation of various areas of the brain was reported (Penfield and Roberts, 1959, p. 133). In some instances, an arrest or hesitation followed by a slowing of speech, or in other instances an acceleration of speech, was observed with electrical stimulation of the thalamic area prior to a surgical ablation procedure for the relief of parkinsonism (Guiot et al., 1961).

Classification of cerebral palsy and characteristics of speech dysrhythmia was also discussed by Ingram and Barn (1961) in their study of 258 cerebral palsied children.

Dysrhythmia among hemiplegics occurred in 14 percent of the cases and was manifested as a combination of arrest or hesitation with stammer; dysrhythmia among ataxics was reported in a high number of cases and was manifested by irregular division of phrases and irregular speech acceleration and deceleration; and dysrhythmia among dyskinesias was present in more than half of the cases and was characterized by involuntary action of the respiratory muscles that moved out-of-phase with muscles of articulation. In the dyskinesias, speech might be suddenly arrested, or unexpected inspiratory activity would cause inspiratory speech episodes. Periodic speech arrest also appeared related to obstruction of the speech airstream at the laryngeal level.

In the case of the dyskinesias, dysintegration of inspiratory and laryngeal open-close reflexes appear to be contributing to the cause of interrupted speech flow.

Dysintegration of Expressive Communication

Efficient expressive communication implies the good coordination of hands, face, and mouth talk that may be used at various communispheral levels. Such expressive communication results from the progressive integration and elaboration of basic listening, basic speech postures, and basic hand and speech movements by speech centers responsible for skilled listening, imitative vocalization, and speech movements. Dysintegration of basic movements and consequent involvement of skilled movements is manifested by dyscoordination of hands-face-mouth talk, by problems in the development of spoken language, and by limitations in full participation at various communispheral levels.

HANDS-FACE-MOUTH TALK

Coordinated talking reflects the integration of hands, face, and mouth talk into a pattern of talking. Problems with coordinated talking includes dysintegration as well as paralytic symptoms.

Dysintegration of Coordinated Talking

Dysintegration of coordinated talking is related to hands, face, and mouth talk dysintegrations reflected by symptoms of atrophy, dystrophy, or hypertrophy of various reflexes.

Hands talk dysintegration describes problems in the use of hand movements for symbolic gestural and adjunctive gestural purposes.

The child with cerebral palsy may not be able with his hands to indicate that he wants to be picked up; that he wants something; or that he wants to be taken somewhere. Also, he may not be able to gesture symbolically "come here," "goodbye," and so on. Adjunctive gestural functions of accompanying speech with supportive hand movements and the use of compensatory hand movements when searching for a word may also be lost or limited in children with cerebral palsy. Atrophy of arm-support or arm-balance reactions or hand-to-mouth feeding movements, or hypertrophy of upper limb flexion-extension patterns associated with nonintegrated long spinal and tonic neck reflexes may form the background for such limitations on hands talk.

Face talk dysintegration describes problems in the use of facial movements to display various emotions. The child with cerebral palsy may not be able with his face to exhibit boredom, fear, sadness, happiness, and so on, either in natural accompaniment with appropriate speech or in a compensatory fashion when speech is lacking. Atrophy of certain basic facial expressions or hypertrophy of a limited number of expressions, like fear expressions, may form the background for such limitations on face talk.

Mouth talk dysintegration describes problems in the coordination of breathing, voicing, articulation, and rhythm speech functions for purposes of transmitting speech symbols.

Children with cerebral palsy may have problems with the coordination of some or with all of these levels of talking.

Paralysis of Coordinated Talking

In addition to dysintegration symptoms, coordinated talking may also suffer because of problems in more direct innervation of the muscles responsible for hands, face, and mouth talk. Such paralysis may seriously limit hand, face, and speech effector movements.

SPOKEN LANGUAGE

Efficient spoken language reflects the integration by cortical speech centers of R-complex and limbic speech. Problems with spoken language includes symptoms of dysintegration as well as those due to direct involvement of central neural mechanisms responsible for spoken language.

Numerous investigators have reported that retardation of spoken language is a frequent symptom in cerebral palsy in various studies:

- In 67 spastic hemiplegics under 13 years, the development of language depended on mental potential rather than on degree of impairment, or preferred hand, or presence of convulsive disorder (Kastein, 1951).
- In 200 cerebral palsied individuals, an average retardation of from three to four years in vocabulary and verbal recall was found (Dunsdon, 1952).
- In 157 cases of cerebral palsy, 66 percent either had no speech or no more than one year of language development (Achilles, 1955).
- In 334 spastic hemiplegics, a delay of nine months in uttering first words and a delay of six months in the use of sentences was found; further, those considered mentally defective spoke their first words 14 months later (Hood and Perlstein, 1956).
- In athetotic and spastic quadriplegic children between two and seven years, all children were found retarded in the appearance of first words and two- and three-word sentences; further, language maturation reflected that of normals but at a reduced rate (Byrne, 1959).
- In the rate of language development of children with cerebral palsy, the average age of onset of speech was about 27 months (Denhoff, 1966).
- In 110 children with cerebral palsy, 70 percent showed delay in speech onset (Kamalashile, 1975).

Dysintegration of Spoken Language

Atrophy of cortical, or logical speech, or hypertrophy or dystrophy of R-complex, or ritual speech, and limbic, or emotional speech, may characterize dysintegration of spoken language.

Ritual speech dysintegration may be characterized by the predominant use of social-gesture speech such as "hi," "bye," "I'm fine," and by memorized speech such as counting, saying the days of the week, and nursery rhymes.

Emotional speech dysintegration may be characterized by the predominant use of emotional utterances such as stock phrases indicating anger, fear, hate, love.

Logical speech dysintegration would be characterized by the predominant use of ritual and emotional speech with little or no use of logical speech forms such as conversation, narration, discussion, and persuasion.

Pathology of Spoken Language

Language disorders among the cerebral palsied may be complicated by the presence of language symptoms that appear more directly related to involvement of the central neural mechanisms devoted to spoken language function.

Language symptoms of children with minimal brain dysfunction, who are relatively free of intellectual, hearing, and psychosocial problems, should prove informative relative to the identification of symptoms of specific neurogenic language disturbance. In that regard, a number of investigators (Strauss and Kephart, 1955; Ingram, 1960; Lewis et al., 1960; Hagberg, 1962; Mysak, 1968) have reported on spoken language differences among children with minimal brain dysfunction. Symptoms reported among these children include retardation or marked reduction in language; confusion among similar sounding words; syllable reversals within words; neologisms; grammatical confusions; omitted or mistakenly used functional words in sentences; lack of meaning associated with verbalization; irregular verbal associations; word-finding problems and circumlocutionary verbalization; near normal comprehension with significant lag in expression; excessive use of gesture; verbal perseveration; and echolalia. Most of these symptoms may be observed in normals who become aphasic following trauma to speech centers in the brain.

Symptoms of excessive use of gesture, verbal perseveration, and echolalia may be reflections of dysintegration of hands talk and imitative vocalization.

Aphasiform symptoms among children with cerebral palsy were observed by a number of investigators. Reports include aphasic symptoms and lingual apraxias (Palmer, 1949); language difficulties resembling aphasia in adults (Cohen and Hannigan, 1956); auditory agnosia and lip and tongue dyspraxia accompanied by profound language-learning disorders (Greene, 1964, p. 81); and acquired aphasia in two congenital cases following severe epileptic attacks (Ingram and Barn, 1961).

In contrast, deviant language among the cerebral palsied was not found when 27 individuals were studied using a matched control group of physically handicapped individuals (Love, 1964); and another investigator (Lencione, 1976, p. 183) believes that ''What appears to be emerging from recent research is that the degree of the speech and language problem in cerebral palsy may be more closely related to 'intelligibility' or motor skills rather than to disorders of language processing.''

Other Causes of Disordered Spoken Language

Language disorders among the cerebral palsied may be attributed to other than dysintegration and pathological involvement of central language centers. Substantial hearing loss, mental retardation, perceptual dysfunctioning, socioemotional problems, and limited stimulation and experience are all factors that may contribute to disturbance in spoken language.

Simple retardation of speech development, usually associated with mental retardation or hearing loss, is the most commonly observed speech disorder among the cerebral palsied (Ingram and Barn, 1961). Among children with hemiplegia, bilateral hemiplegia, diplegia, ataxia, and ataxic diplegia, simple retardation of speech development associated with mental impairment was the most common disorder. Because of the smaller proportion of mental retardation among those with dyskinesias, speech retardation due to mental retardation is less frequent; however, speech retardation due to hearing impairment is higher than in other groups. Also on the Illinois Test of Psycholinguistic Abilities, spastics and athetotics were found to perform better or worse depending on the language task (Myers, 1965).

COMMUNISPHERE

Communispheral development is marked by the progressive integration and elaboration of the child's basic biosphere into intimate, personal, and family communispheres. Communispheral dysintegration may occur at any or at all levels.

Dysintegration of the Intimate Communisphere

Problems in the development of the intimate communisphere (body contact range) may occur for a number of reasons. Because of frequent nursing or feeding difficulty the primal mother-child communication may not be associated with warmth, comfort, and pleasure. Positive eye regard and vocalization from the mother may be limited and strained because of not uncommon maternal feelings of sorrow, anxiety, and guilt. Problems in holding the child in general, or the development of the attitude that the child is sick and should not be handled as much, may also contribute to differences in the development of the intimate communisphere.

Dysintegration of the Personal Communisphere

Problems in the development of the personal communisphere (person-to-person range) may occur because of limitations in the acquisition of back, elbow, or sit speech postures. Head balance problems that accompany difficulty in assuming and maintaining early basic speech postures results in limitations and abnormalities of eye contact, which, in turn, contributes further to problems in the establishment of the personal communisphere.

Dysintegration of the Family Communisphere

Problems in the development of the family communisphere (person-to-small group) are extensions of problems in the development of intimate and personal communispheres. Certainly, problems in acquiring sit or stand speech postures, establishing eye contact, and speaking with sufficient carrying power will all interfere with the function of the person-to-small group communisphere.

The close of this chapter completes part one of the book devoted to providing the foundation for the remaining five chapters. The following chapters are concerned with the book's central purpose—the description and explanation of neurospeech therapy for the cerebral palsied.

REFERENCES

Achilles, R. F. Communicative anomalies of individuals with cerebral palsy: I. Analysis of communicative processes in 151 cases of cerebral palsy. *Cerebral Palsy Rev.,* 16, 15–24 (1955).

Berry, M. F., and Eisenson, J. *Speech disorders: Principles and practices of therapy.* New York: Appleton-Century-Crofts, Inc. (1956).

Blakeley, R. W. Erythroblastosis and perceptive hearing loss: Responses of athetoids to tests of cochlear function. *J. Speech Hearing Dis.,* 2, 5–15 (1959).

Blumberg, M. L. Respiration and speech in the cerebral palsied child. *Amer. J. Dis. Child.,* 89, 48–53 (1955).

Brain, R. W. *Diseases of the nervous system.* London: Oxford University Press (1961).

Byers, R. K., Paine, R. S., and Crothers, B. Extrapyramidal cerebral palsy with hearing loss following erythroblastosis. *Pediatrics,* 15, 248–254 (1955).

Byrne, M. Speech and language development of athetoid and spastic children. *J. Speech Hearing Dis.,* 24, 231–240 (1959).

Canter, G. J. Observations on neurogenic stuttering. A contribution to differential diagnosis. *Br. J. Disord. Commun.,* 6, 139–143 (1971).

Clement, M., and Twitchell, T. E. Dysarthria in cerebral palsy. *J. Speech Hearing Dis.,* 24, 118–122 (1959).

Cohen, P., and Hannigan, H. M. Aphasia in cerebral palsy. *Amer. J. Phys. Med.,* 35, 218–222 (1956).

Crothers, B., and Paine, R. S. *The natural history of cerebral palsy.* Cambridge, Mass.: Harvard University Press (1959).

Cunningham, C., and Holt, K. S. Problems in diagnosis and management of children with cerebral palsy and deafness. *Devel. Med. Child. Neurol.,* 19, 479–484 (1977).

Denhoff, E. Cerebral palsy: Medical aspects. In W. M. Cruickshank (Ed.), *Cerebral palsy.* Syracuse: Syracuse University Press (1966).

Dunsdon, M. I. *The educability of cerebral palsied children.* London: Newnes Educational Publishing (1952).

Farmer, A., and Lencione, R. An extraneous vocal behavior in cerebral palsied speakers. *Brit. J. Dis. Comm.,* 12, 109–118 (1977).

Fisch, L. The functions of listening and its disorders. In *Learning problems of the cerebrally palsied.* London: The Spastics Society (1964).

———, and Beck, D. E. The assessment of hearing in young cerebral palsied children. *Cerebral Palsy Bull.,* 3, 145–155 (1961).

Gerrard, J. Kernicterus. *Brain,* 75, 526–570 (1952).

Greene, Margaret C. Speech and reading disorders in cerebral palsy. In *Learning problems of the cerebral palsied.* London: The Spastics Society (1964).

Grewel, F. Dysarthria in post-encephalitic parkinsonism. *Acta Psychiatrica et Neurologica,* 32, 440–449 (1957).

Guiot, G., Hertzog, E., Rondot, P., and Molina, P. Arrest or acceleration of speech evoked by thalamic stimulation in the course of stereotaxic procedures for parkinsonism. *Brain,* 8, 363–369 (1961).

Hagberg, B. The sequelae of spontaneously arrested infantile hydrocephalus. *Develop. Med. Child. Neurol.,* 4, 583–587 (1962).

Hardy, J. C. Intraoral breath pressure in cerebral palsy. *J. Speech Hearing Dis.,* 26, 310–319 (1961).

Hardy, W. G. Hearing impairment in cerebral palsied children. *Cerebral Palsy Rev.,* 14, 3–7 (1953).

Hood, P. N. and Perlstein, M. A. Infantile spastic hemiplegia: V. oral language and motor development. *Pediatrics,* 17, 58–63 (1956).

Hopkins, T. W., Bice, H. V., and Colton, K. C. Evaluation and education of the cerebral palsied child—New Jersey Study. Washington, D.C.: International Council for Exceptional Children (1954).

Hull, H. C. A study of the respiration of fourteen spastic paralysis cases during silence and speech. *J. Speech Dis.,* 5, 275–276 (1940).

Ingram, T. T. S. Pediatric aspects of specific developmental dysphasia, dyslexia, and dysgraphia. *Cerebral Palsy Bull.,* 2, 254–277 (1960).

Ingram, T. T. S. and Barn, J. A description and classification of common speech disorders associated with cerebral palsy. *Cerebral Palsy Bull.,* 3, 57–69 (1961).

Jackson, J. H. Evaluation and Dissolution of the Nervous System. In J. Taylor (Ed.), *Selected writings of John Hughlings Jackson,* Vol. 2, New York: Basic Books, Inc. (1958).

Kamalashile, J. Speech problems in cerebral palsy children. *Language and Speech,* 18, 158–165 (1975).

Kastein, S., and Hendin, J. Language development in a group of children with spastic hemiplegia. *J. Pediatrics,* 39, 476–480 (1951).

Katz, J., Myrick, D. W., and Winn, B. Central auditory dysfunction in cerebral palsy. Presentation at ASHA Convention, Washington, D.C. (1966).

Lassman, F. M. Clinical investigation of some hearing deficiencies and possible etiological factors in a group of cerebral palsied individuals. *Speech Monogr.,* 18, 130–131 (1951).

Lencione, R. M. Speech and language problems in cerebral palsy. In W. J. Cruickshank (Ed.), *Cerebral palsy.* Syracuse: Syracuse University Press (1966).

———. The development of communication skills. In W. J. Cruickshank (Ed.), *Cerebral palsy: A developmental disability.* Syracuse: Syracuse University Press (1976).

Lewis, R. S., Strauss, A. A. and Lehtinen, L. E. *The other child: The brain-injured child.* New York: Grune and Stratton (1960).

Lorenze, E., and Canero, R. Prognosis for deficiencies in speech accompanying cerebral palsy. *Arch. Phys. Med. Rehab.,* 43, 621–626 (1962).

Love, R. J. Oral language behavior of cerebral palsied children. *J. Speech Hearing Res.,* 7, 349–359 (1964).

Lyons, D. C. An evaluation of the effects of cerebral palsy on dentofacial development, especially occlusion of the teeth. *J. Pediatrics,* 49, 432–436 (1956).

McCall, G. N. Study of certain somesthetic sensibilities in a selected group of athetoid and spastic quadriplegic persons. Unpublished doctoral dissertation, Northwestern University (1964).

McDonald, E. T., and Chance, B. *Cerebral palsy*. Englewood Cliffs, N.J.: Prentice-Hall, Inc. (1964).

Mecham, M. J., Berko, M. J., and Berko, F. G. *Communication training in childhood brain damage*. Springfield, Ill.: Charles C Thomas (1966).

Morley, Muriel, E. *The development and disorders of speech in childhood*. Baltimore: The Williams and Wilkins Company (1965).

Morrison, E. B., Rigrodsky, S., and Mysak, E. D. Parkinson's disease: Speech disorders and released oroneuromotor activity. *J. Speech Hearing Res.*, 13. 655–666 (1970).

Myers, P. A study of language disabilities in cerebral palsied children. *J. Speech Hearing Res.*, 8, 129–136 (1965).

Mysak, E. D. Disorders of oral communication. In M. Bortner (Ed.), *Evaluation and education of children with brain damage*. Springfield, Ill.: Charles C Thomas (1968).

Nakano, T. Research on hearing impairment in cerebral infantile palsied school children. *International Audiology*, 5, 159–161 (1966).

Netzell, R. Evaluation of velopharyngeal function in dysarthria. *J. Speech Hearing Dis.*, 34, 113–122 (1969).

Nober, E. H. Auditory Processing. In W. J. Cruickshank (Ed.), *Cerebral palsy: A developmental disability*. Syracuse: Syracuse University Press (1976).

Palmer, M. F. Speech disorders in cerebral palsy. *Nerv. Child.*, 8, 193–202 (1949).

———. Speech therapy in cerebral palsy. *Pediatrics.*, 40, 514–524 (1952).

Penfield, W., and Roberts, L. *Speech and brain mechanisms*. Princeton: Princeton University Press (1959).

Perlstein, M. and Shere, M. Speech therapy for children with cerebral palsy. *Am. J. Dis. Child.*, 72, 389–398 (1946).

Perlstein, M. A. Neurologic sequelae of erythroblastosis fetalis. *Am. J. Dis. Child.*, 79, 605–606 (1950).

Rutherford, R. A comparative study of loudness, pitch, rate, rhythm, and quality of the speech of children handicapped by cerebral palsy. *J. Speech Hearing Dis.*, 9, 263–271 (1944).

Schneider, D. E. The cortical syndromes of echolalia, echopraxia, grasping, and suckling: Their significance in the disorganization of the personality. *J. Nerv. Ment. Dis.*, 88, 18–35 and 200–216 (1938).

Sheppard, J. J. Cranio-oropharyngeal motor patterns in dysarthria associated with cerebral palsy. *J. Speech Hearing Res.*, 7, 373–380 (1964).

Strauss, A. A., and Kephart, N. C. *Psychopathology and education of the brain-injured child*, Vol. 2. New York: Grune and Stratton (1955).

Travis, L. E. *Speech pathology*. New York: Appleton-Century Co. (1931).

Twitchell, T. E. Variations and abnormalities of motor development. *J. Amer. Phys. Ther. Assoc.*, 45, 424–430 (1965).

Ward, M. M., Malone, H. D., Jann, G. R., and Jann, H. W. Articulation variations associated with visceral swallowing and malocclusion. *J. Speech Hearing Dis.*, 26, 334–341 (1961).

West, R. An agnostic's speculations about stuttering. In J. Eisenson (Ed.), *Stuttering: A symposium* (1958).

———, and Ansberry, M. *The rehabilitation of speech*. New York: Harper and Row (1968).

Westlake, H. *A system for developing speech with cerebral palsied children.* Chicago: National Soc. Crippled Child. and Adults, Inc. (1952).

——, and Rutherford, D. *Speech therapy for the cerebral palsied.* Chicago: National Soc. Crippled Child. and Adults, Inc. (1961).

Wilson, F. B. Differential diagnosis in speech and hearing with the cerebral palsied child. In W. T. Daley (Ed.), *Speech and language therapy with the cerebral palsied child.* Washington, D.C.: The Catholic University of America Press (1965).

Witkop, C. J., and Henry, F. V. Sjögren-Larsson syndrome and histidinemia: Hereditary biochemical diseases with defects of speech and oral functions. *J. Speech Hearing Dis.,* 26, 334–341 (1963).

Wolfe, W. G. A comprehensive evaluation of fifty cases of cerebral palsy. *J. Speech Hearing Dis.,* 15, 234–251 (1950).

Wyke, B. Neurological mechanisms in stuttering: a hypothesis. *Br. J. Disord. Commun.,* 5, 6–15 (1970).

Zentay, P. J. Motor disorders of the central nervous system and their significance for speech. Part I. Cerebral and cerebellar dysarthrias. *J. Speech Dis.,* 2, 131–138 (1937).

Part II

PRINCIPLES AND METHODS OF NEUROTHERAPY

4

Neurotherapies

WHEN ATTEMPTING TO apply knowledge of human neurophysiology to the development of therapy programs for children with neurophysiological disorders, one may focus on normal sequential patterns in neurological maturation; using early reflexes and reactions; facilitating or enhancing the response of the motor unit; selective stimulation of various sensory modalities; or organizing programs that draw from all possible ways of positively influencing the child's nervous system. During the last 35 years or so, a number of individuals have attempted to organize systems of therapy by concentrating on such neurological factors.

This chapter analyzes, compares, and contrasts four major neuro-physiologically oriented approaches to the treatment of cerebral palsy. These approaches are identified as the paleoreflex orientation, the motor unit orientation, the sensory receptor orientation, and the postural patterns orientation. The orientations are discussed primarily from the standpoints of Fay, Kabat, Rood, and the Bobaths. The reason for representing the orientations via the concepts of these authorities is that they are considered the major synthesizers of, and contributors to, these orientations. Admittedly, this author's descriptions of the four orientations may not necessarily be in accord with the current views of the respective authorities, and, indeed, that is not necessary for the purposes of this chapter. For those wishing to explore more directly the ideas of these authorities, a substantial bibliography of their works has been provided among the references at the end of the chapter. This chapter also identifies concepts and techniques that contributed to the development of the neurospeech therapy discussed in the last four chapters of the book.

Paleoreflex Orientation

The paleoreflex orientation may also be called primitive reflex therapy, phyletic heritage or neurophylogenetic approach, neuromuscular reflex therapy, or the neurological organization approach. That which distinguishes this approach from other neurologically oriented therapies is the belief that cerebral palsied children frequently display reflexive movements that may be viewed as phyletic traces of man's origin, and that these movements could be considered as a basis for treatment rather than as symptoms to be eliminated.

THEORY

Fay (1948, 1954a, 1954c) was among the first to describe a neuro-phylogenetic approach to the development of special therapy techniques for the cerebral palsied. Later Doman et al. (1960) described a further development of the idea under the term "neurological organization."

Fay (1948) stated, "Surgical corrections, both orthopedic and neuro-surgical, offer only limited possibilities in specially selected cases. Drugs have real value only as adjuncts to physical therapy and proper correctional measures under careful medical supervision." Fay also said "that specialized forms of physical therapy offer the best means of treatment at our disposal for the child with cerebral palsy today." Thirty years later Fay's assessment of cerebral palsy management remains essentially unchanged.

Fay referred to his special form of therapy variously as neurophysical rehabilitation, reflex therapy, pattern method, and neuromuscular reflex therapy. It was based on observations by neurologists and himself that symptoms of organic lesions involving the pyramidal tract include paralysis, increase of reflexes, ankle clonus, Babinski's sign, and the appearance of reflexes of spinal automatism (described by Babinski as defensive reflexes and by Sherrington as spinal automatisms). Fay believed that cerebral palsy specialists should be aware of the "meaning and value of postural reflexes, reactions of defense, tonic neck reflexes and pattern movements," at least from a clinical standpoint. In explaining his approach (Fay, 1954a), he reminded us that human beings are the highest existing form of vertebrates and that their neurological and structural development reflects development through the ages and includes reptile and amphibian behavior. "Integrated movements, purposeful and more complicated movements concern the medulla, pons, midbrain, and cortex. Skilled movements and controls are housed in the human cortex. Before the human types of cortex and hemispheres arose, the frog could hop, the salamander run, and the great reptiles walked . . . Many of these early movements and reflexes remain in the human being after his brain surface has been injured or destroyed. These residual and retained patterns are the agents that may serve to replace or enhance crude function after higher skilled centers have been lost. Neuromuscular reflex therapy seeks to utilize these primitive responses to aid in ambulation, feeding, and self-care where spastic paralysis or dystonia has produced severe handicaps in the patients' expressive motor function.''

As indicated earlier, the essence of a paleoreflex orientation is the use of primitive responses in therapy. Therefore, before describing the therapy, the phyletic heritage of spinal and tonic neck reflexes, and the basis for therapy are discussed.

Phyletic Heritage of Reflex of Defense or Spinal Automatism

The reflex of defense or spinal automatism may be seen in extensor spasticity. Noxious stimuli such as pinching or scratching of the lower extremity, or sudden flexion of the toes or lateral compression of the foot results in a movement of tonic reflexion or shortening of the lower limb at all joints with dorsiflexion of the ankle and toes. This reflex of defense may also be elicited by bending the toes downward and inward and at the same time pressing the knee outward gently, resulting in a full and spontaneous flexion of the leg and knee.

Amphibian, or homolateral crawling is a pattern movement, of which the reflex of defense, when viewed with the child on his abdomen, may be interpreted as being just a part, according to Fay. Early amphibian crawling, or homolateral pattern movements, are characterized by "a forward thrust of the hand and foot on the same side alternating with a similar movement of the opposite side.'' A pattern movement is reflected in homolateral crawling when a limb is pushed downward in the act of progression and the head turns toward the advancing upper limb. (This, according to Fay, is probably the basis of the tonic neck reflex.)

Reptilian, or cross-pattern crawling is characterized by the upper extremity on one side and the lower extremity on the other advancing simultaneously. The head and eyes are also turned toward the advancing upper limb. This pattern is similar to eventual bipedal, coordinated walking. Homolateral and cross-pattern crawling are considered to be mediated at the level of the pons and emerge between 2 and 10 months (Doman et al., 1960).

The instructive point here is that due to the use of a customary examining position—that is, child in supine and passive, dorsiflexion of the toes and ankle, and flexion of the lower limb at all joints in response to certain stimuli applied to the lower limb—may be interpreted as an isolated withdrawal or defense reflex. However, this very same movement, when viewed with the child in prone and from the standpoint of early crawling, may be interpreted as a part of a functional movement pattern concerned with body progression.

Phyletic Heritage of Tonic Neck Reflexes

Turning the head, neck, and eyes toward the extended upper limb, or one of the tonic neck reflexes, according to Fay, "are probably responses which belong to the upper portion of a segmented 'pattern movement' seen in the embryonal amphibian." The tonic neck reflex, or eye-head-neck-tail movement, as well as various forms of spinal automatism, combine to produce an amphibian pattern of progression. Again, when defense and tonic neck reflexes are analyzed with the child in supine they appear to have little functional significance; however, when the child is in prone "with the head and neck turned to one side and the upper extremity advanced toward the eyes of that side there is frequently an associated drawing up of the lower extremity on the same side, or there may be the crossed (contralateral) reflex seen in pattern movements at the reptilian level with flexion of the opposite knee."

Basis for the Treatment Plan

Instead of viewing these reflexes as symptoms to be gotten rid of, as was the case in the past and for the most part is still the case, Fay saw them as forming the basis of a treatment approach.

"Organizing" the reflexes or eliciting them so that they formed a total pattern movement of an amphibian or reptilian type was recommended. Hopefully, such reflex organization would develop muscles, relax antagonists, and coordinate tone. Fay claimed that total pattern movement, or "patterning," relieved spasticity and even at times emerged into partially controlled coordinated movements in the paralyzed part.

He supported his ideas by reasoning that the child with cerebral palsy may be paralyzed from the standpoint of voluntary movement, but yet may retain many reflex-pattern movements of the extremities. Various pattern movements may persist in the motor levels of the midbrain, medulla, and upper cervical and thoracic portions of the cord. The challenge was to ascertain whether "certain automatic spinal reflex activities can be organized and coordinated with what remains of higher cortical centers . . . to bring about a pattern movement to assist in whatever motor activity the patient may perhaps utilize with the aid of braces and proper exercises of balance and other coordinated activities, to enhance or restore a useless part."

As an example of a pattern of movement having a body progression effect, he referred to the tonic neck reflex as a meaningless expression of limb movement when elicited with the individual on his back; however, when the individual is placed on his abdomen and when the head is rotated from side to side "a serialized initiation of the amphibian type of homolateral extremity response ensues, with semi-automatic reciprocation of the trunk and extremity movements . . . so that a crude progression effect results." It is the head movement in prone that initiates the serialized neck, upper limb, trunk, and lower-limb pattern and unlocks muscles and muscle groups in preparation for body progression activity. Such eye-head-neck movement apparently does not need the cortex to initiate and maintain a large number of cord reflexes that are integrated below the level of the pons. In short, the purposeless jerky movements exhibited in supine are transferred into a purposeful, smoother pattern of progression when the individual is under the postural-vestibular influence of the prone position.

An instructive image of Fay's point is the "supine turtle syndrome" where the turtle's apparently purposeless head twisting and leg movements need only the influence of the prone position to reveal their purposeful pattern of progression.

Overriding impaired higher brain levels was the potential that the "old reflexes" held for Fay; that is, there are ways to make the muscles work even when higher brain levels have been impaired as in certain types of cerebral palsy. He spoke of built-in exercises in the form of normal and pathological responses. In spasticity, for example, individual or groups of muscles may be "exercised" by eliciting normal deep tendon or superficial reflexes and by eliciting various pathological responses. Fay wrote, "It is high time that we began to put certain 'normal' and so-called 'pathological' reflexes to work for the benefit of the patient and not merely record them as curiosities of neurological response."

Jackson's concepts of duplex symptomatology and evolution and dissolution of the nervous system are recalled by Fay's therapy ideas. Jackson described neuropathology as first reflecting a reversal in nervous system evolution or dissolution and as always presenting defect of function or negative symptoms and involuntary movement or positive symptoms. In Fay's view of the symptoms of the child with cerebral palsy, he recognizes the defect of function symptoms or paralysis and the involuntary movement symptoms or old reflexes. He then appears to say that since we cannot overcome the negative symptoms directly let us try to overcome them indirectly by "exercising" the positive symptoms. Such exercises might at least keep muscles moving, relax antagonists, regulate tone, and, in some cases, might even emerge into partially controlled movements.

THERAPY

Fay's reflex therapy is discussed in two main sections: part-movement exercises and pattern-movement exercises.

Part-movement Exercises

Eliciting all normal and "pathological" reflexes, preferably in prone, that might represent portions of patterns of movements characteristic of amphibian and reptilian movements are activities that may be subsumed under part-movement exercises. Fay prescribed eliciting 12 to 20 of these reflexes in succession once or twice daily for spasticity. He claimed such exercise improves spastic muscle function, increases its volume, and the response begins "to automatically integrate into a wider and more organized pattern." The part exercised also exhibits a diminution in the spastic tone and postural disturbance. "It would appear that the spastic type of paralysis, arising when cortical control and suppression is withdrawn, yields to influences of lower primitive centers when these are deliberately aroused and placed in command at the level of function for which they originally functioned." Other authorities would disagree with this interpretation and would say that such stimulation would only strengthen these responses and make them less amenable to higher-center control in the future.

Normal and pathological reflex exercises could include eliciting the following reflexes:

1. Deep tendon reflexes such as the biceps, triceps, brachioradial, knee jerk, and ankle jerk
2. Clonus of the ankle and patellar varieties
3. Superficial or skin reflexes such as the upper, middle, and lower abdominal reflexes, and the plantar, the palmar, and the gluteal reflexes
4. Pyramidal signs such as the Babinski, and other reflexes that produce dorsiflexion of the toes such as the signs of Oppenheim, Gordon, Chaddock, and Gonda; signs of abnormal plantar flexion of the toes as well, such as in those of Rossolimo and Mendel-Bechterew; also, in-the-hand reflexes such as Hoffman's sign and pathological forced grasping
5. Abnormal spinal reflexes such as flexion, extension, and cross reflexes, and bilateral general flexion of the lower limbs

Unlocking reflexes and positions to be used for establishing relaxation and better function of muscles were also described by Fay. "Unlocking reflexes are used to release the spastic part in preparation for more complex patterns of movement."

1. Unlocking the spastic hand is done with the individual in prone, face turned to the opposite shoulder, and the hand in the palm up over the buttocks position. An opening or fanning of the fingers can be accomplished in this position. Passive manipulation of the fingers and wrist for several minutes should arouse a body-image consciousness of the part. The use of mirrors for visual feedback of the movements and

feelings is also recommended. Hopefully, the function of opening the fingers can be learned "and the relaxation component ultimately 'captured' by higher cortical controls for voluntary uses."

2. Unlocking the spastic flexed arm is done with the individual in prone, elevating the elbow to the level of the shoulder cap, having the face turned toward the hand (thumb at the teeth level) "and then drawing the hand and wrist downward, outward, and backward, rotating the humerus 30° with the elbow-tip at the shoulder level, until the hand has passed beyond the mid-perpendicular point of lateral sweep. At this point and throughout the ensuing arc of 45°, the forearm will be found to easily relax and extend, especially as the hand begins to assume the palm-up position on its way to complete the cycle over the adjacent buttocks."

3. Unlocking spastic lower extremities is also done with the individual in prone but may also be done in supine. Clonus, Babinski, and other reflexes may be used to relax the foot and toes; and 5 to 10 minutes of repeated application of the Marie-Foix reflex may temporarily relax adductors. To elicit the Marie-Foix reflex, the toes are bent downward and pressure is applied to the ball of the foot. The leg should flex at the knee and the adductors should relax after a few responses.

In applying the reflex of defense as a form of exercise or unlocking of spastic lower extremities, the clinician may place the child in supine with the knees and big toes pointing outward (frog leap position). One hand is placed with the palm above the knee and the other with the palm over the dorsum of the foot with fingers curved over the toes and the tips against the ball of the foot. Then the toes are bent downward and at the same time pressure is applied to the ball of the foot. The leg should spontaneously flex and the knee should be guided outward as far as possible. After the limb is in full flexion the knee should be rotated back toward the midline and downward pressure applied on the leg from above. In the flex position, the leg may also be returned to its original position by a tap on the patellar tendon. The exercise should be repeated rapidly and maintained rhythmically for a period of 15 minutes in each lower limb and then in combined fashion. "Reduction in the spasticity for the benefit of later 'patterns of movement' and crawling in the prone position is thus accomplished." "It is now possible to 'unlock' and relax certain spastic muscle groups by the use of intrinsic reflex spinal cord mechanisms. The benefits to posture, muscle tone and functional activity depend upon training and utilization of the improved state of spasticity and muscle response and through appropriate measures of physical therapy and 'patterns of movement.' "

Pattern-movement Exercises

Pattern-movement exercises may follow reflex conditioning and unlocking maneuvers. For example, in a case where the right upper extremity has good movement and some voluntary response to cortical control, but the left side is paralyzed and both lower extremities are spastic, the clinician might "initiate a crossed-pattern movement and train the coordinated existing responses of the right upper extremity to set up homolateral or crossed spinal responses to aid the other uncontrolled and paralyzed parts." Many patients who were started on homolateral pattern movements and later mastered them may advance to crossed-pattern movements, which are the basis for coordinated patterns of walking, almost without further work, according to Fay. Also, according to Fay (1954c), "feeding, walking and certain self-care responses are available through 'conditioning' even for the profoundly involved cases, when reflex patterns are used as the base for activating otherwise paralyzed and spastic musculature."

Study of a Fay-oriented Treatment

Doman et al. (1960) reported on a two-year study of 76 children with severe brain injuries who took part in a system of therapy referred to as a program of neurological organization. The program was a modification and extension of Fay's approach.

According to the investigators, the program must include—

(a) the opportunity for the brain-injured to spend prolonged periods on the floor in the prone or quadruped position, so that he may crawl or creep in order to utilize uninjured areas in physiological development; (b) the utilization of patterns of activity administered passively to a child which reproduce the mobility functions for which injured brain levels are responsible; (c) a program of sensory stimulation to make the child body conscious in terms of position sense and proprioception; (d) a program of establishing cortical hemisphere dominance through the development of unilateral handedness, footedness, and 'eyedness'; and (e) the initiation of a breathing program to achieve maximum vital capacity."

The criterion of progress during the study was level of mobility reached based on a system of 13 levels of normal development. The 13 levels were rolling, crawling in a circle or backward, crawling without pattern, homologous crawling, homolateral crawling, cross-pattern crawling, creeping without pattern, homologous creeping, homolateral creeping, cross-pattern creeping, cruising, walking without pattern, cross-pattern walking. The mean improvement of mobility was 4.2 levels. The mean length of mobility at the start of the program was 4.4 and at the end of the program was 8.6. The range of improvement was 0 to 12 levels. The investigators stated that the results of the study were significantly better than those achieved by the investigators when using other methods.

Treatment involved an outpatient program of "neurological organization" that was taught to the parents. The progress of the children was reviewed approximately every two months by the team. With progress, appropriate treatment changes were made. Treatment consisted of two types:

Treatment type I required that all nonwalking children spend all day on the floor in prone and be encouraged to crawl or creep. The only exceptions to this requirement were times to feed, love, or treat the child.

Treatment type II involved "patterning" the child. That is, "a specific pattern of activity was prescribed which passively imposed on the central nervous system the functional activity which was normally the responsibility of that damaged brain level." Children were patterned by three adults for five minutes, four times a day, seven days a week. Patterns were performed smoothly and rhythmically with one adult responsible for head movements while each of the other two adults were responsible for right arm and leg, and left arm and leg movements. Children who could not crawl and those who crawled below cross-pattern level were administered activity pattern I or were patterned in the homolateral pattern; children who could crawl in cross pattern or who could creep were administered activity pattern II or were patterned in cross pattern. Children who walked but not well were also patterned at the cross-pattern level (activity pattern III).

Also "to enhance neurological organization" children, after appropriate evaluation, were placed on a program of (a) sensory stimulation (application of heat and cold, brushing, pinching, and body-image appreciation), (b) establishing brain dominance (unilateral handedness, footedness, eyedness), and (c) improving vital capacity.

Motor Unit Orientation

The motor unit orientation may also be called proprioceptive-cortical facilitation (Gellhorn, 1949), central facilitation (Kabat, 1952a), or proprioceptive neuromuscular facilitation (Voss, 1972, Ch. 5). That which distinguishes this approach from other neurologically oriented therapies is the focus of its adherents on the means of obtaining maximal excitation of motor units of the muscle. The motor unit orientation is discussed primarily from the standpoint of Kabat (1948, 1950a, b, c, 1952a) since he is recognized as the major contributor to this orientation.

THEORY

Contrasted to Fay's concern and interest in the heritage of patterns of movement and how they may be applied in treatment is Kabat's (1952a) concern and interest in applying "powerful facilitating mechanisms and summation of the facilitation to increase excitation at the anterior horn cells." The core of an effective program for paralysis is techniques of central facilitation, according to Kabat. Kabat and Knott (1948), however, in discussing treatment of spastic paralysis, made various recommendations under a section called "reinforcement of voluntary innervation," and one of them included innervating a muscle by voluntary activation "of a more complex primitive pattern, of which the muscle forms a part." They indicated that such primitive patterns may be active after loss of the corticospinal tracts and assumed to be extrapyramidal in origin. As examples of primitive patterns they identified total flexion or extension of the neck, trunk, and lower extremities (apparently describing tonic labyrinthine or otolithic reflexes in prone and supine positions); extensor thrust of the lower extremity, flexion of hip, knee and ankle; and extensor thrust of the upper extremity (apparently describing various spinal and long spinal reflexes). "A variety of technics of reinforcement based on utilization of various reflexes and primitive patterns has been developed and applied successfully in treatment of patients with spastic paralysis." So Kabat and his associates have also made use of paleoreflex techniques.

Kabat described the usual routine in the treatment of paralysis as physical therapy starting with passive motion (a type of "patternless" patterning) and moving gradually to assistive motion, free motion with gravity eliminated, free motion against gravity, and finally resistive motion. Avoidance of fatigue and stretch of the affected muscles is emphasized. Such a program is relatively ineffective since the large majority of motor units of the muscles are left inactive, and since "it is the activity of the motor unit which results in therapeutic benefit to the muscle in the form of hypertrophy and to the nervous mechanism in greater ease of impulse transmission." (Kabat, 1952a).

Maximal activation of the neuromuscular mechanism, of which the motor unit (anterior horn cell, motor nerve fiber, myoneural junction and the hundred or more muscle fibers innervated by the single motor nerve fiber) is the fundamental unit, is the goal of an effective program of neuromuscular reeducation. "By exciting all or almost all of the available motor units of the muscle, each exercise would have the greatest possible therapeutic effectiveness both for the muscle and its nervous mechanism." The goal of maximal excitation of the motor units of a muscle with each voluntary effort depends "on the bombardment of the anterior horn cells with impulses from the motor mechanisms in the central nervous system." Therapy for paralysis, therefore, should be aimed at the central nervous system and only indirectly at the muscles (Kabat, 1952a).

THERAPY

Five techniques of central facilitation—resistance, stretch, reflexes, mass movement patterns, reversal of antagonists—were identified by Kabat (1952a).

Resistance

Resistance increases the response of muscles in voluntary contraction. Building muscle power and causing hypertrophy through the principle of maximum resistance is a well-known principle among weight lifters and body builders. Manual resistance (rather than weights, pulleys, etc.) allows the greatest range of technical procedures for facilitation. Greater response in voluntary contraction of affected muscles is obtained through combining a variety of facilitating techniques with resistive exercise.

Maximal resistance for isotonic contraction is the use of opposing force that is almost equal to but somewhat less than the force of the movement so that with maximum exertion the client succeeds in the movement through as much of the range as possible; maximal resistance for isometric contraction is the use of opposing force that is somewhat greater than the force of the movement so that with maximum exertion the client holds a position as strongly as possible (Kabat, 1950b). The mechanism by which resistance increases the power of muscular contraction was demonstrated by Gellhorn (1949). The voluntary motor mechanism is facilitated by proprioceptive stimulation arising from the increase in tension in the muscle resulting from muscle contraction against resistance.

Manual resistance may be selectively applied to (a) maintain a maximal contraction throughout a range of motion; (b) increase the active range of motion; and (c) guide voluntary motion in the desired direction. The selective application of resistive work may also contribute to the establishment of complex patterns such as sitting and standing balance.

From a functional or dynamic viewpoint, the effectiveness of resistive techniques appears related to what may be termed the "emergency or challenge principle," that is, the firing of suprathreshold motor units when the organism is threatened or challenged—the use of back-up or reserve power, so to speak.

Stretch

It is known that afferents favor the contraction of elongated muscles. Resistance applied to a stretched muscle may elicit a stronger response than when applied to a shortened muscle. But Kabat (1952a) has noted that in some cases, such as in athetosis, "voluntary contraction in the shortened range of the muscle against resistance is usually greater than in the lengthened range."

Facilitation (Kabat, 1952a) through rapid stretch is especially effective when using techniques such as sudden breaking of a hold followed immediately by active motion against resistance, and also the hold, relax, and then active motion maneuver. Facilitation of a paralyzed muscle may also be achieved through the stretch of another muscle that is part of the same mass movement.

Range of motion and facilitation of voluntary contraction of the agonist muscle may be inhibited through stretch of an antagonist, especially if the antagonist is spastic. Greater facilitation of the agonist should occur when using a position in which stretch of the antagonist is avoided.

The facilitation effect in the stretch technique also appears related to threat of the organism; in general, stretching a muscle implies possibly tearing it and so requires a response from the organism. More specifically, stretching of mandibular extensors to the rupture point in animals could be life threatening, and hence the nervous system responds by facilitating the shortening of the muscles.

Reflexes

Voluntary neuromuscular response may be facilitated through the use of reflex excitation, or in Fay's language, reflex conditioning. The procedure involves the simultaneous stimulation of the reflex and the voluntary motion in the same muscle group.

Proprioceptive reflexes that can facilitate voluntary effort include: tonic neck reflexes, righting reactions, positive supporting reaction, the von Bechterew reflex (mass flexion reflex of the lower extremity following passive flexion of the big toe), and the palatal and pharyngeal reflexes. For example, arm extension and flexion may be facilitated by voluntary use of the asymmetrical tonic neck reflex, or leg extension via eliciting the positive supporting reaction, or velar elevation via eliciting the palatal reflex (Kabat, 1950b).

Complex patterns of muscular response such as those required for sitting, kneeling, and standing balance may also be facilitated through postural and righting reactions.

Such reflex excitation, conditioning, or facilitation is related to the "coordinative structures principle." That is, if voluntary motor activity or programming is affected, and if reflexes form the basic units of the motor program, then, hopefully, eliciting the basic units should contribute to organizing or reorganizing the motor program.

Mass Movement Patterns

Kabat is convinced "that the treatment of isolated muscles or isolated motions is ineffective and unsound" (Kabat, 1952a). Voluntary activities are almost never characterized by the use of a single muscle or isolated individual motion. Also, a mass movement pattern of an entire extremity against resistance serves as a powerful facilitation of the voluntary response of a paralyzed muscle. "The facilitation in a mass movement pattern can occur not only through overflow from functioning proximal muscles to paralyzed distal muscles in the extremity but also in the reverse direction."

Kabat also believes that diagonal-spiral mass movement patterns are usually more effective in facilitation than straight mass movement patterns. He bases this on the observation that activities requiring great effort like chopping wood, running, using a shovel, throwing a ball, and swimming use primitive, complex patterns of motion that are diagonal and spiral, not straight. "These primitive patterns of motion in which combinations of motions are associated in a more complex pattern, are present in infants" (Kabat, 1952b). Mass movement patterns are instinctive natural patterns in the CNS.

Diagonal-spiral movements are observed when a young child rolls to his side by way of the body-on-body righting reaction, or when he assumes sitting from supine by way of the partial rotation pattern.

For even greater facilitation, combinations of mass movement patterns may be used. For example, voluntary movement in a paralyzed lower limb may be facilitated by a combination of mass movement patterns of the leg with the stronger opposite arm in a primitive running pattern.

Mass movement patterns appear intact and relatively undisturbed in patients with severe paralysis from various lesions of the corticospinal tracts, anterior horn cells, or cerebellum. Only patients with athetosis appear to show disruption and disturbance of the natural mass movement patterns. The basal ganglia, therefore, appear to have an important role in the mechanism of mass movement patterns. Working on mass movement patterns with athetotics, however, may result in decrease in involuntary motion and improvement in voluntary control.

Resistive maneuvers in mass movement patterns may be applied in mat work in activities such as crawling, rolling over, and sitting up.

Maximal stimulation of mass movement patterns not only facilitates voluntary movements but has also resulted "in marked and prolonged relaxation of spasticity, muscle spasm, and Parkinsonian rigidity" (Kabat, 1950a). Activation of inhibitory mechanisms for muscle tonus via excitation of mass movement patterns is apparently the reason for this relaxation.

Kabat's mass movement technique suggests principles such as the "coordinative principle," "back-up or redundancy principle," and "primitive pattern principle." That is, facilitation of involved muscles via mass movement patterns may be based on the fact that you "ride" on the larger coordinated movement that characterizes almost all voluntary activities; or there is redundancy in muscles and movements like in other parts and functions of the body and when you call into play more and larger muscles the redundancy manifests itself. Or, some of the diagonal-spiral patterns are suggestive of righting reactions or even lower-order cross-pattern crawling movements in the upright position and such movements may be controlled by undamaged lower integration centers.

Reversal of Antagonists

"The contraction of the antagonist against resistance immediately preceding resistive exercise of the agonist is a valuable technique of facilitation" (Kabat, 1952a).

Such facilitatory patterns of motion occur naturally in work and sports activities. An antagonist motion immediately preceding the main action may be seen in sports, for example, pitching a baseball, kicking a football, and swinging a golf club, a tennis racket, a baseball bat, and so on; and in work movements, for example, swinging an axe, using a shovel, or a pick, and so on. "The stronger the contraction of the antagonist, the greater the facilitation of the agonist muscle." When the agonist is paralyzed and the antagonist is comparatively unaffected, the technique is especially effective. "Reversal of antagonists is usually applied in mass movement patterns against maximal resistance and can be summated with other facilitation techniques."

A number of specific techniques may be applied of rapidly alternating contraction of antagonistic muscle groups against maximal resistance.

Rhythmic stabilization represents a technique of rapid alternation of isometric contraction of antagonists against maximal resistance; for example, "the patient holds the wrist in the neutral position and the therapist rhythmically applies resistance alternately to the radial extensor then the ulnar flexor." Following facilitation via rapid alternating isometric contraction of the antagonist muscles, then "maximal isotonic contraction of the agonist is performed repeatedly against resistance." For greater response, rhythmic stabilization is employed in mass movement patterns and summated with other facilitation techniques (Kabat, 1952a).

Patients with lower motor neuron, corticospinal tract, and basal ganglia involvements respond to rhythmic stabilization; however; those with cerebellar dysfunction do not, according to Kabat. The cerebellum, therefore, is apparently an important part of the central mechanism for rhythmic stabilization. Just as mass movement patterns activate the extrapyramidal system, rhythmic stabilization excites the cerebellar system.

Isotonic reversal of antagonists is characterized by alternating active motion of the antagonists against maximal resistance. The technique may be employed through a part or through the entire range of joint motion.

Isotonic reversal of antagonists with isometric contraction is done against maximal resistance while "the patient performs isotonic contraction of the antagonist through the range, then isometric contraction of the antagonists in the shortened range, followed immediately by active motion of the agonist through the range succeeded by holding with the agonist."

Quick reversal of antagonists involves isotonic slow motion of the antagonist against maximal resistance and through the range, "then suddenly the motion is reversed and the agonist is contracted and assisted as rapidly as possible to the shortened position, immediately following which there is an isometric contraction of the agonist against maximal resistance." The quick reversal technique has been especially useful in work with cerebellar lesions. Good examples of the normal use of quick reversal of antagonists is chopping wood and the golf swing (Kabat, 1950c).

Kabat stated that manual resistive exercise is based on summation of a number of facilitation techniques in each exercise; for example, mass movement pattern, one of the reversal of antagonists techniques, and resistance are used routinely. Stretch and a suitable reflex to improve response may also be added. That is, "in order to produce truly maximal voluntary motion, simultaneous application of a combination of facilitating techniques is used routinely" (Kabat, 1950b).

The "coiled spring principle" is suggested by the reversal of antagonists technique. It's as though, through the technique, muscles are calling upon central mechanisms for a maximum effort and are taking advantage of a form of "nervous energy momentum."

Physiologic Mechanisms Underlying the Techniques

Kabat (1952a) discussed the physiologic mechanisms underlying therapeutic facilitation techniques as follows:

It is apparent that voluntary motion and proprioceptive afferent impulses and reflexes are very closely related and interdependent. It seems possible that the motor cortex initiates voluntary motion by stimulating the reflex mechanism through which the motion is actually performed in coordinated mass movement patterns. This hypothesis would conform to the evolutionary concept that the higher centers of the brain have become dominant and modify and control the function of the lower centers rather than eliminate them.

Such a statement recalls the theories of Jackson, Fay, and more recently, those expressed by Easton (1972), among others.

Referring to animal experiments and to his observations on facilitation of voluntary motion in patients with paralysis, Kabat stated:

The underlying physiologic mechanism of resistance, stretch and mass movement patterns is essentially proprioceptive. Postural and righting reflexes and related facilitation techniques are also proprioceptive in nature. The facilitating effect of reversal of antagonists is due to successive induction [fundamental principle demonstrated by Sherrington of the functioning of the reflex centers in the spinal cord whereby previous activities in the antagonist centers is followed immediately by a period of facilitation of the agonist pattern], proprioceptive stimulation [through resistance and stretch], and cocontraction [cocontraction rather than reciprocal innervation results from increased intensity of cortical stimulation as well as from strong proprioceptive facilitation—in cocontraction both antagonists contract simultaneously with stronger contraction of the agonist group]. A cerebellar mechanism appears to be involved in rhythmic stabilization.

Again referring to animal studies Kabat is convinced that "proprioceptive stimuli are not only required for coordination, guidance and control of voluntary motion, but are essential for any voluntary response at all."

Neurologic Hypotheses Arising from Treatment

Kabat's (1950b) hypothesis was "that the fundamental function of the cerebellar hemisphere is to facilitate voluntary isometric muscular contraction." This hypothesis is based on the study of a large number of individuals with cerebellar disease (a) whose cerebellar syndrome of intention tremor, hypotonia, dysmetria, rebound and marked fatigability appeared to be fundamentally related "to a deficiency in power, range, and particularly endurance of isometric voluntary contraction of individual muscles" and (b) whose cerebellar syndrome of asynergia responded to techniques (quick reversal combined with mass movement patterns against maximal resistance) designed to develop power, range, and duration of isometric contraction.

The function of the corticospinal system is to initiate voluntary motion and inhibit spasticity. And since the basic patterns of voluntary motion are mass movement patterns, and since proper functioning of mass movement patterns are dependent on the integrity of the neostriatum (caudate nucleus and putamen), the performance of voluntary motion requires that the corticospinal system function together with the extrapyramidal system responsible for mass movement patterns.

The paleostriatum (globus pallidus and substantia nigra) facilitates voluntary isotonic muscular contraction. This hypothesis is based on the study of individuals with Parkinson's disease (paleostriatum implicated) whose parkinsonian symptoms of weakness, slowness, fatigability, lack of range, and difficulty in initiating isotonic voluntary motion responded to techniques (mass movement patterns, rhythmic stabilization, and slow reversal of antagonists) designed to improve voluntary isotonic contraction.

Sensory Receptor Orientation

The sensory receptor orientation has also been referred to as the sensorimotor approach (Stockmeyer, 1967, 1972). What distinguishes this approach from other neurologically oriented therapies is its concentration on sensory stimuli and sensory receptors. The sensory receptor orientation is discussed primarily from the standpoint of Rood (1954, 1962) since she is recognized as its major contributor.

Rood (1954), like so many other clinicians working with children with cerebral palsy, expressed dissatisfaction with generally available techniques. Her position was that more attention should be paid to neurophysiological aspects. This echoed the beliefs of Fay, Kabat, and the Bobaths who were busily at work at the time on the neurophysiological aspects of the problem. After considerable study, Rood was convinced that more effective treatments based on neurophysiological principles could be developed.

She expressed the rather commonly held belief that "Motor patterns are developed from fundamental reflex patterns present at birth which are utilized and gradually modified through sensory stimuli until the highest control is gained on the conscious level.'' She believed, therefore, that if ''it were possible to apply the proper sensory stimuli to the appropriate sensory receptor as it is utilized in normal sequential development, it might be possible to elicit motor response reflexly and by following neurophysiological principles, establish proper motor engrams. The movement which results in response to a summation of various reflexes is 'boosted' up to higher centers for final reception at the sensory cortical level'' (Rood, 1954).

THEORY

Two important factors that contributed to the development of the Rood approach were (a) her critical analysis of more traditional techniques (Rood, 1954) and (b) her study of developmental patterns of movement and posture (Stockmeyer, 1967).

Critical Analysis of More Traditional Techniques

A number of neurophysiological principles appeared to be violated, according to Rood, by the use of traditional techniques such as passive movement in preparation for voluntary movement; braces and splints to obtain, maintain, or restrain movement; conscious relaxation for control of voluntary movement; exercise techniques; and positioning and handling.

Proper motor engrams, ''available for reproduction in motor action at the cortical level, are based on the summation of many sensory impressions arising within the physical structures of the part.'' Passive movement work does not contribute to the development of these sensory impressions because it eliminates stimuli arising from the effect of gravity, provides opposing stimuli arising from the therapist's hands, and eliminates the balancing force of muscle acting proportionately against each other. ''Assistance by the therapist can more effectively be given by applying sensory stimuli which will cause motor reaction through the nervous system and so lay the foundation for the proper engram. The appropriate stimulus is determined by the type of receptor in the particular muscle involved in the desired action.''

Control of movement via braces and splints is often actually prevented by them because their application may produce sensory stimulation of touch, pressure, and stretch that may result in undesirable muscle contraction.

Physiologic relaxation normally follows action. Conscious relaxation for control of voluntary movement, a traditionally accepted technique, is considered nonphysiologic ''and therefore voluntary cessation of motion is abnormal and the most difficult means of achieving relaxation.'' The principle of tension reduction through vigorous exercise is well known to joggers, swimmers, cyclists, disco dancers, and so on.

Physiologic relaxation or diminution in spastic tone was described by Fay following his reflex conditioning exercises. Prolonged relaxation of spasticity, muscle spasm, and parkinsonian rigidity was reported as one of the effects of Kabat's mass movement maneuvers.

Cephalocaudal development represents the normal developmental pattern. Rood (1954) believed that a common error on the part of many therapists was to emphasize exercise work on the lower extremities. "Eye, head, and neck control precedes control of other parts of the body, thereby indicating that motor control develops in successive levels away from the brain just as sensory stimuli reach the brain afferently through successive levels."

Developmental Patterns of Movement and Posture

Two major sequences in motor development that are distinct and yet inseparable because of their interaction are those of skeletal functions and vital functions. Neck, trunk, and extremity functions comprise the skeletal function sequence, while respiration and food intake functions and their combination in speech development comprise the vital function sequence. Relatedness of the two sequences are based on a number of factors, for example, both sequences are dependent for their effectiveness on the degree and distribution of proximal tone, and both sequences have their origins in the trigeminal reflexes (the first response of the embryo occurs as a result of perioral stimulation). Differences of the two sequences "lie partly in the identification of some components of the vital function sequence as being voluntary somatic functions and other components as being involuntary autonomic functions, while all parts of the skeletal function sequence are classified as voluntary somatic functions."

In treatment, the skeletal and vital function sequences are approached as interacting mechanisms as they are associated in development; however, for the sake of exposition, the two sequences are presented separately.

The vital function sequence is composed of eight steps:

1. Inspiration—The inspiratory center in the medulla is continuous in its function. Inspiration is the most important vital function since the first one is truly the "breath of life."
2. Expiration—Crying, sneezing, and coughing are three of its forms. Before the adaptive, discriminating functions of taste and smell develop, sneezing and coughing serve as protective reactions against unpleasant stimuli.

    In time, respiratory function also comes under voluntary control, at least up to a point, and an individual is able to voluntarily cease breathing, or alter inspiratory-expiratory cycles at will.
3. Sucking of fluids, or more accurately the suckling reflex—This is a grasping, or pursuit reflex, designed for ingestion of food. When

suckling, the tongue is grooved and performs a holding contraction during each stroke.

4. Swallowing of fluids—The swallowing reflex is activated by food stimuli, or other stimuli applied to areas supplied by the trigeminal. Swallowing is facilitated by the sequence of muscle activity (orbicularis oris, buccinator, superior constrictor) during suckling. Two forms of swallowing may be recognized: visceral and somatic. The visceral form is characterized by preceding mouth opening and forward movement of the tongue, while the somatic form is characterized by fixation of the tip and action at the base of the tongue.

   Suckling and swallowing are interrelated and, in fact, synreflexic and interact with respiratory functions. The suckling center establishes the pattern for respiration by coordinating suckling, swallowing, and breathing. Suckling and swallowing are therapeutically facilitated in the supine-withdrawal pattern or the neck-cocontraction pattern because of their functional relationship to a flexion pattern.

5. Phonation—Phonation is viewed as a form of controlled expiration. Prerequisite for normal phonation is the respiratory control associated with suckling. Phonation may be therapeutically facilitated in the pivot prone position if a good suckling pattern were established, since the open-mouth position is functionally related to an extensor pattern.

6. Chewing—The postural function of the chewing muscles of maintaining the mandible in place against gravity is dependent on the muscles working against resistance during chewing. Food particles (swallowing solids develops in association with chewing) act as a stimulus to tongue action, which is coordinated with chewing.

7. Swallowing of solids—This develops in association with chewing.

8. Speech articulation—This represents the skill level of the sequence. "The motor act involved in speech is dependent upon the contributions to coordinate movement of all previous steps in the designated order."

Respiration, suckling, swallowing, chewing, and reflexive utterances are co-developing during at least the first 10 months of life. Therefore, step eight could be misleading unless a distinction is made between reflexive and voluntary "articulation" in the very young child. Also, dispute may exist over whether breathing and velopharyngeal closure mechanisms, the tongue, lips, and mandible are primarily eating organs that have emerged secondarily as speech organs, or whether, because of the importance of speech, they have emerged primarily as speech organs that serve secondarily as eating organs. On that basis, Rood's vital function sequence would require reinterpretation.

Such a view would also help explain why some clients display relatively good eating function but relatively poor speech function, or relatively good speech function but relatively poor eating function.

The skeletal function sequence reflects development of two primary motor functions: mobility and stability. Two additional responses needed for coordinated movement develop from the combining of mobility and stability: mobility superimposed on stability in a weight-bearing position ("heavy work movement pattern superimposed on cocontraction") and mobility superimposed on stability in a non-weight pattern ("skill").

Stockmeyer (1967) says: "The developmental sequence can be analyzed to determine the stages which demonstrate the acquisition of the four levels of function and what sensory information is related to responses at the various levels. In evaluation and treatment planning the therapist identifies the functions lacking, the stages which lay the foundation for the more advanced activity and the stimuli which may facilitate the responses of each stage."

1. Functional mobility develops during the first three stages of the skeletal function sequence: the withdrawal-supine, roll-over, and pivot-prone stages.
   a. The withdrawal-supine pattern is a total flexion response characterized by neck flexion; shoulder flexion, adduction, internal rotation; elbow flexion, forearm pronation with wrist and finger extension; hip flexion, abduction and external rotation; and knee flexion and foot dorsiflexion with toe extension. It could be viewed as a response to protect the anterior neck, face, and lower body and extremities. It is a reciprocal pattern with activated flexors and inhibited extensors and reflects integration of the tonic labyrinthine and asymmetrical tonic neck reflexes. (The pattern is reminiscent of the protective startle reflex characterized by an adductor-flexor reaction of the body when individuals are startled or surprised.)

      The pattern is facilitated in patients who do not have a reciprocal pattern or who are dominated by extensor tone or an asymmetrical pattern.
   b. The roll-over pattern is characterized by flexion of upper and lower extremities on the same side. Activation of the extremities and of lateral trunk muscles effects rolling at this stage. The pattern is facilitated in those who show tonic reflexes in supine, do not use lateral trunk flexors, or need mobilizing of extremities.
   c. The pivot-prone, or prone-extension pattern, represents Peiper's symmetrical chain reflex in the abdominal position dependent on the labyrinthine on-head righting reaction. The full range of extension of the neck, trunk, lower extremities, and proximal regions of

the upper extremities characterizes its display. Its primary role as a preparation for stability is considered more important than its mobilizing role.

Muscles active in patterns of functional mobility can be kinesiologically distinguished from stabilizers in a number of ways. They are the muscles associated with flexor patterns. They are usually most active when the distal lever is free and not weight bearing. They work to initiate movement and perform brief bursts of activity, and are the muscles that play a major role in distal patterns during skill.

Receptor functions associated with mobility patterns (especially flexion) appear related to processes of protection. Areas of the face, palms of the hands, and soles of the feet that have a high concentration of specific skin receptors respond first to tactile stimuli by avoidance responses. "It is speculated that low threshold skin receptors, those with 'A' size fibers, are closely tied in function to the superficial phasic muscles which provide protective mobility at first, and later in development contribute to fine manipulatory skill." Also, Rood postulates that mobilizers respond differently to forms of proprioceptive stimuli and contain different concentrations of proprioceptors than stabilizers.

2. Functional stability develops during stages three through eight: pivot prone, cocontraction neck, on elbows, all fours, standing, walking. It is "that motor function which fixes portions of the body so that weight bearing can be done."

   c. The pivot-prone pattern (one of Peiper's chain refleves) was considered under mobility development but its most important function is as the first pattern in stability development. It is considered an essential prerequisite for all weight-bearing patterns. Peiper believes the chain reflex which is dependent on the labyrinthine on-head righting reaction contributes to bringing the body into the upright position, that is, into sitting and standing. "More dynamic weight bearing functions cannot be done normally without the pivot prone pattern as a basis for stability."

   d. The neck cocontraction pattern precedes all other concontraction patterns, in accordance with the principle of cervicocaudal and cervicorostral development, and it is demonstrated when the head is brought from the face vertical position in pivot prone to the face horizontal position. Such head balance is prerequisite for stability of the eyes and for feeding and speech to develop to the skill level.

   e. The prone-on-elbows pattern reflects the advance from the prone extension pattern to weight bearing on elbows. Also "unilateral weight bearing on one upper extremity while the other is engaged in exploratory activities is more important in the development of stability than the bilateral weight bearing."

f. The quadruped pattern demonstrates the peak of the stability-developing stage of the upper trunk and upper extremities. Initially, the lower trunk and lower extremities may lag behind in the development of stability but eventually the entire trunk assumes a horizontal position. "Weight shift will occur to free some extremities for movement and the added weight on one extremity increases the stability response of that extremity."

g. The standing and walking patterns follow the quadruped with intervening activities, but these intervening activities are not considered major steps in stability development. At first standing is static and bilateral and becomes unilateral upon weight shifting. Unilateral weight bearing in standing and walking adds significantly to stability development.

Muscles active in patterns of functional stability can be kinesiologically distinguished from mobilizers in a number of ways. They perform "heavy work"; do prolonged holding while distal reciprocal skill is taking place; work primarily in a stretched position; and play a major role in proximal functions during skill.

Receptor functions associated with stability patterns are related to maintained responses that are dependent upon maintained sensory input. Speculations on a gamma motor system explanation for using skin stimuli to facilitate stabilizing functions are as follows: (a) increased contact of the surfaces of the body causes adaptation of specific skin receptors and increased reception of the general skin receptors ("C" size fibers); (b) discharges from these afferent neurons are transmitted in the spinothalamic system; (c) the reticular-activating system is influenced by collateral inflow from the spinothalamic tracts; and (d) reticulospinal influence, in turn, affects the gamma motor neuron which, in turn, changes sensitivity in the muscle spindle receptor to stretch and in feedback from the spindle to the central nervous system. "Sensitivity to stretch in the deep extensor groups of the trunk, neck, and shoulder girdle and lower extremities is thought to be developed in the pivot prone pattern." Also the stretch that weight bearing puts on the tonic intrinsic muscles of the hands and feet appears to facilitate cocontraction of the entire extremity and is specially important to the development of stability.

3. Mobility superimposed on stability is the third level in the development of coordinate movement and "is characterized by an increase in proximal rotatory functions, an increase in stability and the development of heavy work movement."

Movement superimposed on stability in the neck cocontraction pattern is that of moving into the face vertical position, rotating the head and holding the position; in the on-elbows pattern is that of pushing backward, then forward, and then rocking from side-to-side; in the quadruped pattern is that of forward and back and side-to-side rocking type movements; and in the standing pattern is that of side-to-side weight shift.

Muscles active in mobility superimposed on stability represent the combined functions of proximal mobilizers and all stabilizers. Kinesiologically, heavy work movement is movement of the body in a weight-bearing position in preparation for unilateral weight bearing; an increase in demand on the stabilizers resulting in cocontraction; and the freeing of the extremity away from the weight shift for skill functions.

Receptor functions associated with mobility superimposed on stability is facilitation of cocontraction patterns. A major source for this facilitation is assumed to be feedback from the high threshold proprioceptors in the spindle and joint. Stimuli arise from rocking-bouncing stretch on stabilizers and joint compression from unilateral weight bearing.

4. Skill development is the fourth level and as used by Rood refers to "coordinate movement in man rather than an exceptional degree of motor control." Extremities are prepared for skill functions only after development in their support role. Freedom of the distal part of the extremity from the supporting surface and movements superimposed on stability characterizes patterns at the skill level.

The skill level of the on-elbows pattern shows significant gains in speech articulation (prespeech articulation) and eye control, upper extremity weight bearing in a unilateral position, trunk rotation due to the unilateral weight bearing and freeing of the opposite limb; of the quadruped pattern shows one upper extremity reaching forward to grasp and explore while the other assumes weight, creeping, and associated trunk rotation; of the standing pattern shows freeing of the upper extremities for manipulation and freeing of one lower extremity for movement; and of the walking pattern shows stance, push off, pick up, and heel strike activities.

Once standing and walking are stable, the upper limbs are completely free for manipulative behaviors. Since the rostral portion of the head with its highly specialized distance receptors leads the body in space, the sensorimotor development of this area reaches the skill level before all other bodily parts.

Also, the same progression through four levels of muscle function are followed by the somatic components of the vital function sequence (autonomic components cannot be analyzed in this way). Tongue function is given as an example of progression to the skill level within the vital function sequence. The progression is (a) tongue protrusion in spontaneous suckling (mobilizing response to reject noxious stimuli), (b) tongue grooved and holds during suckling stroke (stabilizing function), (c) fixation of tongue tip and heavy work movement of tongue base during swallowing (movement superimposed on stability), and (d) tongue movement during chewing in response to food stimulus (beginning skill level) and tongue movement during speech articulation without environmental stimulus (higher skill level).

The muscles active in skill patterns are both mobilizers and stabilizers. Stabilizers are required to provide refined regulation of mobility, and the essential mobilizers for skilled movements are the most distal and rostral ones.

Receptor functions associated with skill patterns are discriminatory sensory functions. Just as "movement has levels or steps through which it progresses to arrive at skill, sensory functions must progress in a complimentary manner."

THERAPY

Some general principles of treatment as well as some specific techniques with the cerebral palsied are presented next.

General Principles of Treatment

Some general principles of Rood's approach were identified by Stockmeyer (1967) as follows:

- Natural or therapeutically devised stimuli are employed to facilitate, inhibit, or activate responses.
- Stimuli are applied to complement correct-response feedback.
- Motor responses are sought according to developmental sequence in terms of components of the patterns and patterns that represent stages in the sequence.
- Activation of normal automatic responses should be done without conscious effort from the client.
- Voluntary effort on the part of the patient to enhance a response should be used only when the therapist is sure the response will be more normal.
- Evaluation and treatment planning begin by identifying the pattern to be activated and the appropriate eliciting stimuli.
- Influencing the alpha and gamma motor neurons involved in a specific response is the ultimate purpose of all therapeutic stimuli.
- Receptors that facilitate mobilizers are influenced by quick, changing

stimuli, and receptors that facilitate stabilizers are influenced by continuous uninterrupted stimuli.

Techniques and Examples of Their Application

The sensory stimulation method of treatment makes use of various stimuli: chemical, thermal, tactile, and proprioceptive. Quick tactile and cold stimuli, acceleration and deceleration during movement of the head, tendon tapping, quick stretch and moderate resistance during movement are examples of stimuli used to facilitate mobility; while fast brushing or maintained touch, maintained ice (3 to 5 sec.), heavy resistance to maintained contraction in the shortened range, maintained stretch of a stabilizer at one joint, and consistent pressure on the muscle belly are examples of stimuli used to facilitate stability.

Examples of the development of the vital function sequence through selective sensory receptor stimulation follow.

Respiration may be improved by use of cold stimulus. "Emergency demands" that result in deeper inspiration are under the control of the sympathetic system that can be activated by cold. Cold in the form of ice is applied to the area of sensory distribution of the muscle fibers of the diaphragm, T6 and T12, whose segmental or myotomal (myotome designates a group of muscles innervated from a single spinal segment) distribution is the same as for the somatic antagonistic abdominal muscles. To avoid overflow, the restricted area T7 to T10 is selected. The supine position is recommended because it requires maximum work by the diaphragm in overcoming the resistance of the abdominal viscera. "If the anterior supraclavicular muscles are tense from spasticity or nervous tension, ice applied to the sternocleidomastoid and scaleni while the patient is in the upright antigravity position, will cause relaxation of these muscles and put greater demand on the already stimulated diaphragm" (Rood, 1954). In this example, cold is used for visceral stimulation and for somatic relaxation.

Tongue mobility may be facilitated by both chemical and somatic stimuli. Protrusion may be activated by bitter substances, or retraction in preparation for suckling may be activated by the use of sweet and pleasant stimuli. Also, quick touch stimuli to the alveolar ridge may stimulate tongue movement.

Mouth opening may be facilitated by quick ice stimuli to the lips.

Suckling, swallowing, and chewing patterns, considered as stability-developing patterns, may be prepared for facilitation by fast brushing and ice (3 to 5 sec.) over the skin area of stabilizers, in addition to resistance and pressure over muscle bellies.

Velar activity may be stimulated with the use of a sterile camel's hair brush.

Facial muscle activitation is accomplished through trigeminal nerve stimulation by vinegar or ammonia.

Examples of the development of the skeletal function sequence through selective sensory receptor stimulation follow.

The withdrawal-supine pattern, or components of, may be facilitated through stretch and resistance. Flexion is facilitated by placing stretch on the suboccipital extensors and deep lumbar extensors. Resistance is applied to the upper extremity flexion, internal rotation, and adduction pattern.

The roll-over pattern may be facilitated by mobilizing the right upper extremity, having the hand open and flattened on the surface, and once the hand is in place applying pressure through the elbow to the heel of the hand in an attempt to keep wrist flexors inhibited.

The pivot-prone pattern is facilitated through resistance to the lateral aspect of the trunk. Upper extremity response may be encouraged through a toy motivator. Pressure on shoulder girdle muscles may facilitate holding.

The neck cocontraction pattern may be facilitated by joint compression from the top of the head. Pressure to the thoracic extensors may also facilitate the response.

The on-elbows pattern is held and pressure is applied to facilitate concontraction of the shoulder girdle. Proximal extension and external rotation at the shoulder is encouraged.

Examples of approaches to the different types of cerebral palsy through selective sensory receptor stimulation follow.

Children with hypotonia are treated by (a) facilitating reciprocal mobilizing responses to low threshold tactile stimuli, then (b) applying pressure, stretch, and resistance to prepare for the pivot prone, and (c) progressing the child to weight bearing after pivot prone is accomplished, and so on through the skeletal function sequence.

Children with spasticity (superficial mobilizers are holding and inhibiting the antagonistic reciprocal pattern and stabilizers) are treated by (a) stimulating by fast brushing the high threshold skin receptors over the stabilizers, followed by (b) high threshold stretch and joint compression for cocontraction of stabilizers. The establishment of stability responses inhibits holding by superficial muscles and spontaneous movement may occur.

Children with athetosis and ataxia are viewed as lacking the regulatory influence of cocontraction of stabilizers and often exhibit contact withdrawal. Athetotics are treated by (a) using slow stroking (less than two times per second) or neutral warmth on the skin area innervated by the posterior primary rami in order to reduce excessive movement and (b) using maintained contact, deep prolonged rubbing of the hands and feet, and fast brushing of the outer ring of the trigeminal nerve dermatome to reduce avoidance reactions.

Postural Patterns Orientation

The postural patterns orientation may also be referred to as the neuro-developmental approach (Bobath, B., 1963, Bobath, K., and Bobath, B., 1972). That which distinguishes the approach from other neurologically oriented therapies is its concentration on the development of normal postural reactions and on modifying primitive movement patterns. Discussion of the postural patterns orientation is basically from the standpoint of Bertha and Karel Bobath since they are the founders of the approach. Also, in view of the long series of writings by these two workers and in recognition of the inevitability of changes in some concepts over the years, the material here is based on their more recent works. This author also attempted earlier interpretations of the approach (Mysak, 1959; Mysak and Fiorentino, 1961) and produced objective film studies of the application of techniques based on the approach (Mysak, 1960, 1962).

As with other workers in the area of cerebral palsy, who turned to the study of neurophysiological concepts of treatment, the Bobaths were dissatisfied with the traditional approach that accepted the fundamental irreversibility of the CNS lesion and its effects in cerebral palsy. This approach is designed primarily to help the child make the best possible use of his abnormal motor patterns by (a) direct teaching of motor developmental tasks, (b) the use of special devices, braces, and so on, and (c) the common use of orthopedic surgery when untreated abnormal motor patterns result in secondary muscle and bone deformities.

Instead, the Bobaths believe it to be potentially more beneficial to the child with cerebral palsy (a) if his condition were viewed as a release of primitive postures and movements from the inhibition normally exerted by higher centers of the CNS, (b) if many of his symptoms were considered changeable and not all irreversible, (c) if more physiologic techniques were employed to facilitate the emergence of certain motor patterns, and (d) if much of the secondary muscle and bone deformities were considered preventable by the application of special techniques and activities.

THEORY

A postural reactions orientation to the definition of cerebral palsy, to motor development, and to sensorimotor learning have all contributed to the development of the treatment techniques, just as the use of treatment techniques over time have contributed to ideas on definition, development, and sensorimotor learning.

Definition of Cerebral Palsy

From a postural reactions orientation a child with cerebral palsy is viewed as one who because of a brain lesion suffers arrested or retarded motor development reflected by (a) involvement of head control and of postural reflex mechanisms, (b) retention of infantile total reflex patterns of movement, and (c) eventual abnormal muscle tone and posture and movement. Associated primary and secondary sensory disturbances in audition, vision, and proprioception are common.

Development of Basic Postural Patterns

For purposes of diagnosis and assessment and for treatment planning and management from a postural patterns orientation, it is important to understand motor development in terms of "the underlying modification of the baby's primitive reflex behavior with the gradual appearance of certain automatic postural and adaptive reactions which make these activities possible and which are responsible for the child's physical and mental growth" (Bobath, K., 1963). New activities are developed upon previous patterns that are progressively modified and elaborated. Regardless of the great variety of activities of the normally developing child "there are a few basic motor patterns of postural control and adjustment which develop simultaneously at certain stages and which seem to underlie and make possible the great number of new and complex functional abilities which the child develops at any particular stage. It is more useful to facilitate the basic motor patterns which the child can then use and translate into a whole group of new activities" (Bobath, B., 1967).

At four months basic postural patterns include the labyrinthine on-head righting reaction, the Landau reaction (not fully developed), symmetrical postural behavior, and the neck righting reaction.

This development is reflected by midline orientation of the head and hands in supine, head control and forearm support, and rolling to sides and back to supine.

At six months basic postural patterns include a stronger labyrinthine on-head righting reaction reinforced by the optical on-head righting reaction, a strong Landau, modification of the primitive total flexion and extension patterns, modification of the neck righting reaction, the arm-support-forward reaction, and equilibrium reactions in prone.

This development is reflected by symmetrical extension with abduction of arms and legs, reaching out with extended arms and weight support forward on extended arms and hands, raising the head in supine, and pulling into sitting.

At eight months basic postural patterns include a stronger Landau; a stronger body-on-body righting reaction; arm-support-sideways as well as forward; equilibrium reactions in prone, supine, and sitting; and well-established labyrinthine and optical on-head righting reactions.

This development is reflected by segmental rotation along the body axis, supine to prone and back to supine lying, sitting up from prone, and perfect sitting balance.

At ten months basic postural patterns include incipient equilibrium reactions in standing, established equilibrium reactions of trunk and legs in sitting, arm-support-backward as well as forward and sideways, and a fully established Landau.

This development is reflected by standing and hand-walking, picking up objects from the floor, and sitting up from supine using a partial rotation pattern.

Without the development of basic postural patterns the development of functional skills would either be impossible or at least limited and abnormal. Such patterns also form the background for more voluntary movement throughout life. An early effort at relating basic postural and motor patterns, basic oromotor and articulatory patterns, and basic hand and intentional hand movements was illustrated in tabular form by the author (Mysak, 1959; Mysak and Fiorentino, 1961).

Also the concept of basic postural patterns or key motor patterns appears as a companion concept to Rood's skeletal function sequence.

Movement and Learning

Movement or normal sensorimotor experience is essential to various aspects of child learning and development (Bobath, B., 1971b).

Movement experiences and perceptual development begins first with self-discovery (body movements and movements of the hands to face, body, knees, feet) and then hands and finger awareness (hands to mouth and together), texture, shape, and temperature awareness of objects (touching, mouthing), lips and tongue awareness (hands, and moving food), personal size awareness (reaching for objects, crawling over and under things), and environmental awareness (crawling, creeping, and walking).

Movement and speech development is shown by early child communication through movement and gestures. Also preceding speech is the development of coordinated movements that allow the child to walk and use his hands in manipulation and self-help activities. A reciprocal relationship between speech and play also may be seen during various speak-play games.

Movement and socio-emotional development is reflected by the child's gradual movement away from mother and toward greater independence. His early movements are in response to handling during washing, dressing, and feeding. Then, as his movement capacity develops, he wants to do things himself—to feed, dress, and wash himself.

Movement and motor skill development follows the establishment of basic postural patterns, walking, and use of the hands. Following such basic abilities are the more difficult skills of running, jumping, catching a ball, speaking, writing. "The change and adaptation of existing movement patterns to new activities throughout any performance depends on sensory input, vision, hearing, touch, pressure, and proprioception . . . Repetition will make the performance more automatic, quicker and smoother, requiring less effort" (Bobath, B., 1971b).

For a discussion on the possible role of primary and secondary sensory involvements and sensory feedback disturbances on speech and perceptual development among the cerebral palsied, the reader is referred to an early article written by the author (Mysak, 1959).

THERAPY

Patient criteria, general goals, and general principles of and cautions in therapy, and techniques and examples of therapy are discussed here.

Patient Criteria

A postural-patterns orientation has been shown to benefit a wide range of children with cerebral palsy as well as certain adult neuropathologies. This author has applied a version of the approach with children who were braced for years, who had contractures, who were considered poor therapy candidates because of emotional factors, who were seven, nine, fourteen, twenty-four at the start of therapy, who were considered spastic, athetotic, or mixed, and so on. Among individuals who represented such a variety of ages, types, and conditions the author found an impressive amount of good response to therapy in terms of improved general muscle tonus, more normal protective and balance reactions, and advances in head control, sitting, standing, or walking.

However, a number of reasons were offered on why the cerebral palsied might benefit more if treatment were to begin by about nine months of age (Bobath, B., 1971b), or at least by one or two years. Among these reasons are: adaptability and plasticity of the infantile brain, preventing the adoption of abnormal sensorimotor patterns for use in various functional movements, preventing secondary mental retardation based on "sensorimotor deprivation," preventing the development of abnormal postural activity and tone (or at least being more easily changed), and preventing contracture and deformity.

General Goals of Therapy

The general goals of a postural-patterns orientation to therapy may be stated as follows:

1. Prevention of abnormal postural activity and movement and hence reducing or stabilizing abnormal muscle tone
2. Stimulation of normal postural and motor patterns and muscle tone

3. Progression to learning normal movements and skills
4. Prevention of contractures and deformities

Principles of Therapy

A number of general principles and ideas associated with treatment may be identified:

1. The special handling technique of inhibition, that is, of reflex inhibiting postures, has evolved from static reflex inhibiting postures (passive reversal of abnormal pattern, with therapist holding and controlling every part of the body) to reflex-inhibiting movement patterns (Bobath, B., 1969). The active inhibiting technique allows the therapist to modify part of the abnormal pattern at key points of control; to reduce spasticity throughout the body; to establish a more normal postural set; and to request or stimulate and guide active movements. That is, inhibition and activation of movements are combined. Examples of modified inhibitory patterns follow:
   a. Extension of neck and spine and external rotation of the arm at the shoulder with extended elbow (proximal keypoints) is a main pattern used to counteract flexor spasticity in the trunk and arms.
   b. Abduction with external rotation and extension of hips and knees is a main inhibiting pattern to counteract both extensor and flexor spasticity in the leg.
   c. Rotation of the shoulder girdle against the pelvis and the pelvis against the shoulder girdle is another main inhibiting pattern.
      Reduction of spasticity may also be achieved through the manipulation of the "distal keypoints" of ankles and toes and wrists and fingers.
      Other such inhibiting patterns must be developed to counteract the abnormal patterns of individual children.
2. The special handling technique of facilitation is defined as one that "obtains inherent automatic movement patterns in response to handling in contrast to movements performed at request." Examples of techniques of facilitating righting and equilibrium reactions (Bobath, K., and Bobath, B., 1964) follow:
   a. Patterns of the neck righting and body righting reactions are used to facilitate movements of the body from the head or shoulders. Key points of control are the head (one hand lightly under the chin and the other against the back of the head) and the shoulder girdle (hands underneath armpits spreading fingers so as to control scapulae and upper arms). Such rotation patterns can be used to facilitate rolling over, sitting up, getting on hands and knees, crawling, creeping, kneel-standing, half kneeling, standing, and

walking. For example, head-initiated roll over from supine is done by flexing the head forward and rotating it to the side, and as the child moves into side lying, slow head extension and chin lift until the child moves into prone.

b. Patterns of labyrinthine, body, and optical on-head righting reactions are used to facilitate head control and righting. Such head control and righting may be facilitated in prone, supine, side lying, sitting, standing. For example, head control and righting may be facilitated by lifting the child from side lying with one arm while the opposite arm moves into a supporting position with concomitant adjustment of head position.

c. Patterns of equilibrium reactions are facilitated by displacing the child's center of gravity. Various patterns of head righting and support and balance movements of the limbs may be seen. A primarily protective pattern is seen in the arm-support reaction where forward weight transference elicits forward extension of the arms (six months), sideways weight transference elicits a sideways extension (eight months), and backward weight transference a backward extension (ten months). This reaction may also be facilitated in sitting and kneeling. In self-supported sitting, head righting as well as support and balance movements are seen. Tipping the child's body by applying pressure to one side of the trunk should result in head righting, arm-support reactions toward the side of weight transfer, and arm-balance reactions toward the opposite side. For an excellent discussion and illustrations of facilitation techniques, the reader is referred to the Bobath's article on the topic (Bobath, K. and Bobath, B., 1964).

3. Through special handling techniques abnormal patterns of posture and movement and hence tonus can be changed.

4. Treatment techniques are designed to elicit active movements in the form of normal postural reactions.

5. Changes in patterns of posture and movement should be attempted without the patient's conscious participation.

6. Special handling techniques should be individually selected and based on a careful initial assessment and frequent reassessments of the child.

7. Only techniques to which the child shows immediate improvement in tone and active movement, or at least improvement after a short trial, should be continued.

8. "Normalizing" muscle tone (reduce in spastics, reduce and steady in athetotics) is accomplished by weakening and gradually inhibiting tonic reflexes through modifying patterns produced by them. (In contrast, paleoreflex and motor unit orientations make use of tonic reflexes under special circumstances.)

9. Contingent on normalizing muscle tone, righting and equilibrium reactions should be elicited in developmental sequence.

10. Abnormal coordination of muscle action is the problem in cerebral palsy, not weakness or paralysis of muscles.

11. Special additional techniques of proprioceptive and tactile stimulation are used in cases of true muscle weakness. (To avoid producing spasticity or spasms, stimulation must be carefully graded.)

12. Through special handling techniques the fundamental motor patterns that normal children develop during the first two years of life are stimulated.

13. Postural adjustment movements in response to therapeutic handling are guided and controlled by the therapist.

14. Guidance and control of the child's motor output should be gradually and systematically withdrawn in accordance with progress in treatment.

15. More normal movement patterns are not taught, but their appearance is facilitated.

16. Allow the child to experience the most normal sensorimotor patterns, or, in treatment, do not allow abnormal performance of movements and skills.

17. Teach the mother ways of special handling in order to minimize the child's experiencing abnormal postures and movements.

18. Close cooperation of physical and occupational therapists, the speech clinician, the special teacher, and the parents in furthering the goals of treatment is essential.

Cautions in Therapy

The application of certain treatment techniques over a period of years inevitably leads to the development of a list of "do's and don'ts." Some of the "dont's" may be a function of the particular children worked with, or the method of application of the technique, and so on. Many are based on neurophysiological dynamics. A number of "pitfalls" in treatment have been identified by B. Bobath (1971b).

Normal developmental sequences cannot be followed in detail in treatment because it would take too long and is unnecessary, and because some normal movements appear to reinforce patterns of spasticity or spasm. For example, kicking may increase extensor and adductor spasticity in the legs; "bridging" (lifting pelvis in supine) movements may increase neck and shoulder retraction and extensor spasms of the trunk; crawling, without work on extension in prone lying and standing, may reinforce a pattern of flexion at the hips and knees and dorsiflexion of the ankles; "pulling" along the floor in prone (crawling activities) may increase extensor spasticity of the legs and flexor spasticity and pronation of the arms; and "tailor" sitting may reinforce flexor spasticity and inversion of the ankles.

Cautions against allowing the involved child to engage in motor activities associated with normal children may appear contradictory to a developmental approach to treatment.

Motor patterns should not be sequentially stimulated in treatment because normal development is characterized by simultaneous development of motor patterns. That is, the therapist must not concentrate for long periods on head control and when that is accomplished move to sitting, and so on. By simultaneous is not meant co-equal development of motor patterns but more like a figure-ground development of motor patterns. The figure-ground concept is characterized by a primary activity going on against a background of activities. During overall development, the figure motor pattern may recede and one of the ground motor patterns may emerge and vice versa. Further clarification of this concept of motor development may come from creating a motor movement-symphony movement analogy.

A symphony may have four related movements, varying in form and execution, and played by string, wind, and percussion sections of an orchestra. The four musical movements may be viewed as the four motor movements of roll over, crawling, creeping, and walking. The string, wind, and brass sections may be viewed as playing different motor stages within the movements of roll over, crawling, creeping, and walking. During any one time in the symphony, all sections may be playing in any one movement, or one or another section may be dominant, and versions of parts of any of the four movements may be heard in any one movement. So, too, with motor movements, at any one time in development, stages within or any of the four motor movements may be seen, or one or another may be dominant, but as in the symphony, all motor movements develop harmoniously toward the grand motor finale of skilled movements, that is, running, skating, dancing from basic standing and walking; sewing, drawing, typing, piano playing from basic reach-grasp-release; and speech articulation from basic suckling, swallowing, and chewing.

Specific examples of the figure-ground development may be seen at six months where the child may stand supported, has no sitting balance, but uses his hands for support forward in sitting, can "swim" in prone lying, and reaches out for objects; and at eight months where he enjoys sitting balance, assumes sitting from prone unassisted, creeps and starts to pull himself up into standing; and at nine months where he creeps, may do erect arm walking, or walks when held by both hands.

So at this early stage the therapist may stimulate and reinforce simultaneously forms of sitting, creeping, standing, and walking activities.

Certain techniques must not be used in spastic conditions because the use of, for example, "effort, irradiation, mass patterns, and especially tonic reflexes to strengthen muscles will only reinforce the few existing abnormally increased tonic reflexes" (Bobath, B., 1969). (This constitutes a warning against the use of certain techniques found in the paleoreflex and motor unit orientations.)

Eclectic application of techniques must be done with caution because without full knowledge of the techniques and their underlying concepts, techniques may be used "which may actually cancel themselves out" (Bobath, K., and Bobath, B., 1967).

Certain children are poor candidates for the postural patterns form of treatment such as those with extensive surgery, those who have experienced long-term immobilization in casts, and those who must wear braces for long periods of time between therapy sessions (Bobath, K., and Bobath, B., 1967).

Planning Therapy

A therapy plan is based first on a developmental assessment of the child "in terms of the acquisition and gradual perfection of the postural reflex mechanism . . . Treatment is then directed towards inhibiting the abnormal postural reflexes which interfere with the baby's motor activities, and facilitating the innate normal abilities in keeping with his chronological age" (Bobath, B., 1967).

Second, if motor development is generally retarded the treatment plan is more broadly based, if development shows a scattered profile treatment is planned to "fill in the gaps."

More specific bases for the therapy plan are:

Begin treatment at that stage of development following where the child's motor behavior appears fairly normal.

Provide missing stages of development for those children who show developmental scatter.

Inhibit abnormal postural patterns that appear to interfere with the child's activities in various test positions.

Prevent abnormal postural patterns that may cause familiar contractures and deformities (persistent asymmetries of neck and trunk, flexion-pronation of elbows and wrists with fisted hands, adduction-inward rotation of legs, tilting of pelvis, kyphosis, or kyphoscoliosis).

Postural tonus modifications are based on how tonus responds to passive movements of the child, active movements, particular positions, and balance demands.

Special goals for the spastic child usually includes (a) an abundance of active movement, (b) much but carefully provided sensory stimulation, and (c) gradual increase of speed and range of movements.

Special goals for the athetotic child usually include (a) maintaining normal posture for progressively longer periods, (b) weight-bearing work with or without resistance, and (c) reducing excessive range and speed of movements.

Special goals for the hypotonic baby usually include (a) tactile and proprioceptive stimulation (carefully graded) to increase postural tone against gravity, (b) alignment of head with body, and body with limbs, and then (c) facilitating righting of posture against gravity and balance reactions.

Special tactile and proprioceptive stimulation is planned for children with (a) ataxia and some athetotics where hypotonia and impaired reciprocal innervation make postural control and guidance of movements difficult, (b) athetosis or spasticity where postural tone is too low following successful inhibition of hypertonus, and (c) reduced tone resulting from reduced sensory input. The special techniques "serve to increase postural control and to regulate the disturbed interplay of agonists, antagonists, and synergists" (Bobath, K., 1971). According to K. Bobath, the techniques are probably similar to Kabat's (1952a) maximal resistance (recruiting) and rhythmic stabilization (summation) techniques. Special techniques also mentioned by the Bobaths (Bobath, K. and Bobath, B., 1964) include tapping, pressure, and weight bearing.

Stimulation of Basic Postural Patterns

As indicated the treatment plan for any one child is developed after a careful developmental assessment. From this information the most important basic postural patterns that need to be accomplished are selected as therapy goals. Following are some of these patterns and some techniques designed to elicit them in young children (Bobath, B., 1967).

Pattern of extension is characterized by whole body extension in prone-lying, upper part supported by upper limbs and hands, and lower limbs abducted and outwardly rotated. It may be viewed as a combination pattern based on the Landau and arm-support-forward reactions. It may also be viewed as a precursor pattern for standing. This pattern and Rood's prone-on-elbows pattern (a stage in functional stability) may be considered similar or identical.

Techniques for helping the child achieve this pattern may include: (a) eliciting the Landau, or preparing for its elicitation by placing the child in prone lying with the head up, (b) placing the child in the prone-on-elbows pattern and applying pressure on the sacrum to stimulate spine extension and head raising, (c) if the child is small enough, extending the child's body with abducted legs in outward rotation on an oversized beach ball with the feet placed against the therapist who then provides intermittent pressure on the soles to stimulate support tonus, and then lowers the child over the ball into standing (arms are held up and extended to counteract flexor spasticity), and (d) the above technique can be similarly executed in a supine-lying position.

Pattern of head righting against gravity provides head control when the child's body is passively or actively moved. It represents the first phase in sitting from prone or supine, and prepares for equilibrium reactions that emerge only when head control is established. This pattern and Rood's pivot prone and neck cocontraction patterns may be considered related.

Techniques for helping the child achieve head righting include: (a) pull child into sitting from supine and facilitate head flexion during pulling by stimulating the grasp reflex, flexing and adducting arms, and approximating hands to mouth, (b) place the child in a seated position with the back against the therapist's raised lap (therapist in flexed supine position), and extending the arms in outward rotation (child's hands in a grasp position around therapist's thumbs) thus extending the trunk and neck, (c) place the child in prone with the upper chest on a roll thus extending the spine and abducting the child's extended arms, (d) place the child in the sitting position on the lap with the legs abducted, and extending the head and spine against gravity by abducting the child's extended arms, and (e) place the child in supine, extend and adduct the arms and hold them alongside of the calves of the flexed legs and pull into sitting.

Symmetrical postural pattern is characterized by the head in midline with shoulder girdle and pelvis level. Prone lying, side lying, and sitting patterns may be stimulated. Such patterns allow the child to bring the hands to the midline, put them into the mouth, and to explore the body. Such postures are preparatory to the development of the skills of feeding, dressing, washing, and so on. This pattern is similar to Rood's withdrawal-supine pattern.

Techniques for helping the child assume symmetrical posture patterns include: (a) place the child in side lying with shoulders forward and hands together and to the mouth (fetal-like), then roll the child to supine holding the pattern, and (b) place the child in sitting, legs abducted, spine forward, head and hands in midline, and hands and objects to the mouth.

Pattern of protective extension of upper limbs and hands is seen first forward, then sideways, and finally backward. The pattern prepares for a number of functions: support and balance in sitting, pushing up into sitting from prone or supine, out-reach and grasp, getting on to hands and knees for creeping, and pushing up to standing. It remains throughout life as an important protective mechanism against falling.

Techniques for helping the child assume arm-support patterns include: (a) for the forward form, place the child in a forward sitting position on the floor with extended arms and hands brought forward between the feet, (b) for the sideways form, place the child in sitting on a table or chair, tip the child laterally and facilitate extension of the arm on that side by extending and abducting the opposite arm, (c) for the backward form, place the child in sitting, retract the shoulders, move the hands backward and extend the dorsal spine to facilitate the movement.

Pattern of long sitting is characterized by a forward-leaning trunk, abducted legs, well-flexed hips, and hands on feet. The pattern prepares the child for sitting and standing up.

Techniques for helping the child assume long sitting include: (a) placing the child into supine, bringing the hands and feet into contact, and bringing both toward the face, and (b) holding the child in the air, by gripping approximately in the angle made by the knees, legs abducted, and trunk well forward.

Patterns of rotation within the body axis are reflected by body-on-body righting reactions. The pattern prepares for rolling over from supine, sitting up from prone, side-sitting, and getting on hands and knees in order to stand. Part of these patterns is related to Rood's roll-over stage of functional mobility development.

Techniques for helping the child achieve these rotation patterns include: (a) in supine, allow the child to lateralize or lateralize the head, then release the shoulder girdle and the pelvic girdle in sequence, (b) in sitting, encourage rotation of the trunk while facilitating the arm-support-backward reaction on one side.

Patterns of equilibrium reactions are characterized by limb extension and abduction support movements toward the side of weight transference and limb extension and abduction balance movements toward the opposite side. They are essential for sitting, standing, and walking balance.

Techniques for eliciting these reactions include: (a) place the child on a roll in sitting with legs abducted, move roll slowly until balance reactions are stimulated, (b) hold the child from behind by the knees in standing and gently move the upper body forward, backward, and sideways until balance reactions are stimulated.

The techniques described in this section are only examples. Many more techniques are possible for working for the various postural patterns described. Many need to be devised to serve the particular needs of any individual child.

Analysis and Synthesis of Orientations

Following is an attempt to analyze and, where possible, synthesize the four orientations. The organic nature and controlled studies of the orientations and practical considerations in their application are topics discussed here.

Organic Nature

The word organic is used here in the philosophical sense that the orientations have a complex but necessary interrelationship.

Neurodynamically, the orientations have focused on interrelated and interdependent aspects of human neurophysiology: (a) the paleoreflex orientation, on the growing acknowledgement of aspects of recapitulation in human neuro-ontogenesis; (b) the sensory receptor orientation, on the essentiality of sensory input and feedback for motor output; (c) the motor unit orientation, on the essentiality of the motor unit for human movement, and (d) the postural patterns orientation, on the essentiality of postural patterns from which to derive and form the background for all voluntary and skilled functional activity. In short, the orientations reflect concentrations on different aspects of the same organic whole.

Other factors common to the orientations are that:

Workers want to elicit motor patterns that involved individuals have problems with or cannot perform through simple modeling, instruction, or simple practice.

Fundamental research in neurophysiology, done mostly by others and mostly on animals, is used to support and develop the orientations. From that sense workers representing the orientations are basically synthesizers and not originators.

Reflexes are apparently acknowledged as the basic unit of motor activity.

Developmental sequences form the basis of most of the treatment plans.

Sensory input and feedback modification appear as common therapeutic agents. In considering the modification of sensory stimuli as a possible common denominator of many neurophysiological approaches, Taft et al. (1962) stated, "For optimum facilitation, each organism may require stimuli of the proper intensity, sequence, duration, modality, frequency and time. If this is true, then many varieties of therapeutic stimulation may be required to produce optimum results."

Controlled Studies

A reasonable response to the controversy that surrounds neurophysiological vs. traditional approaches, as well the comparative effectiveness of various neurophysiological orientations, is why comparative studies haven't been done? After all, over 30 years have passed.

Taft et al. (1962) pointed out a number of reasons why attempts at such studies are rarely planned, or results of which are rarely reported. Among the variables that are almost impossible to control are subjects, therapy effects, and intervening factors. More specifically, how does the researcher form experimental and control groups of children with such diverse and changeable lesions? Since habilitation studies involve processes over time, how does the researcher differentiate between maturative versus therapeutic effects? And since subjects within such studies exist within particular environments, how does the researcher control the variables of intervening home and school stimulation, parental attitudes, motivation and so on. A great number of additional hard-to-control variables are sure to occur to the reader. Despite all these problems some studies have been attempted and reported. For example, the Doman et al. (1960) study and the film studies by the author (Mysak, 1960, 1962).

Practical Considerations

During the more than 30 years of the application and development of neurophysiologically-based treatment techniques, the four basic orientations have gained adherents and have reported enough success to warrant their continuation and development. If, in fact, the orientations are different in any substantive way, how are the reported degrees of success by all four approaches explained? One explanation is that they are somewhat different ways of doing the same thing and hence each may enjoy varying amounts of success. From another standpoint, Taft et al. (1962) point out that because children with cerebral palsy may have lesions of almost infinite type and combination, ". . . the residual nervous system of every patient is anatomically and physiologically different and has the capacity to work in its own unique functional manner." Given that the cerebral palsied represent a wide range of sensorimotor involvements, it is reasonable to expect that varieties of therapeutic stimulation may bring results with different cases and different times. So, depending on the particular child or children with whom one works, certain techniques may or may not produce results, or may only produce partial results. "In the light of the concept of modified sensory input, all specific methods of treatment may have value at one time or another, but none can be all things to all patients" (Taft et al., 1962).

Again, given that cerebral palsy does represent a wide variety of disorders, and that no particular medical, surgical or rehabilitative approach has provided "all things to all patients," it behooves all workers to become aware of and to understand each others potential contributions to the care of the cerebral palsied, and to be prepared to recommend the most appropriate approach for any individual child.

Finally, the organic nature of the orientations, the problems and attempts with controlled studies, the practical considerations in therapy for any one child, and the writer's personal research and clinical experiences have in the past invited the writer to the eclecticism found in the next four chapters on neurospeech therapy.

REFERENCES

Bobath, B. *Abnormal postural reflex activity caused by brain lesions.* London: Heinemann (1971a).

———. A neuro-developmental treatment of cerebral palsy. *Physiotherapy,* 242–244 (1963a).

———. A new treatment of lesions of the upper motor neurone. *Brit. J. Phys. Med.,* 2, 26–29 (1948a).

———. A study of abnormal postural reflex activity in patients with lesions of the central nervous system. *Physiotherapy,* 40 (1954).

———. Control of postures and movements in the treatment of cerebral palsy. *Physiotherapy,* 39, 99 (1953).

——. Motor development, its effect on general development, and application to the treatment of cerebral palsy. *Physiotherapy,* 1–7, November (1971b).

——. The importance of the reduction of muscle tone and the control of mass reflex action in the treatment of spasticity. *Occup. Ther. and Rehab.,* 27, 371–383 (1948b).

——. The treatment of motor disorders of pyramidal and extra-pyramidal origin by reflex-inhibition and by facilitation of movements. *Physiotherapy,* 41, 146–153 (1955).

——. The treatment of neuromuscular disorders by improving patterns of co-ordination. *Physiotherapy,* January (1969).

——. The very early treatment of cerebral palsy. *Develop. Med. Child Neurol.,* 9, 373–390 (1967).

——. Treatment principles and planning in cerebral palsy. *Physiotherapy,* 1–3 (1963b).

Bobath, K. An analysis of the development of standing and walking patterns in patients with cerebral palsy. *Physiotherapy,* 48, 144 (1962).

——. *The motor deficit in patients with cerebral palsy.* London: Heinemann (1966).

——. The neuropathology of cerebral palsy and its importance in treatment and diagnosis. *Cerebral Palsy Bull.,* 1, 13–33 (1959).

——. The normal postural reflex mechanism and its deviation in children with cerebral palsy. *Physiotherapy,* November, 1–7 (1971).

——. The prevention of mental retardation in patients with cerebral palsy. *Acta Paedopsychiatrica,* 30, 141–154 (1963).

——. Tonic reflexes and righting reflexes in the diagnosis and assessment of cerebral palsy. *Cerebral Palsy Rev.,* 16, Sept.–Oct. (1955).

Bobath, K., and Bobath, B. An assessment of the motor handicap of children with cerebral palsy and of their response to children. *Occup. Ther.,* 21, 19 (1958).

——. A treatment of cerebral palsy based on the analysis of the patient's motor behavior. *Brit. J. Phys. Med.,* 25, 107–117 (1952).

——. Cerebral palsy: Part I: Diagnosis and assessment of cerebral palsy; Part II: The neurodevelopmental approach to treatment. In P. H. Pearson and C. E. Williams (Eds.), *Physical therapy services in the developmental disabilities.* Springfield, Ill.: Charles C Thomas (1972).

——. Control of motor function in the treatment of cerebral palsy. *Physiotherapy,* 43, 295 (1957).

——. Spastic paralysis: Treatment by the use of reflex inhibition. *Brit. J. Phys. Med.,* 13, 121–127 (1950).

——. The diagnosis of cerebral palsy in infancy. *Arch. Dis. Child.,* 31, 408 (1956).

——. The facilitation of normal postural reactions and movements in the treatment of cerebral palsy. *Physiotherapy,* August (1964).

——. The neuro-developmental treatment of cerebral palsy. *J. Amer. Phys. Ther. Assoc.,* 47, 1039–1041 (1967).

Doman, G., Delacato, C. H., and Doman, R. J. *The Doman-Delacato developmental mobility scale.* Philadelphia: The Rehabilitation Center at Philadelphia (1960).

Doman, R. J., Spitz, E. B., Zucman, E. Delacato, C. H., and Doman, G. Children with severe brain injuries: neurological organization in terms of mobility. *J.A.M.A.,* 174, 257–262 (1960).

Easton, T. A. On the normal use of reflexes. *American Scientist,* 60, 591–599 (1972).

Fay, T. Basic consideration regarding neuromuscular and reflex therapy. *The Spastic Quarterly,* 3, 5–8 (1954a).

———. Effects of carbon dioxide (20%) and oxygen (80%) inhalations on movements and muscular hypertonus in athetoids. *Amer. J. Phys. Med.,* 32, 338 (1935).

———. Observation on rehabilitation of movement in cerebral palsy problems. *W. Virginia Med. J.,* 42, 77 (1946).

———. Origin of human movement. *Am. J. Psychiat.,* 111, 644–652 (1955).

———. Rehabilitation of patients with spastic paralysis. *J. Internat. Col. Surgeons,* 22, 200 (1954b).

———. The neurophysical aspects of therapy in cerebral palsy. *Arch. Phys. Med.,* 29, 327–334 (1948).

———. The use of pathological and unlocking reflexes in the rehabilitation of spastics. *Am. J. Phys. Med.,* 33, 347–352 (1954c).

Gellhorn, E. Proprioception and the motor cortex. *Brain,* 72, 35–62 (1949).

Kabat, H. Central facilitation: The basis of treatment for paralysis. *Permanente Foundation Med. Bull.,* 10, 190–204 (1952a).

———. Central mechanisms for recovery of neuromuscular function. *Science,* 112, 23–24 (1950a).

———. Studies on neuromuscular dysfunction, XIII: New concepts and techniques of neuromuscular reeducation for paralysis. *Permanente Foundation Med. Bull.,* 8, 121–143 (1950b).

———. Studies on neuromuscular dysfunction, XI: New principles of neuromuscular reeducation. *Permanente Foundation Med. Bull.,* 5 (1947).

———. Studies on neuromuscular dysfunction, XII: Rhythmic stabilization, a new and more effective technique for treatment of paralysis through a cerebellar mechanism. *Permanente Foundation Med. Bull.,* 8, 9–19 (1950c).

———. Studies on neuromuscular dysfunction: Role of central facilitation in restoration of muscle function in paralysis. *Arch. Phys. Med.,* 33:521 (1952b).

Kabat, H., and Knott, M. Principles of neuromuscular reeducation. *Phys. Ther. Rev.,* 78, 107–111 (1948).

Kabat, H., McLeod, M., and Holt, C. Neuromuscular dysfunction and treatment of corticospinal lesions. *Physiotherapy,* 45, 251 (1959).

Mysak, E. D. Study films of a neurophysiological approach to cerebral palsy habilitation: Parts I and II. Films released by Newington Children's Hospital, Newington, Conn. (1960, 1962).

———. Significance of neurophysiological orientation to cerebral palsy habilitation. *J. Speech Hearing Dis.,* 24, 221–230 (1959).

———, and Fiorentino, M. R. Neurophysiological considerations in occupational therapy for the cerebral palsied. *Amer. J. Occup. Ther.,* 15 (1961).

Rood, M. S. Neurophysiological reactions as a basis for physical therapy. *Physical Ther. Rev.,* 34, 444–448 (1954).

———. The use of sensory receptors to activate, facilitate, and inhibit motor response, autonomic and somatic in developmental sequence. In C. Sattely (Ed.), *Approaches to treatment of patients with neuromuscular dysfunction.* Dubuque, Iowa: William C. Brown Company (1962).

Stockmeyer, S. A. An interpretation of the approach of Rood to the treatment of neuromuscular dysfunction. *Am. J. Phys. Med.,* 46, 900–961 (1967).

———. A sensorimotor approach to treatment. In P. H. Pearson and C. E. Williams (Eds.), *Physical therapy services in the developmental disabilities.* Springfield, Ill.: Charles C Thomas (1972).

Taft, L. T., Delagi, E. F., Wilkie, O. L., and Abramson, A. S. Critique of rehabilitative technics in treatment of cerebral palsy. *Arch. Phys. Med. and Rehab.,* 43, 238–243 (1962).

Voss, D. E. Proprioceptive neuromuscular facilitation: The PNF method. In P. H. Pearson and C. E. Williams (Eds.), *Physical therapy services in the developmental disabilities.* Springfield, Ill.: Charles C Thomas (1972).

5

Neurospeech Therapy:
General Factors

NEUROSPEECH THERAPY MAY also be called the neuroevolutional, the neurointegrative, or the neuroeclectic approach. Each form emphasizes the related concerns of the approach with phylo-ontogenetic factors, with integration centers of the CNS, and with eclecticism in the application of techniques. The choice of neurospeech therapy with which to designate the approach is based on the desire to use the simplest term to represent the overall neurological focus in speech habilitation of the cerebral palsied. To expand on the eclectic factor, the author wants to acknowledge again his indebtedness to the large number of individuals who provided fundamental and clinical research information—Jackson, Sherrington, Magnus, Weisz, Zador, Walshe, Rademaker, Schaltenbrand, McGraw, Prechtl, Peiper, Thomas, Penfield, Twitchell, and Easton—and to those who generated substantial amounts of theory and therapy information—Fay, Kabat, Rood, and especially the Bobaths. Their work made an indispensable contribution to the ideas expressed here.

This chapter forms the basis for the next three chapters devoted to neurospeech therapy: evaluation of basic and skilled movements; stimulation of basic movements; and stimulation of skilled movements. General goals of therapy, program requirements, and bases and principles of therapy are the topics discussed here.

183

Goals and Definition

In the most general terms, the goal of neurospeech therapy is to stimulate the highest level of speech system neuro-ontogenesis. It is fundamentally a sensory approach designed to stimulate integration and elaboration of spinal and brainstem sensorimotor integration centers by midbrain and midbrain plus cortical and cerebellar sensorimotor integration centers. In Jacksonian terms, it is a therapy designed to stimulate the process of nervous evolution starting from a particular child's level of nervous system arrestment, retardation, or dissolution.

More specifically, the goals of neurospeech therapy are to stimulate:

1. Integration and elaboration of lower-center listening behaviors by centers that mediate skilled listening behaviors.
2. Integration and elaboration of lower-center tone, posture, and movement (TPM) patterns by centers that mediate basic speech postures.
3. Integration and elaboration of lower-center TPM patterns by centers that mediate hand movements related to speech activities.
4. Integration and elaboration of lower-center TPM patterns by centers that mediate skilled speech movements.

Apropos of the neurospeech therapy goals are the following statements by Jackson (1958, p. 91):

> What on the lowest level are centres for simplest movements of the limbs become evolved in the highest centres into the physical bases of volition. . . . what on the lowest level are centres for simple reflex actions of eyes and hands are evolved in the highest centres into the physical bases of visual and tactual ideas, . . . what on the lowest level are centres for movements of the tongue, palate, lips, etc. as concerned in eating, swallowing, etc. are in the highest centres evolved into the physical bases of words, symbols serving us during abstract reasoning.

In sum, the goals of neurospeech therapy reflect what may be called the vertical-lateral dominance theory of speech central nervous system (SCNS) maturation. The theory is based on the progressive and successive integration of lower sensorimotor integration centers by higher centers and, finally, the integration of the right hemisphere by the left hemisphere.

Program Requirements

Program requirements are discussed from the standpoints of selection of candidates, formation of a therapy team, parents role, neurophysiological hygiene, records, and criteria for discontinuance of therapy.

SELECTION OF CANDIDATES

The author has applied the therapy to children and adults representing a wide range of types, ages, and conditions with varying degrees of beneficial effect.

Types

The reason why children with cerebral palsy may benefit from the therapy regardless of the type of cerebral palsy that they represent may be based on comments made by Twitchell (1965): "From the neurophysiological view, the separation of patients into various categories—such as spasticity, rigidity, athetosis, tremor—is wholly artificial." He continues by stating that regardless of classification, the physiological substrata for spasticity and for athetotic phenomena, as examples, can be demonstrated in all patients. "Strict adherence to the various classifications of cerebral palsy are artificial and based on unphysiological tenets." Twitchell also advanced his belief that the defect in voluntary movement and in reflex mechanisms in cerebral palsy have a common basis which "is a defect in sensory-motor integration with conflict between hypertrophied infantile reflexes." He urged that "more attention be paid to the physiological basis for the motor deficit in each individual patient so that treatment could be oriented to that individual patient rather than to some arbitrary grouping."

Age

Whenever possible, beginning therapy during the prespeech, or primary speech period, that is, with children aged below one year, is to be desired; however, infants up to two years of age remain prime therapy candidates. Among the reasons offered by B. Bobath (1971) for an early start of therapy, and which are applicable here, are: adaptability and plasticity of the infant brain, preventing "rutting" of abnormal sensorimotor patterns, and helping to prevent contractures and deformities. Also, since primary language acquisition is believed to occur between 2 and 13 years of age, therapy done with children within that age range (or at least at the lower end of the range up to almost 10 years) continues to profit from concomitant maturative processes.

Ideal

As a result of earlier studies and continued clinical experiences, the following should be considered characteristics of "ideal" candidates for neurospeech therapy:

The factor of etiologic category should be considered. According to Josephy (1949), the cerebral palsies may be subsumed under at least three categories: Heredo-degenerative (e.g., Marie's ataxia, Friedreich's ataxia, tuberous sclerosis, Schilder's disease, juvenile general paresis, etc.), cranial malformations (e.g., hydrocephaly, microcephaly, macrocephaly, defect of corpus callosum, congenital cerebellar ataxia, hypertelorism, macrogyria, pachygyria, etc.), and residue of destructive processes (e.g., vascular impairment, trauma, infection). All else being equal, candidates should be drawn from the residue of destructive processes group where, theoretically, the children began with a normal CNS and not one undergoing degenerative processes or one demonstrating developmental malformation.

A number of general factors have also proved important in predicting response to the therapy. Children should—

1. be without history of previous treatments, or at least prolonged previous treatments (parents' and child's past therapy orientation and philosophy may be so different as to make adjustment to a different approach difficult);
2. show demonstrable signs of lower-center TPM (without extremes of muscle tone);
3. show initial response to therapy maneuvers designed to stimulate integration of lower-center TPM;
4. be within or close to the normal range for height and weight;
5. be emotionally tractable and motivated toward self-improvement;
6. be able to receive daily treatment on an out-patient basis, or better yet, two treatment sessions daily on an in-patient basis; and
7. be those whose daily life postures can be reduced to approximately their neuromaturational levels without causing adverse parental or child reactions.

THERAPY TEAM

A neurospeech therapy program may be applied by a single speech pathologist educated and trained in the procedures. However, since the goals include the development of at least some basic speech postures and speech-associated hand movements, as well as skilled speech movements, it would be ideal if at least one neurophysiologically oriented physician as well as a physical and an occupational therapist could participate in evaluational and therapy activities.

PARENTS ROLE

Parents should be willing and capable of instituting particular neurophysiological hygiene practices, learning about therapy goals, and applying certain therapy techniques. They represent the home transfer part of the therapy effort and are essential. Participation in periodic parent-clinician conferences on therapy progress is also recommended.

NEUROPHYSIOLOGICAL HYGIENE

At least five guiding principles of neurophysiological hygiene should be considered: appropriate neurophysiological bases, facilitation of individuation, body progression responsibility, communication responsibility, and the challenge-assistance ratio.

Appropriate Neurophysiological Bases

Appropriate bases refers to those fundamental postures and movements of which the child's CNS is capable of mediating. Such fundamental postures and movements should be determined for each child and the child should be required to spend the major portion of his active day functioning from those motor bases. For example, the child may enjoy the support and balance reactions required to allow the back, the elbow, or floor-sit speech postures. These then are the fundamental postures from which he should interact with his environment. To have the child spend substantial time in, or to have him attempt to develop skill behavior from unphysiologic patterns, that is, patterns that may be beyond his neurophysiological capacity, for example, chair-sit, stand, or walk patterns, should be discouraged.

Body Progression Responsibility

Responsibility for body progression refers to the requirement that the child progress from point-to-point in a room or out of doors independently. Each child's ability for independent progression should be evaluated. Is the child capable of some form of crawling or creeping progression? Whatever the progression level, the child should be given every opportunity each day to move from point to point using the highest form of which he is capable. It is understood that there may be time constraints in certain situations and that the child may have to be carried or wheeled. If the child's mode of progression results in highly irregular tone, posture, and movement, more appropriate modes should be sought.

Facilitation of Individuation

To facilitate individuation, the goal should be that parents, relatives, friends, and professional workers do all in their power to get the child to emerge from the "what can you do for me" stage, to the "what can I do for myself" stage, and, whenever and wherever possible, to the "what can I do for you" stage. Again, whether it be moving through space, self-care activities, and so on, the child must be allowed to do everything possible for himself and to begin doing whatever he can for others. All must guard against the tendency to infantilize the child.

Communication Responsibility

It is necessary to make sure that each child intra- and intercommunicates on whatever levels are available at any one time. Whether or not some level of actual talking is possible, "inner talking" or thinking in words should be encouraged as well as whatever form of "outer talking" is possible. The child may be able to use body, hands, or face forms of communication, and such should be encouraged. While working on improving their speech skills, children may also need to use compensatory forms of communication such as language boards, and so on. The point here is that "significant others" should not anticipate needs or speak for the child without giving the child every opportunity for making himself understood on some level and by some means.

Challenge:Assistance Ratio

A therapeutic challenge:assistance ratio exists when the ratio is in favor of challenge. More specifically, a therapeutic environment is one in which the handicapped child is regularly exposed to situations where carefully measured challenge always exceeds carefully measured assistance. This guideline addresses the theory that the residual CNS almost always reflects lower than actual potential, and the way to get at all of the child's residual neurophysiology is by challenging it. Frequently, a ratio that favors assistance may be observed as well as the "vicious spiral" that such a ratio usually engenders. Many individuals in the environment of handicapped children feel sympathy and want to help. And the more they assist the child who is unable to do too much to begin with, the less the child needs to or tries to do; and the less the child tries to do, the more the individual assists, and so on. The path of those with such "good intentions" is often strewn with many casualities of habilitation efforts.

RECORDS

Those who undertake neurospeech therapy should be prepared to keep various types of records. Such records are important for therapy planning, teaching, and research purposes.

Videotapes

Pretherapy videotape records should be made of the highest level of speech posture, speech-associated hand patterns, and skilled speech samples. These samples can be collected during appropriate times in the administration of the Neurophysiological Speech Index described in the next chapter.

The highest level of speech posture that the child can assume and adequately maintain through support and balance reactions should be recorded. For example, if the child can assume a floor-sit speech pattern, he should be shown (a) moving from the supine into the sitting position and (b) demonstrating support and balance reactions in sitting.

Speech-associated hand patterns should be recorded during speech attempts. For example, is there speech-associated hand activity at all? Are there only bilateral movements, or are there unilateral movements? Also, are the arm movements differentiated from the head and trunk? Is the forearm differentiated from the upper arm, and the hand differentiated from the forearm? And, finally, does the child use symbolic and/or adjunctive gestural patterns?

Skilled speech samples of sustained maximum phonation, laryngopraxis, laryngodiadochokinesia, articulopraxis, and articulodiadochokinesia, and of conversational speech should also be included.

Respiratory Function

Pretherapy records of vital capacity and of thoracic and abdominal breathing records during vegetative and speech breathing activities should be collected as well.

Videotape and respiratory function data should be collected at least every three months and at the termination of therapy.

DISCONTINUANCE OF THERAPY

At least four criteria for discontinuance of therapy are worthy of consideration: (a) six-to-nine-month plateau period, (b) adverse emotional reactions in the child, (c) irregular attendance, and (d) lack of home follow-up of therapy and neurophysiologic hygiene.

The criterion of a six-to-nine-month plateau period before discontinuing therapy has proven to be a rather fair test period of whether any more progress can be expected via neurospeech therapy techniques. Almost all good candidates show initial progress and some show continual progress over two, three, four, and more years. However, some children may show progress only up to a certain point and for one or more reasons may stop. For example, it may be that some of these children have reached the limits of their residual neurophysiological potentials. But it has also been found that some of these children, after a three- or four-month "clinic holiday," may again show gains. For this reason, at least one return to a full therapy program is advised before terminating neurospeech therapy in plateau cases.

Adverse emotional reactions and irregular attendance may be considered related criteria. Some children appear unable to adjust to a therapy program that is as intensive and incorporates the kind of challenge-assistance ratio as does the neurospeech therapy program. Often these are the children who have experienced long periods of the "we-will-adjust-the-environment-to-you approach." Of course, there may be a number of other reasons—such as parent-child problems or clinician-child problems—why children may show the kind of adverse emotional reactions that dictate against continuance of therapy.

Because neurospeech therapy by definition is an intensive form of therapy, irregular attendance is incompatible with the approach and is another cause for discontinuance of therapy.

Lack of home follow-up of therapy and of neurophysiologic hygiene recommendations are again incompatible with the definition of the neurospeech therapy approach. Parental involvement is considered integral to the concept of intensive therapy and neurophysiologic hygiene is considered integral to a neurophysiologic approach. Consistent problems with either are considered a basis for discontinuing therapy.

Bases and Principles

It is incumbent upon clinicians to base their therapeutic procedures and techniques upon the best available knowledge arising from basic and applied research as well as from clinical experience. It should also be understood, therefore, that the rationale we use today to explain why certain procedures and techniques appear effective may not be adequate tomorrow because of new basic and applied research findings. Also, there may be procedures and techniques that appear effective, but for which the clinician finds explanation difficult in terms of presently available basic and applied information. With that said, this section of the chapter attempts to identify a number of "principles" that undergird neurospeech therapy techniques, or that may be used to explain why they appear to be effective. Some of the principles enjoy support from basic and applied research, while others emerge as a result of clinical experience. They are the principles of emergent specificity, reflexization of movement, figure-ground motor stimulation, and the integration-elaboration of sensorimotor patterns. Each of the following sections of the chapter present pertinent information from which each of these therapy principles emerge.

PHYLO-ONTOGENESIS

At least three phylo-ontogenetic concepts contribute to the development of a neurospeech therapy program: the phylogenesis of man and speech, of sensorimotor behavior in general, and of expressive communication.

Phylogenesis of Man and Speech

Speech phylogenesis is related to the development of the bipedal posture, manual dexterity, the liberation of the mouth from use in crude grasping and manipulative activities, and the development of the communisphere. The ontogenetic reflection of this phyletic heritage is noted when observing the development of true speech in the infant. True speech development in the infant approximately co-occurs with the development of bipedal head, neck, and trunk balance; the use of a preferred hand; the integration of various cranio-oropharyngeal reflexes such as protective, feeding, and emotional reflexes; and the growing need to communicate.

Evolution of Sensorimotor Behavior

Sensorimotor behavior in the developing child proceeds from generalized, uncoordinated responses toward increased specificity, differentiation, and selectivity of behavior. Related developmental concepts include: (a) the simpler the function, the more rapid its development; (b) the more complex the function, usually the slower its development; (c) the coordination of large muscles, as, for example, those required for assuming and maintaining basic speech postures, precedes the coordination of small muscles, as, for example, those required in skilled movements of the speech effectors; and (d) the life of an organism is marked by so-called readiness periods when it profits most from certain kinds of environmental stimulation.

Evolution of Expressive Communication

A number of stages are recognized in the phylo-ontogenesis of expressive communication in humans as detailed in Chapter 1:

Body talk is hypothesized as a form of expression in early humans as well as in the early child or infant. This stage is marked by relatively undifferentiated whole body movements such as might have characterized pre-fight stances of early humans, or may characterize feelings of discomfort in the young infant.

Hands talk describes the stage of integration and elaboration of body talk and the gradual emergence of bilateral and unilateral hand gestures. Here is an early emergence of specificity that may have been characterized by "go-away," "come-here," and "that's-mine" gestures in early humans and by those as well as by "pick-me-up" and "I-want" gestures in the infant.

Face talk describes the stage of integration and elaboration of body and hands talk and the gradual emergence of a repertoire of facial expressions (including head movements). Such face talk may have been characterized by the following dichotomies of basic facial expressions in early humans: happy-sad, security-fear, expectancy-surprise, and excitement-boredom; and by the same basic facial expressions in the young child, but with added range, or a continuum of expressions within each dichotomy.

Mouth talk describes the stage of integration and elaboration of body, hands, and face talk and the gradual emergence of a repertoire of utterances. Such mouth talk may have been characterized by the following forms in early humans: emotional vocalization (utterances associated with pain, fear, anger, excitement, pleasure), onomatopoeic vocalization (animal sounds, natural sounds of running water, thunder, and so on), and the use of some simple, arbitrary code of utterances (forms of no, yes, give me, and so on).

Principle of Emergent Specificity

From the base of phylo-ontogenesis may be drawn the therapy principle of emergent specificity. The principle informs the clinician that speech waits upon the emergence of the individual to the upright posture, the differentiation of the arms and hands, the freeing of the mouth from crude grasping and manipulative activities, and the concomitant emergence of mouth from body talk. The decision to divide Chapters 7 and 8 on procedures and techniques in neurospeech therapy into one devoted to basic movements and one devoted to skilled movements was based on the principle of emergent specificity.

REFLEXES AND SENSORIMOTOR DEVELOPMENT

The relationship between the development of reflexes and basic speech postures and basic speech movements represents another basis for neurospeech therapy.

Basic Speech Postures

The emergence of basic speech postures such as the back, elbow, sit, or stand patterns, depends on the integration and elaboration of spinal and brainstem reflexes by righting reactions and the co-occurring integration of righting reactions by equilibrium reactions. For example, assumption of the elbow speech posture is dependent on the integration of tonic neck and tonic labyrinthine reflexes, and the emergence of body-on-body and on-head righting reactions. Stabilization of the posture is dependent on support and balance reactions in the prone-on-forearms position.

Basic Speech Movements

Just as with the development of other kinds of motor skills, skilled speech movements emerge from and are superimposed upon certain fundamental postural patterns and movements. Skilled movements of the speech effectors or speech breathing, phonation, resonation, and articulation emerge from basic protective, emotional, and vegetative reflexes, and reflexive vocalization; and are performed on a background of basic facial and hand movements and basic speech postures and movements.

Principle of Reflexization of Movement

From the relationship between reflexive maturation and motor development may be drawn the therapy principle of reflexization of movement. The clinician does not attempt to teach fundamental postural patterns but must elicit the righting, support, and balance reactions that allow the child to assume and maintain the patterns. So too, the clinician must elicit the reflexive voicing and primary talking that reflect integration of more basic protective, emotional, and vegetative reflexes and from which will emerge skilled speech movements.

SIMULTANEOUS DEVELOPMENT OF SENSORIMOTOR PATTERNS

Children do not develop basic speech postures and movements in strict sequential fashion, nor do they develop basic speech movements or skilled speech movements in strict sequential fashion.

Basic Speech Postures

As pointed out in a section of the postural-patterns orientation, discussed in Chapter 4, a child at six months may stand with support, but may not enjoy independent sitting balance; at eight months he may enjoy sitting balance, may assume sitting from prone, may creep, and may pull himself up into standing; and at nine months he may creep, do erect arm walking, or walk when held by both hands. So at this early period we observe co-developing head balance, sitting, creeping, standing, and walking. However, the sequence, with respect to the concept of figure-ground motor activities, would be head balance against all the other ground motor patterns, then sitting against the others, then standing against the others, and, finally, walking against the others. In other words, observation of motor development reveals the emergence of a figure motor pattern simultaneously with "rehearsal" or "practice" of future major motor levels.

Accordingly, a child may be observed to co-develop the basic speech postures of back, elbow, sit, and stand patterns, with, at any one time, one of the speech postures predominating.

Basic Speech Movements

Similarly, basic speech movements develop in a figure-ground relationship. For example, basic protective, emotional, and vegetative movements may be observed as co-developing, but with certain movements or combinations of movements predominating. Apropos of speech effector motor patterns, respiratory, phonatory, resonatory, articulatory patterns may be observed at any one time in the infant but with the figure motor pattern emerging theoretically in a respiratory to phonatory, to resonatory, and, finally, to articulatory sequence. Also, reflexive vocalization may include at any one time a range of glottal, linguavelar, linguapalatal, lingua-alveolar, linguadental, labiodental, and bilabial sound forms, but with the figure pattern emerging in a back-to-front fashion in contrast to the approximate pattern found during the skilled period of speech sound development.

Principle of Figure-Ground Motor Stimulation

From the observation of figure-ground development of motor patterns, or the co-development but not co-equal development of motor patterns, may be drawn the therapy principle of figure-ground motor stimulation. Translated into practical therapy procedures, the principle invites the clinician to stimulate, for example, a range of basic speech postures, but with focus on a sequentially appropriate pattern; or a range of basic speech movements, but with focus on a sequentially appropriate pattern.

SENSORY DYNAMICS

Sensory stimuli such as radiant, acoustical, mechanical, thermal, and chemical energies may activate, inhibit, or guide movements. In other words, sensory dynamics are marked by input, integration, and feedback phases. Since primary as well as secondary sensorimotor deficits are found in cerebral palsy, secondary deficits are also included here.

Input

It could be said that without sensory input there would be no movement. Exteroceptor stimuli of various forms such as visual, auditory, tactile, and olfactory, proprioceptive stimuli, and interoceptive stimuli such as pain, hunger, and discomfort may all activate, facilitate, or inhibit movement depending on the type, strength, duration, and frequency of the stimuli and its level of integration. Sensory input is basic to awareness of the external as well as internal environments of the individual. It is primary to learning about one's self as well as one's environment.

Integration

Sensory inflow is processed at different levels or combinations of levels of integration centers. For example, a special form of pain stimulus, an itch, may be processed at the spinal level, and elicits the scratch reflex while simultaneously being integrated at the cortical level where the individual wonders about the cause of the itch. Also, depending on the level of integration of sensory input, the same input may elicit different responses. For example, the proprioceptive input arising from head lateralization if integrated at the level of the brainstem may result in the manifestation of the asymmetrical tonic neck reflex, while if integrated at the midbrain level may result in the neck righting reaction. In terms of Jackson's evolution of the CNS, as stimuli are integrated at progressively higher levels, responses become progressively less automatic, less organized, and more complex. The essence of the neurospeech therapy approach is to stimulate the progressive integration of sensorimotor integration centers by higher ones until the highest possible level of sensorimotor integration has been achieved.

Concepts related to integration and which have therapeutic implications are sensory routing and integration, rerouting of sensory inflow, and incomplete integration.

Sensory routing and integration may explain some symptoms of cerebral palsy and may also explain the effects of certain therapeutic maneuvers. Theoretically speaking, the abnormal motor patterns of many cerebral-palsied children may be viewed as a consequence of irregular sensory routing. That is, due to the lesion in any one particular case of cerebral palsy, lower-level integration centers, such as spinal and brainstem levels, may become dominant and resistant to integration by higher centers. Because of this lower-center "domination," afferent inflow may be "drawn" or routed into lower-order synaptic channels. Another way of expressing the concept is that the abnormal motor patterns of many cerebral-palsied children may be seen as the result of "short-circuiting" of afferent inflow into lower-order synaptic channels; or as reflecting infantile sensorimotor integration. Such infantile routing of sensory inflow may take place despite the presence of intact or partially intact higher integration centers. Hence, such "draining off" of sensory inflow would not allow the child to manifest all of his sensorimotor potential. Such a concept invites clinicians to attempt to develop therapeutic techniques that might cause rerouting of sensory inflow to higher integration centers. When such techniques are effective, the concept also explains the rather rapid responses to the application of neurospeech therapy techniques in many children.

Rerouting of sensory inflow is a concept that gains support from the early work of Magnus (1924). His "law of shunting" offers a possible way of counteracting the short-circuiting of inflow just described. His hypothesis was that the state of contraction and elongation of muscles determines the distribution of excitatory and inhibitory processes within the CNS, and, therefore, the subsequent motor outflow; or, more simply, sensory inflow favors the contraction of elongated muscles.

Another way of discussing the concept of rerouting may be through the modern concept of muscle monitoring and control systems. (See McMahon and Greene, 1978, for a good description of the muscle control system.) Figure 5.1 represents a simple illustration of the basic components of the muscle control system. Higher motor centers supply electrochemical impulses or commands to the lower motor cells in the spinal cord and, in turn, these alpha motoneurons transmit the commands to the muscle fibers. Information about the consequent muscle activity is transmitted back to the CNS via two important stimulus-sensitive receptors: the spindle-organ receptor, or stretch receptor, that is primarily sensitive to muscle length and the Golgi tendon-organ receptor that is primarily sensitive to muscle force. Impulses from the receptors are fed back to the CNS via fibers of nerve cells of the dorsal-root ganglion of the peripheral nervous system. Pathways that

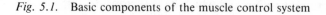

Fig. 5.1. Basic components of the muscle control system

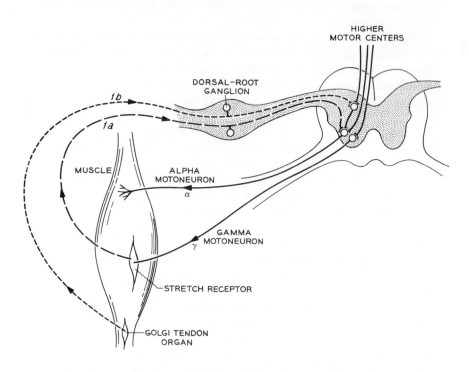

serve the stretch receptors are designated la and those that serve the tendon-organ receptors are designated lb. These feedback signals are not only returned segmentally to the respective lower sensory cell and eventually to the responsible alphamotoneuron, but may be received at the highest levels of the CNS. Stretch receptors are not only sensitive to changing length but also to the rate of change; hence, they provide position as well as velocity information. Also, the spindle organ, which is composed of muscle cells, may be innervated directly by gamma motoneurons and act as muscles. Also, higher motor centers acting through gamma motoneurons can adjust the length of the spindle organ or recalibrate it, thus tuning it for large-scale changes such as body-position changes.

The patellar reflex may be used as an example of the feedback control of reflexes, in this case, the stretch-reflex arc. The physician's hammer applied below the knee cap imposes muscle lengthening, which results in concomitant spindle-organ lengthening with its associated sensory report of length and rate of length changes of the muscles being fed back over the la pathway to the respective alpha motoneuron, which, in turn, results in the observed muscle shortening or kick reaction. The rate-of-change feedback from the muscle gives rise to a damping effect.

The central function of the Golgi tendon-organ was originally thought to be only a safety one, that is, to inhibit alphamotoneuron activity whenever a muscle force capable of injuring a muscle is sensed. However, there are those who think that the tendon-organ feedback may also influence the stretch reflex so that muscle stiffness rather than length or force is controlled. That is, muscle stiffness may be maintained at a constant level through the regulation of spindle organ and tendon organ feedback (McMahon and Greene, 1978).

This simplified discussion of muscle control systems did not really touch on the various suprasegmental influences on feedforward and feedback phenomena. So much speculation remains on all aspects of movement and its control that additional discussion of the phenomena at this point in time may not be too productive.

In any event, the discussion of the law of shunting and the fact that afferent inflow favors the contraction of elongated muscles and the discussion of the stretch-reflex arc are interesting and useful companion discussions. They form a background for discussion of their practical implications in the therapy concept of rerouting sensory inflow.

If, in fact, important amounts of cerebral palsy symptomatology are based on lower-center routing and integration of sensory inflow, how might the clinician influence such dynamics? How can the clinician influence the distribution of excitatory and inhibitory influences within the CNS from without? The discussion here suggests that at least the clinician can elongate or stretch muscles. Flexed muscles can be extended, inwardly rotated muscles can be outwardly rotated, and so on. Such maneuvers can modify the length of spindle organs and hence the feedback from the muscles. The clinician may attempt to act as a "surrogate" gamma motoneuron system. The clinician may learn to elongate sets of multimuscle groups in ways that favor the contraction of certain muscles and the elongation of others. Influencing the alpha and gamma motoneurons involved in a specific response may be viewed as the ultimate purpose of all therapeutic stimuli by the motor unit, sensory receptor, and, for that matter, all the neurotherapy orientations.

Clinicians who attempt to reroute sensory inflow to higher integration centers hope that by providing novel feedbacks from the peripheral musculature, tendons, and joints they will invite novel and higher center responses. Figuratively speaking, they ask novel "sensory questions" of a sensorimotor system that at least contains the innate potential to answer at the highest integration levels, and hope for replies from those higher centers. Therapeutic stimuli are those that represent patterns of sensory questions that invite such replies.

Such rerouting is impossible to trace experimentally in a client, but the concept enjoys a form of clinical support. For example, a child in prone may not be able to raise the head and support the trunk in the elbow speech posture because of the influence of spinal and brainstem integration centers manifested by primitive limb-withdrawal patterns and a general increase in flexor tonus. The clinician may design a sensory question in the form of extending the child's limbs and trunk and outwardly rotating the shoulders, and thereby feeding back sensory stimuli from tactile and proprioceptive receptors that result in a new motor reply consisting of upper limb support movements and a head righting and balance reaction. Such a reply implies the integration by a higher center of rerouted and/or novel sensory input.

Incomplete integration refers to incomplete motor expression by a higher integration center because of the presence of increased muscle tone (usually associated with lower-center integration). Theoretically, certain sensory inflow may actually reach centers responsible for the righting, support, and balance movements required for assuming and maintaining various speech postures, but the condition of heightened muscle tone may prevent their expression. With this concept in mind, when a particular maneuver, like the one described above, proves therapeutic, which almost always means positive changes in tonus, it will be impossible to know whether the result should be attributed to rerouting of sensory input or to completing integration processes.

Feedback

The feedback phase of sensory dynamics is basic to motor control and to all motor learning. It has been said that movements are not learned but only their associated sensations, or movements excited by exteroceptors are guided by proprioceptors. The author (Mysak, 1976, Ch. 8) described the speech system as an error-sensitive, error-measuring, self-adjusting, goal-directed one. Speech control and monitoring is dependent on feedback, especially auditory and proprioceptive feedbacks, and important therapy techniques may be based on stimulating self-adjusting mechanisms in the speech system. The roles of feedback in stimulating and integrating certain reflexes and reactions and in learning are discussed here.

A discussion of the role of nonauditory feedback in the control of speech movements serves as an introduction to this portion of the chapter on the roles of feedback in stimulating and integrating certain reflexes and reactions and in sensorimotor learning.

In an attempt to determine the role of peripheral afferent feedback to speech motor control, Abbs and Eilenberg (1976, pp. 139–68) reviewed what they considered to be key studies of afferent feedback and voluntary motor control for speech and nonspeech activities. They hoped their discussion might help resolve the controversial issue of the role of afferent feedback mechanisms in the control of speech movements.

Many investigators of voluntary motor control believed that sensory information available from spindle, tendon, and joint receptors is part of a slow-monitoring system responsible for the control of involuntary postural or tonic motor activity, and/or for providing peripheral state information as a basis for CNS efferent commands, but sensory information was not crucial to voluntary movement control. However, more recent experiments of voluntary movement in humans showed that anesthetization of gamma efferent innervation of elbow flexors, for example, resulted in loss in fine motor control. With respect to elbow flexors then, it appeared that the gamma loop acts to "optimize the initiation of movement, via agonist facilitation, and damp movement via antagonist facilitation." Such findings provide support for "afferent contribution to voluntary movement control, even in systems (unlike speech) where visual feedback information is available" (Abbs and Eilenberg, 1976, p. 154).

Controversy also remains on the role of nonauditory afferent feedback in the control of speech movements. Early studies of interference with nonauditory afferent feedback and its effect on speech control suffered from at least the following design problems (Abbs and Eilenberg, 1976, 157–58): (a) assessing speech motor changes via perceptual judgment of speech errors, (b) lack of specificity of the afferent channel anesthetized, (c) lack of consideration of compensatory capabilities of the speech system, and (d) use of nerve block procedures that may have caused motor weakness as well as sensory deprivation.

Data on more recent studies of the role of afferent feedback in the control of speech movements are related to studies of articulatory movement coordination and of experimental disruption of particular aspects of the speech motor control system (p. 158). Observation as well as investigation shows that acoustically similar speech output may be achieved by different motor configurations involving lips, jaw, and tongue. Studies that show "patterns of speech movement that vary in adaptation to the state of the peripheral system, would tend to support the notion that the central mechanism prepares the system for certain target behaviors and that the peripheral mechanisms are charged with carrying out these general goals employing afferent feedback" (p. 160). Also, an experimental disruption study (Abbs and Eilenberg, 1976), that is, interruption of gamma efferent innervation to the masticatory system, resulted in disturbance in control of jaw movements, but interestingly, perceptually normal speech performance.

Such information adds to the growing data on the importance of sensory feedback not only to automatic tonic and postural adjustments, but also to control of voluntary movement.

The stimulation of new movement patterns through feedback recalls the concept of patterning discussed in the paleoreflex orientation. It is hoped that by providing the sensory feedback pattern associated with a desired but not yet available motor pattern that eventually the sensory feedback stimulation will excite the corresponding motor feedforward activity. The author has previously referred to this concept in terms of the stimulation-development principle of emergent reflexes and reactions. Simply put, if a

particular reflex like the rooting reflex has not emerged, or has only partially emerged, the clinician applies the appropriate stimulus, for example,
touch or stroke stimulus to the cheek, and physically initiates and guides the
expected head lateralization toward the source of the stimulus. It is a technique that forms the necessary sensory-motor loop. By such attempts at
closing the sensorimotor loop associated with the rooting reflex, it is hoped
the appropriate integration center has been stimulated, and hence a new
motor response established.

The integration of primitive movement patterns through feedback is a
concept that is based on mismatching sensorimotor feedbacks. If, for example, a child is unable to assume the back pattern speech posture because of
the presence of tonic reflex and tonic labyrinthine reflexes in supine, the
clinician may stimulate the integration of these infantile patterns by
mismatching the respective sensorimotor loops. For example, the reflex
loop of the tonic labyrinthine reflex in supine is characterized by (a) sensory
impulses from the labyrinths to the brainstem signaling the supine position
of the child, (b) the integration of the sensory stimuli by the brainstem
center resulting in increased extensor tone throughout the body including
the neck (making head raising via the labyrinthine on-head righting reaction
impossible), and (c) the generation of associated sensations feeding back to
the CNS confirming the increased extensor tone and the extensor posture.
Repetition of such looping could be viewed as strengthening the chain
synaptic arrangement representing the tonic labyrinthine reflex acting in the
supine position.

The integration of the tonic labyrinthine reflex by on-head and body-on-
body righting reactions may be attempted by the mismatching maneuver.
That is, with the child in the supine position, the clinician modifies the
generalized extensor pattern with a gentle flexor pattern and thereby feeds
back to the CNS an incongruent sensory pattern. Such a mismatching
maneuver may (a) "disturb" the function of the brainstem integration
center, (b) activate the midbrain integration center through feedback
associated with on-head and body-on-body righting patterns, and (c) actually elicit on-head and body-on-body righting movements.

Integration of primitive movement patterns like, for example, the mouth-
opening reflex, in response to a stimulus presented to the child's visual field
or a touch stimulus to the lips, may also be integrated by applying the appropriate stimulus and physically resisting the expected response. Such
maneuvers need to be carried out over a period of time before results may
be achieved.

The establishment of new motor patterns through feedback or the
establishment of higher-center synaptic bonds is accomplished basically by
repetition of activity. The concept under consideration is sensorimotor
learning or physiological memory (Russell, 1958). Once a new motor pat-

tern is stimulated, the job of the clinician is to ensure its continuance. Since it has been said that one of the most powerful features of all nervous functioning is for nerve cells to repeat patterns of activity, the way for a clinician to "imprint" a new and desirable pattern and make it a part of the individual's motor repertoire is by virtue of repetition of evocation. So the more often one can elicit normally emerging righting, support, and balance reactions, for example, and provide the CNS with the concomitant feedback from these patterns, the greater the chances are that these patterns will be "remembered" by the CNS and become part of the child's motor repertoire.

The adjustment of available and new movement patterns through correct-response feedback is related to guidance by the clinician of an available but partially developed pattern, or a newly emerging and not quite developed pattern. In either case, the clinician wants to guide externally these movements whenever they are elicited or appear spontaneously so as to ensure more normal feedback to the CNS. If, for example, a child is attempting to form the /f/ phoneme and is having difficulty making the required labiodental contact, the clinician should assist the child so that a more normal contact and consequently more normal feedback is provided. It is hoped that such correct-response feedback should lead eventually to correct response performance. Such maneuvers bring to mind Young's (1965) motokinesthetic approach to correction of misarticulation.

Secondary Sensorimotor Deficits

Even though the preceding portions of this section of the chapter have implicitly or explicitly addressed themselves to the problem of secondary sensorimotor deficits in cerebral palsy, the topic deserves some specific attention.

The underlying theme of this whole section on sensory dynamics is that sensory and motor phenomena are but two phases of the larger sensorimotor integration process. For the sake of exposition, the phases may be described separately but it must be kept in mind that such separate considerations are not functional. Hence, it should be a given that sensory dynamics are crucial to motor dynamics.

In short, then, sensory deficits may disturb (a) motor development, because movements are not learned but only their associated sensations and (b) motor control, because proprioceptors are essential to the guidance of movements elicited by the exteroceptors. Depending on the degree of primary sensory loss in any given case of neuropathology, motor development and control are affected accordingly. In cerebral palsy, however, secondary sensory involvements may further compound the problem.

Secondary sensory aberrations may arise from short circuiting of sensory inflow; from abnormally toned muscle environments for receptors; as well as from anxiety-induced delays in feedback. To counteract such secondary deficits, techniques need to be developed and applied that tend to regularize muscle tone, reroute sensory inflow, and reduce anxiety in the child through the development of support and balance patterns.

Principle of Integration-Elaboration of Sensorimotor Patterns

From the base of sensory dynamics with its input, integration, and feedback phases may be drawn the therapy principle of integration-elaboration of sensorimotor patterns. The principle requires the development of therapeutic integration maneuvers. Maneuvers must be designed that will stimulate the successive integration of lower-center patterns by higher-centers, and the subsequent elaboration and differentiation of these simpler patterns by the higher centers. Such maneuvers require the selection of the most appropriate sensory stimuli to elicit the desired motor pattern, and the development of therapy concepts such as were mentioned in the section on sensory dynamics, including ideas on rerouting sensory inflow and on providing various kinds of corrective sensory feedback.

ADDITIONAL GENERAL GUIDES FOR THERAPY

In addition to the principles of emergent specificity, reflexization of movement, figure-ground motor stimulation, and integration-elaboration of sensorimotor patterns, a number of additional guides for neurospeech therapy may be drawn from clinical experiences and the neurotherapies described in Chapter 4.

Neurophysiological Relaxation

Reduction of hypertonicity, whether plastic, spastic, or intermittent, is best accomplished through therapeutic activities rather than through attempts at "conscious relaxation." For example, Fay's reflex conditioning exercises and Kabat's mass movement patterns are examples of techniques that may tend to reduce or "normalize" tone. The author routinely uses a technique called "pretzeling" (described in Chapter 7) to induce physiologic relaxation among other effects. The technique is characterized by carefully placing the head, trunk, and limbs in atypical and various positions with the child in prone, supine, and side-lying positions and thereby eliciting automatic adjustive and righting responses from the child. Such pretzeling should be graded in difficulty, with the clinician assisting the child to resume a more normal posture only when necessary. The "workout" should be done rhythmically and over a period of many minutes, depending on the child's status. Some of the normalization of muscle tone is attributed to the great amounts of proprioceptive feedback provided by the clinician's maneuvers and the child's subsequent adjustive responses.

Automatic Movements

When attempting to stimulate the child to assume and maintain through righting, support, and balance reactions various basic speech postures, for example, back, elbow, or various sitting postures, the clinician should not request the child to assist the attempts through voluntary efforts. Righting, support, and balance reactions naturally emerge as automatic movement patterns and hence should be elicited accordingly. Voluntary efforts in this particular instance may interfere with the establishment of these sensorimotor patterns. Only after it becomes clear that certain of the adjustive reactions cannot be elicited automatically or facilitated by the clinician should the clinician consider requesting the child to engage in voluntary, compensatory efforts at effecting the desired responses.

Assistive Devices

Braces, splints, straps, special chairs, and so on are incompatible with the strict application of the neurospeech therapy approach. The incompatibility is based on at least three factors: (a) Such devices may generate irregular touch, pressure, and stretch stimuli and consequent irregular muscle responses. (b) They allow for, and thereby encourage, placing the child in postures that cannot be maintained by the child's own CNS mechanisms for support and balance activities. The imposition of such "nonphysiologic" postures may increase irregular muscle tone and contribute to the development of contractures and deformities. (c) Finally, just as they are "supportive" they tend to inhibit the development of automatic adjustive movements that are basic to maintaining certain postures and balance and prerequisite to developing skilled movements like speech. All three factors tend to be interrelated and interdependent.

There may, of course, be good medical reasons for the use of various assistive devices at particular times in the child's overall treatment. At such times, neurospeech therapy techniques should be suspended or modified.

REFERENCES

Abbs, J. H., and Eilenberg, G. K. Peripheral mechanisms of speech motor control. In N. Lass (Ed.), *Contemporary issues in experimental phonetics.* New York: Academic Press (1976).

Bobath, B. Motor development, its effect on general development, and application to the treatment of cerebral palsy. *Physiotherapy,* 1-7, November (1971).

Jackson, J. H. Evolution and dissolution of the nervous system. In J. Taylor (Ed.), *Selected writings of John Hughlings Jackson,* Vol. 2. New York: Basic Books, Inc. (1958).

Josephy, H. The brain in cerebral palsy, a neuropathological review. *Nerv. Child,* 8, 152-159 (1949).

Magnus, R. *Koerperstellung.* Berlin: Springer (1924).

McMahon, T. A., and Greene, P. R. Fast running tracks. *Scientific American,* 239, 148 (1978).

Mysak, E. D. *Pathologies of speech systems.* Baltimore: Williams and Wilkins (1976).

Russell, W. R. The physiology of memory. *Proc. Roy. Soc. Med.,* 51, 9–14 (1958).

Twitchell, T. E. Variations and abnormalities of motor development. *J. Amer. Phys. Ther. Assoc.,* 45, 424–430 (1965).

Young, E. H. Moto-kinesthetic approach to the prevention of speech defects, including stuttering. *J. Speech Hearing Dis.,* 30, 269–273 (1965).

6

Neurospeech Therapy: Evaluation of Basic and Skilled Movements

EVALUATION OF EACH child's status relative to basic and skilled speech movements is fundamental to each child's therapy plan. The guide for such an evaluation includes information found in the first three chapters and the Neurophysiological Speech Index (NSI). This chapter is devoted to the definition of the index, instructions for estimating the index, and the presentation of a sample form.

Neurophysiological Speech Index

The Neurophysiological Speech Index is a clinical index of the development of the child relative to a "neurophysiological speaking age" that nearly all normal children achieve by 18 to 24+ months of age. This index represents the child's neurophysiological readiness for speech.

The NSI may be used to estimate the progress of normal children toward the neurophysiological speech age; or it may be used to estimate the delay, retardation, or arrest in development of children with suspected or actual brain dysfunction. The NSI may also be used to judge progress in neurospeech therapy by young children with brain dysfunction.

Evaluation Instructions

The NSI is a composite of the Basic Movements Index (BMI) and Skilled Movements Index (SMI). Brief descriptions of these basic and skilled movements are provided in this instruction section; however, for additional information the reader should refer to appropriate sections of Chapters 1 and 2. Rating instructions are found here and on the NSI form at the end of this chapter. Guides for calculating the various subindices, the BMI and the SMI, and finally, the NSI are also found in appropriate sections of the NSI form.

BASIC MOVEMENTS INDEX

Subindices of the BMI include the Basic Listening Index (BLI), Speech Postures Index (SPI), Hand Movements Index (HMI), and Basic Speech Index (BSI).

Basic Listening Index (BLI)

Ratings are made of protective, listening, and tuning reflexes. Parental reports of these events should be considered for rating and noted under the form's "remarks" section.

Protective reflexes include the extensor startle (Moro reflex), eye opening, eye closing, mouth opening, and cry reflexes in response to unexpected loud sounds, including human speech. Regular or r_1 ratings* are applied to normal infants when these reflexes are present; however, r_2 ratings** are applied when these reflexes persist in older infants, or in older infants and children with brain dysfunction.

Listening reflexes, or early listening reactions, include cessation of crying, suckling, and body stilling in response to the human voice. Regular ratings are applied to young infants, as well as older ones, whenever the human voice elicits these responses. These responses may be elicited by calling the subject repeatedly, progressively increasing the loudness level, and/or decreasing the distance between the tester and the subject.

Tuning reflexes serve to sensitize or maximize the efficiency of the auditory system and include changes in heartbeat, respiration, and hormonal flow in response to various sounds, as well as the human voice. Changes in respiration may be instrumentally detected with the aid of a pneumograph, or clinically detected by the use of bimanual palpation; changes in heartbeat may also be detected through palpation, but changes in hormonal flow are not easily detected and therefore are not judged here. Regular ratings are applied here, irrespective of the child's age.

---

*r_1 ratings are based on expected reflexes in infants.

**r_2 ratings are based on the presence of persisting infantile reflexes in older infants and children.

Speech Postures Index (SPI)

Depending on the age of the child, reactions associated with back, elbow, sit, and stand patterns are rated according to r_1 or r_2 criteria. Parental reports should be considered in rating aspects of speech postures.

Back patterns, the earliest speech postures, include various forms of symmetrical supine or semireclining speech postures. The infant form includes head in alignment with the body, lower limbs gently flexed and abducted, with the possibility of the hands being brought together and to the mouth. Among the older forms are found the basic semireclining posture with occiput-in-hands, hands-on-crown, and hands-on-knees positions. The infant form is evaluated and rated by placing the child in the prone-lying position, and requesting or waiting for the child to assume supine-lying, or by modeling the sequence of movements for the child to imitate. As the child moves, the tester evaluates the presence of neck righting and labyrinthine on-head righting reactions. The reactions may also be tested specifically. The presence of stabilizing equilibrium reactions in supine is also assessed.

Elbow patterns include symmetrical and asymmetrical forms. The basic infant form is the child in prone with extension of the neck and trunk; with lower limbs extended, abducted, and outwardly rotated; and with good head balance and support of the upper body on forearms. The head-in-hands cradle posture is another form of elbow pattern. Unilateral forms of these positions may be observed. Prone-on-upper-arm forms include face-in-hand cradle, occiput-in-hand cradle, and chin-in-three-finger cradle positions. The basic infant form is rated by placing children in supine and requesting that they roll over and onto their forearms, or by modeling the sequence of movements for children to imitate. As the child assumes the prone-on-forearms position, the body-on-body righting reaction and the arm support-forward movements are rated. Complete rating of elbow patterns includes the testing of upper limb movement, of Landau and chain-in-prone reactions, and of equilibrium reactions in prone, side lying, and on-forearms.

Sit patterns are the most common speech postures. Floor-sit, squat-sit, and chair-sit postures are forms of sit patterns. Floor-sit patterns are observed first and include side-sit, long-sit, and tailor-sit varieties. Chair-sit patterns include chin-in-hands cradle and chin-on-fist varieties. Chair-table sit patterns include forearms-on-table and chin-in-hands cradle positions. Early floor-sit patterns are rated. The child is placed on her back and asked to assume a sitting position, or the sequence of movements is modeled for the child to imitate. As the child assumes the position, the tester evaluates for the presence of the complete rotation pattern and for the quadrupedal righting reaction. Full scores are given for the more advanced partial rotation or symmetrical sitting patterns. Side-sit, long-sit, or tailor-sit patterns are acceptable. A complete rating of the sit patterns includes testing for on-fours and in-sitting equilibrium reactions.

Stand patterns are the highest form of speaking postures. The earliest form is supported standing, or standing while holding on to something, then free standing, and, finally, dynamic standing such as walking, running, and dancing. Free standing speech postures are rated. The child is placed in the supine position and requested to assume the standing position, or the sequence of movements is modeled for the child to imitate. The child is rated for assuming the on-knees position, then the half-kneel position, and, finally, the standing position; or for moving from the quadrupedal position into the simian stance and then into the standing position. A complete rating of the free-standing speech posture includes testing for upper body, sideways, step position, and one-leg standing, and hopping equilibrium reactions. Appropriate head-lead and eye-movement tuning reactions during the assumption of standing are also rated.

Hand Movements Index (HMI)

Regular ratings are applied to protective, progression, and vegetative reflexes. Parental reports should be considered in rating these reflexes.

Protective reflexes, such as arm-support-forward, sideways, and backward and arm-balance reactions, may have been elicited during testing for elbow and sit speech postures. Arm-support and balance reactions are tested in the floor-sit or chair-sit postures. The child is first tipped forward by gentle pushing from behind, then sideways by applying pressure under the child's arms at the side of the thorax, and then backward by applying pressure to the chest or at the level of the shoulders. Positive responses consist of extensor-abductor support and balance movements of the arms and hands.

Progression reflexes include upper-limb movement, upper-limb placing, arm walking, and quadrupedal hopping. Upper-limb movement is tested by placing children in prone and extending their upper limbs alongside the trunk; head turning, flexion of arms and forearms, and a forward movement of the upper limbs constitutes a positive response. Upper-limb placing is tested by pressing the back of the child's hand against the edge of a surface like a table; flexion of the limb, bringing the hand above the surface, followed by limb extension in a supporting movement, represents a positive response. Quadrupedal hopping is tested with the child in the on-fours position while the tester attempts to push the child off balance; automatic support movements of the limbs that follow the displaced body constitute a positive response. Arm walking may be tested with the child in prone or on-fours. The tester raises the child's lower body at the level of the knees and slowly moves the body forward; extension of the upper limbs in a support reaction followed by reciprocal movements of the upper limbs in a walking pattern constitutes a positive response. Functional testing of these reflexes may be accomplished by observing the child during crawling (upper-limb movement) and creeping (arm walking, placing, and hopping reactions). Ratings of these movements during functional activity is the preferred procedure.

Vegetative reflexes include hand-to-mouth movements and hand-to-mouth feeding. Parental reports are especially useful here. Ratings may be determined by observing whether the child uses a hand-to-mouth movement during play or a hand-to-mouth feeding pattern when presented with a cookie, for example.

Basic Speech Index (BSI)

Ratings are made of protective, emotional, and vegetative reflexes and of reflexive vocalization. Again, depending on the child's age, reflexes are rated according to r_1 or r_2 criteria; however, r_1 criteria are used irrespective of age when evaluating protective, emotional, and breathing reflexes and movement vocalization.

Protective reflexes include glottic closing and opening, sneeze, cough, palatal, and jaw-jerk reflexes and lip and tongue protective reflexes. The glottal closing reflex may be stimulated by having the child inhale ammonia or vinegar, or inferred from "pushing or pulling sounds" made when the infant pushes away from or pulls toward someone or something. The glottic opening reflex may be elicited by pinching closed the child's nostrils or inferred from the "inspiratory sound" heard following the expiratory phase of vigorous crying. Ratings of the glottic closing and opening reflexes and of the coughing reflex may be based on parental report. The palatal reflex is elicited by a touch stimulus (Q-tip stick) applied to the velum. The jaw-jerk reflex is elicited by placing the index finger of one hand across the mental prominence of the mandible and briskly tapping the finger with the ends of the middle three fingers of the other hand. Reflexive lip puckering in response to the corners of the lips being steadily spread apart and reflexive lip spreading in response to lateral compression of the lips constitute the lip-protective movements. Reflexive tongue protrusion in response to the tongue tip being steadily forced backward into the mouth by the examiner's middle finger or tongue depressor constitutes the tongue protective movement. Bitter substances applied to the tongue tip may also elicit reflexive tongue protrusion.

Emotional reflexes include cry, smile, and laugh reflexes. Rating of the cry reflex may be based on parental report. A parent or the examiner may attempt to elicit smile and laugh behavior or ratings of these may also be based on parental report. Ratings are based on sensitivity and the fullness of display of these reflexes.

Vegetative reflexes include breathing reflexes and breathing and feeding reflexes and eating. Rating of one type of inspiratory reflex may be based on parental report of the presence of yawn, or the tester may attempt to elicit it by simulating a yawn within the visual field of the child. Inspiratory reflexes may also be elicited by restricting the child's airway to one nostril, by having the child hold his breath for as long as possible, and by having the child exhaust his breath. Vegetative bpm should also be rated.

Rooting, lip, mouth opening, biting, tongue, suckle, chewing, and swallow reflexes comprise the chain of feeding reflexes. Rooting is elicited by placing a finger at the corner of the child's mouth and lightly stroking outward; a full response is lowering of the respective half of the child's lower lip and movement of the tongue and head toward the stimulus. Rooting may also be tested by stimulation of the perioral area on either side or on the upper and lower lips. The lip reflex is elicited by a touch or a tap applied to the middle of the child's lips; a full response is movement of the lips including closure and pouting activity. Mouth opening may be elicited by introducing a nipple or finger in the visual field of the child, by moving the stimulus toward the mouth, or by touching the lips. The tongue reflex may be tested by applying a touch stimulus (end of a Q-tip stick) to the lateral margin of the tongue; the expected response is movement of the tongue in the direction of the stimulus. Biting or mandibular grasping may be elicited by placing a small tongue depressor between the child's teeth or gums; moving the depressor in an up and down fashion may facilitate holding behavior. Suckle behavior may be elicited by placing a finger, nipple, or Q-tip in contact with the child's lips, tongue tip and blade, or palate; gentle movement of the stimulus may facilitate the suckle reflex. Chewing, or alternating flexion and extension of the mandible, may be stimulated by stroking the anterior or lateral gingival area with a finger, biscuit, or small tongue depressor. Swallowing may be elicited by stroking the palate, fauces, or back of the tongue with a Q-tip.

A functional evaluation of the chain of feeding reflexes may be accomplished by observing the sequence of reflexive components that occur when a nipple or food source is brought toward the mouth or touches the child's perioral or cheek areas. Ratings for the chain of feeding reflexes are based on r_1 criteria during the first months of life; ratings are based on r_2 criteria when observed after about two years of age, or when observed in hypertrophied forms.

Actual eating movements are also inspected and rated, according to the s rating criteria. Among the movements evaluated are: positioning, or whether children can independently position or reposition themselves efficiently toward the food source; transporting, or whether the child can independently bring the bottle, spoon, morsel, or cup to the mouth; grasping, or whether the child can appropriately grasp the food with the lip, tongue, or teeth depending on the type of food source; preparing, or whether the child suckles liquids adequately or chews solids adequately; and, finally, swallowing.

Reflexive vocalization includes movement vocalization, hand-to-mouth vocalization, and "happy-play" vocalization. Ratings of movement vocalization may be based on parental reports of whether the child produces struggle vocalization when attempting to overcome resistance to the raising of the head, rolling over, or sitting up; and work vocalization when working to push, pull, or squeeze objects. Vocalization during hand-to-mouth play or during eating is also checked. The occurrence of vocalization during pleasant sensations (cooing), such as bathing or rocking, or the use of vocalization for play purposes (babbling) are behaviors that may also be rated on the basis of parental report.

SKILLED MOVEMENTS INDEX

Subindices of the SMI include the Skilled Listening Index (SLI), Imitative Vocalization Index (IVI), Skilled Speech Index (SSI), and the Expressive Communication Index (ECI).

Skilled Listening Index (SLI)

Ratings according to the s rating criteria are made of selective inhibition of startle, localizing, and speech perception.

Selective inhibition of startle may be rated on the basis of parental report that indicates that the child does not show flexor-startle in response to unexpected and familiar sounds but startles in response to unexpected and unfamiliar sounds, even though less loud. A higher rating is given if the child accommodates rapidly to repeated and unexpected loud sounds presented by the tester; a lower rating is given if the child demonstrates difficulty in adapting to repeated and unexpected loud sounds. At this time, the earlier extensor-startle pattern has developed into the mature flexor-startle pattern.

Localizing responses, in response to interesting environmental sounds, include head rolling to the right or left when the child is in supine, and head lowering or raising or turning to the right or left when the child is sitting. Localization downward usually precedes localization upward, and localization toward the right usually precedes localization toward the left when the child is sitting. Numerous opportunities to localize should be provided to the child by varying the loudness level of the stimulus and by varying the distance between the child and the stimulus.

Speech perception responses include the localizing of the mother's voice and appropriate responses to the child's name, "no," "bye-bye," and "give me" requests. Ratings may be based on parental report with full scores given for consistency of response. The mother may also be asked to attempt to elicit the desired response in the testing situation.

Imitative Vocalization Index (IVI)

Ratings according to the s-rating criteria are made of two forms of auto-echolalia and three forms of true echolalia. Echolalia is considered to be primary talking. Parental reports may supplement test results. A parent or the tester should attempt to elicit the various levels of primary talking.

Auto-echolalia, I represents imitative replies from the child in response to the speaker speaking pre-words made spontaneously by the child.

Auto-echolalia, II represents imitative replies from the child in response to the speaker speaking pre-words that are similar to those made spontaneously by the child.

True echolalia, I represents imitative replies from the child in response to the speaker speaking pre-words not yet made by the child.

True echolalia, II represents imitative replies from the child in response to the speaker speaking true words.

True echolalia, III represents imitative replies from the child in response to words spoken earlier by the speaker, that is, deferred echolalia.

Assignment of full or lesser scores to the various levels of primary talking is based on consistency, and, later, accuracy of the child's replies.

Skilled Speech Index (SSI)

Ratings are made of speech breathing and of effector system coordination.

Speech breathing includes multisyllabic utterances (babbling, speaking), thoracic activity, abdominal-thoracic asynchrony, speech I-fraction, and oral inspiration. Ratings are made according to the s-rating criteria. Whenever possible, these activities should be rated when the child is in a sitting posture. Rating of multisyllabic utterances may be based on parental report, or the rating may be based on attempts by the mother or tester to elicit such utterances in the testing situation. Observation and bimanual palpation of the abdominal-thoracic area during multisyllabic utterances or during crying should allow for rating of the presence of oral inspiration and thoracic participation during inspiration and abdominal-thoracic asynchrony during expiration. The shift of a vegetative I-fraction of about 40 or 50 percent to a crying or speaking I-fraction of about 10 or 15 percent may be estimated and rated through observation and palpation or through the use of pneumography.

Effector coordination includes differentiation, praxis, and diadochokinesia. Differentiation is rated by evaluating the child's capacity to activate part of the speech effector system in isolation from the rest of the system and is done according to the d-rating criteria. Full scores are given if the child can phonate various vowels or combinations of vowels without moving the head, flex and extend the mandible in isolation from head movements, protrude and spread the lips in isolation from head movements, and protrude and retrude the tongue in isolation from head movements. Full scores are then given for the more difficult differentiation tasks, such as moving the mandible in isolation from the lips and tongue, the lips in isolation from the mandible and tongue, and the tongue in isolation from the mandible and lips. Articulator-from-articulators differentiation tasks usually require cooperation from children who are older than two years.

Praxis is rated by evaluating the child's ability to produce two-syllable combinations and done according to the p-rating criteria. The syllable combinations include various bilabial, labiodental, linguadental, lingua-alveolar, linguapalatal, and lingualvelar combinations, for example, /bʌ-vʌ, vʌ-ðʌ, dʌ-dʒʌ, /dʒʌ-gʌ/. Each combination should be repeated three times. Combinations involving front-to-middle, middle-to-back, back-to-middle, and middle-to-front are tested, and full scores are given for coordination and accuracy, not for speed. Also, full scores are dependent on the child giving at least three, two-syllable and three, three-syllable combinations. Whenever possible three-syllable combinations should be tested. All syllable combinations should contain only those sounds that the child can articulate.

Diadochokinesia is rated by evaluating the child's speed of repetition, duration of repetition, and rhythmicity of repetition, in accordance with the f-rating criteria. Respirodiado is rated by having the child pant as quickly as possible for a five-second period; laryngodiado is rated by having the child phonate a vowel in an on-off fashion as quickly as possible for a ten-second period; velodiado is rated by having the child alternate production of /mʌ/-/bʌ/ for a ten-second period; and articulodiado is rated by having the child produce /pʌ/, /tʌ/, and /kʌ/ as quickly as possible for a ten-second period each. Rates of two or three per second are acceptable for three-year-old children. Full scores are earned not only for rate, but also for durational and rhythmicity factors.

Expressive Communication Index (ECI)

Ratings are made of hands talk, face talk, effector talk, and communisphere level in accordance with the s-rating criteria.

Hands talk includes the use of hands in adjunctive gestural and symbolic gestural modes. Rating of the symbolic gestural mode may be based on parental report or tester observation of whether the child employs appropriate gestures for "pick me up, pay attention, give me, I don't want, and all gone" kinds of communications. Scores are based on consistency and fullness of display of the gestures.

Rating of the adjunctive gestural mode is based on parental report or tester observation of whether the child uses hand gestures in a supportive manner during normal speech attempts and in a facilitatory manner during difficult speech attempts. Scores are based on fullness of display of the gestures.

Face talk includes the use of the face to express ranges of basic emotions, such as ranges of happy-sad, security-fear, and excitement-boredom emotions. Scores may be based on parental report as well as on tester observation.

Effector talk or spoken language includes the use of ritual, emotional, and logical speech. Rating of ritual speech is based on parental report or tester observation of the child's use of social-gesture speech such as "hi," "bye," "I'm fine," and "OK," and memorized speech such as counting, nursery rhymes, prayers, and days of the week. Rating of emotional speech is based on parental report or tester observation of the child's use of "anger, fright, or love talk." Ratings of more advanced logical speech includes the ability of the child to use descriptive, conversational, narrative, and persuasive speech forms and may be based on parental report or tester observation. Scores for emotional and logical forms of speech depend on the ease with which the forms are recognized and the frequency of their use.

Communispheral ranges include intimate, personal, and family. Ratings of these ranges are based primarily on parental report, and scores depend on the frequency and amount of talking within the various communispheres.

At this stage of the development of the NSI, it should be used primarily as a guide for planning therapy and judging its progress and secondarily as an index of the child's neurophysiological speech age.

Evaluation Form

Name _____ Age_____ Sex_____

Examiner _____ Date_____

Basic Movements Index	Rating	Remarks
I. *Basic Listening* (neonatal) A. *Protective Reflexes*	r	
1. Extensor startle (Moro reflex)		
2. Eye opening		
3. Eye closing		
4. Mouth opening		
5. Cry		
B. *Listening Reflexes*	r	
1. Cessation of crying		
2. Cessation of suckling		
3. Body stilling		
C. *Tuning Reflexes*	r	
1. Changes in respiration		
2. Changes in heartbeat		
Total Score		

$$(B)\text{asic }(L)\text{istening }(I)\text{ndex} = \quad \frac{\text{Tot. Score}}{\text{Max. Score}} = \frac{}{30} =$$

	Rating	Remarks
II. *Speech Postures* A. *Back Patterns*	r	
1. Elemental righting reactions (a) neck (0–6 mo.)		
(b) labyrinthine-on-head, prone (1–3 mo.–)		

r_1 rating (infant): average reflex = *3;* diminished reflex = *2;* exaggerated reflex = *1;* absent reflex = *0.*

r_2 rating (older): absent reflex = *3;* diminished reflex = *2;* average reflex = *1;* exaggerated reflex = *0.*

Basic Movements Index (cont.)	Rating	Remarks
(c) labyrinthine-on-head, supine (4–6 mo.–)		
2. Stabilizing equilibrium reaction (a) supine (7–10 mo.–)		
B. *Elbow Patterns*	r	
1. Elemental righting reactions (a) body-on-body (6–8 mo.–2 yrs.)		
(b) upper limb movement (0 mo.–)		
(c) arm-support-forward (4–6 mo.–)		
2. Tuning midbrain reactions (a) Landau (6 mo.–2–3 yr.)		
(b) chain-in-prone (1 mo.–2 yrs.)		
3. Stabilizing equilibrium reactions (a) prone (4–6 mo.–)		
(b) side-lying (6–8 mo.–)		
(c) on-forearms (6–8 mo.–)		
C. *Sit Patterns*	r	
1. Elemental righting reactions (a) complete rotation sitting (10–12 mo.–2–3 yrs.)		
(b) quadrupedal (6–8 mo.–)		
2. Stabilizing equilibrium reactions (a) on-fours (8–10 mo.–)		
(b) in-sitting (10–12 mo.–)		
D. *Stand Patterns*	r	
1. Elemental and stabilizing equilibrium reactions (a) on-knees (13–15 mo.–)		
(b) half-kneel (13–15 mo.–)		
(c) simian stance (12–18 mo.–)		

Basic Movements Index (cont.)	Rating	Remarks
(d) upper body standing (12–18 mo.–)		
(e) sideways standing (12–18 mo.–)		
(f) step-position standing (12–18 mo.–)		
(g) one-leg standing (15–18 mo.)		
(h) hopping (15–18 mo.–)		
2. Tuning cortical reactions (1–3 mo.–) (a) head-movement lead		
(b) eye-movement lead		
Total Score		

$$\text{(S)peech (P)ostures (I)ndex} = \frac{\text{Tot. Score}}{\text{Max. Score}} = \frac{}{78} =$$

III. Hand Movements A. Protective Reflexes	r	
1. Arm-support-forward (6 mo.–)		
2. Arm-support-sideways (8 mo.–)		
3. Arm-support-backward (10 mo.–)		
4. Arm-balance reactions (6 mo.–)		
B. Progression Reflexes	r	
1. Upper-limb movement (0 mo.–)		
2. Upper-limb placing (3–4 mo.–)		
3. Arm walking (2–6 mo.–)		

Basic Movements Index (cont.)	Rating	Remarks
4. Quadrupedal hopping (8–10 mo.–)		
C. *Vegetative Reflexes*	r	
1. Hand-to-mouth movements (2–3 mo.–)		
2. Hand-to-mouth feeding (6 mo.–)		
Total Score		

$$\text{(H)and (M)ovement (I)ndex} = \frac{\text{Tot. Score}}{\text{Max. Score}} = \frac{}{30} =$$

	Rating	Remarks
IV. *Basic Speech*		
A. *Protective Reflexes* (neonatal)	r	
1. Glottic closing		
2. Glottic opening		
3. Sneeze		
4. Cough		
5. Palatal		
6. Jaw jerk		
7. Lip protective		
8. Tongue protective		
B. *Emotional Reflexes*	r	
1. Cry (0 mo.–)		
2. Smile (4–6 wks.–)		
3. Laugh (16 wks.–)		
C. *Vegetative Reflexes*	r	
1. Breathing reflexes		
(a) yawn		
(b) airway restriction		
(c) breath holding		

Basic Movements Index (cont.)	Rating	Remarks
(d) breath exhaustion		
2. Breathing—approx. 20–45 bpm (6 mo.–2 yrs.)		
3. Feeding reflexes (neonatal)		
(a) rooting		
(b) lip		
(c) mouth opening		
(d) biting		
(e) tongue		
(f) suckle		
(g) chewing		
(h) swallow		
4. Eating (6 mo.–)	s	
(a) positioning		
(b) transporting		
(c) grasping		
(d) preparing		
(e) swallowing		
D. Reflexive Vocalization (neonatal)	r	
1. Movement vocalization (a) struggle movement		
(b) work movement		
2. Hand-to-mouth vocalization (a) play		
(b) eating		

s rating: good show = 3; fair show = 2; poor show = 1; no show = 0.

Basic Movements Index (cont.)	Rating	Remarks
3. Happy-play vocalization (a) cooing (0 mo.–4 mo.)		
(b) babbling (4 mo.–8 mo.)		
Total Score		

$$(B)asic\ (S)peech\ (I)ndex\ =\ \frac{Tot.\ Score}{Max.\ Score}\ =\ \frac{\quad\quad}{105}\ =$$

Basic Movements Indices	Values
Basic Listening Index (BLI)	
Speech Postures Index (SPI)	
Hand Movements Index (HMI)	
Basic Speech Index (BSI)	

Total

$$Basic\ Movements\ Index\ (BMI)\ =\ \frac{Total}{4}\ =$$

Skilled Movements Index	Rating	Remarks
I. Skilled Listening	s	
A. Selective Inhibition of Flexor- Startle (3–6 mo.–)		

B. Localizing
   1. Head-roll, supine
      (9–12 wks.–)		

2. Head down, sitting (3 mo.–)		
3. Head to right, sitting (3 mo.–)		

C. Speech Perception
   1. Localization of maternal voice
      (6 mo.–)		

2. Response to name, "no," "bye-bye" (9 mo.–)		

Skilled Movements Index (cont.)	Rating	Remarks
3. Response to "give me" (12 mo.–)		
Total Score		
(S)killed (L)istening (I)ndex =	$\dfrac{\text{Tot. Score}}{\text{Max. Score}} = \dfrac{}{21} =$	
II. *Imitative Vocalization*	s	
A. *Auto-echolalia, I* (0 mo.–4 mo.)		
B. *Auto-echolalia, II* (4 mo.–8 mo.)		
C. *True echolalia, I* (8 mo.–12 mo.)		
D. *True echolalia, II* (12 mo.–16 mo.)		
E. *True echolalia, III* (16 mo.–18 mo.)		
Total Score		
(I)mitative (V)ocalization (I)ndex =	$\dfrac{\text{Tot. Score}}{\text{Max. Score}} = \dfrac{}{15} =$	
III. *Skilled Speech* A. *Speech Breathing*	s	
1. Multisyllabic babbling (7–8 mo.)		
2. Thoracic participation (6–7 mo.)		
3. Abdominal-thoracic asynchrony		
4. I-fraction, 15 percent (10 mo.)		
5. Oral inspiration		
B. *Effector Coordination* 1. Differentiation	d	
(a) larynx from head		
(b) mandible from head		
(c) lips from head		
(d) tongue from head		

d rating: isolated movement = 3; movement plus one = 2; movement plus two = 1; movement plus three or more = 0.

Skilled Movements Index (cont.)	Rating	Remarks
(e) mandible from lips and tongue		
(f) lips from mandible and tongue		
(g) tongue from mandible and lips		
2. Praxis	p	
(a) two syllable combinations (1–3 yrs.–)		
(b) three-syllable combinations (3–5 yrs.–)		
3. Diadochokinesia—2–3 per sec. (3 yrs.)	f	
(a) respirodiado		
(b) laryngodiado		
(c) velodiado		
(d) articulodiado		
Total Score		

$$(S)killed\ (S)peech\ (I)ndex = \frac{Tot.\ Score}{Max.\ Score} = \frac{\_\_\_\_\_}{54} = \_\_\_$$

IV. Expressive Communication A. Hands Talk (infant)	s	
1. Symbolic gestural (a) "pick me up" (reaches up)		
(b) "pay attention" (tugs on clothes)		
(c) "give me" (pointing, reaching)		
(d) "I don't want" (pushes away)		
(e) "all gone" (hands-supinated-separated)		
2. Adjunctive gestural (a) supportive		

p rating: produces three-syllable combinations = 3; two-syllable combinations = 2; single syllables = 1; no syllables = 0.

f rating: adequate rate, rhythm, duration = 3; adequacy of two criteria = 2; adequacy of one criterion = 1; no criteria met = 0.

Skilled Movements Index (cont.)	Rating	Remarks
(b) facilitatory		
B. *Face Talk* (infant)	s	
1. Happy-sad		
2. Security-fear		
3. Excitement-boredom		
C. *Effector Talk* (1 yr.–4 yrs.)	s	
1. Ritual speech (a) social-gesture		
(b) memorized		
2. Emotional speech (a) anger		
(b) fright		
(c) love		
(d) hate		
3. Logical speech (a) description		
(b) narration		
(c) conversation		
(d) persuasion		
D. *Communispheres*	s	
1. Intimate (body contact)		
2. Personal (person-to-person)		
3. Family (person-to-small group)		
Total Score		

(E)xpressive (C)ommunication (I)ndex = $\dfrac{\text{Tot. Score}}{\text{Max. Score}}$ = $\dfrac{}{67}$ =

Skilled Movements Indices	*Values*
Skilled Listening Index (SLI)	_____
Imitative Vocalization Index (IVI)	_____
Skilled Speech Index (SSI)	_____
Expressive Communication Index (ECI)	_____

Total

$$\text{Skilled Movements Index (SMI)} = \frac{\text{Total}}{4} =$$

Estimation of Neurophysiological Speech Index

INDICES	VALUES
Basic Movements Index (BMI)	_____
Skilled Movements Index (SMI)	_____
TOTAL	_____

$$\text{Neurophysiological Speech Index (NSI)} = \frac{\text{Total}}{2} =$$

7

Neurospeech Therapy: Stimulation of Basic Movements

THIS SECOND CHAPTER on neurospeech therapy is devoted to a discussion of the procedures and techniques used for stimulating basic listening movements, speech postures, hand movements, and basic speech movements. Since skilled speech movements emerge from basic listening, hand, and speech movements, and since skilled movements are performed on the background of stable speech postures, the stimulation of these basic postures and movements is fundamental to neurospeech therapy.

Preparatory Maneuvers

As a "warm-up" to pursuing specific therapeutic goals in basic movements, at least four types of preparatory maneuvers are recommended: pretzeling, reflex conditioning, supplementary techniques, and body-image formation. The general purposes of these maneuvers are to enrich sensorimotor experiences; induce physiological relaxation; regularize tone, posture, and movement; and facilitate integration and elaboration of reflexive units.

Related to the concept of preparatory maneuvers is "environmental enrichment" (Twitchell, 1965) and the development of sensorimotor responses. Effects of such enrichment, or special sensorimotor experiences, are interpreted as follows:

1. The low threshold at birth for the instinctive suckling response remains at this low level only if the infant is immediately allowed to suckle.
2. Infants who sleep in the prone position usually develop sitting, standing, and walking more quickly than infants who sleep in supine, and this is apparently due to the more constant stimulation of righting reactions resulting from body contact in the prone.
3. Infants who are usually placed in standing postures on their mother's lap, thus restimulating the positive supporting reactions, usually begin to stand and walk earlier than those who are not.
4. Environmental enrichment also appears to hasten spontaneous prehension in the developing infant.

PRETZELING

Pretzeling maneuvers describe the imposition on the child of disequilibrating postures or the application of "therapeutic discomfort." Such therapeutic discomfort is resolved by the child when he moves into more normal postures. Pretzeling may be performed with the child in supine, prone, side lying, or sitting. Benefits that may be derived from pretzeling maneuvers are physiologic relaxation, or tension reduction through vigorous movement; tactile, otolithic, and general proprioceptive stimulation eliciting automatic movement responses; and body-part awareness and body-part self-adjustment contributions. All possible postures should be imposed, such as postures of extension-flexion, elevation-depression, inward-outward rotation, dorsiflexion-ventroflexion, and compression-traction. Pretzeling should be imposed with a gradual increase in range and directions; speed of posturing should also increase from slow to a moderate speed. Pretzeling activities should be routinized so that a program is established and a "workout" is provided that is smooth and rhythmical. Also, postures should be imposed to the point where they elicit a spontaneous countermovement from the child; if the countermovement does not occur it should be assisted or facilitated.

Supine Pretzeling

Pretzel postures in supine include: (a) crossing legs at the level of the ankles and knees; (b) flexing one leg under or over the other extended leg; (c) bending up both legs under the buttocks; (d) placing hands under the buttocks; (e) placing hands behind the head; (f) crossing arms across the chest; and (g) various combinations of lower and upper limb pretzeling in supine.

Prone Pretzeling

Pretzel postures in prone include: (a) crossing legs at the level of the ankles and knees; (b) flexing one leg under or over the other extended leg; (c) flexing both legs until heels approach or touch buttocks; (d) crossing one or both arms under the chest; (e) extending both arms fully above the head and crossing them; (f) crossing arms across the neck so that hands approach or come into contact with the opposite ears; and (g) various combinations of lower and upper limb pretzeling in prone.

Side Lying Pretzeling

Pretzel postures in side lying include: (a) crossing legs at the level of the ankles or knees; (b) flexing both legs until feet approach or make contact with the buttocks; (c) placing under-body hand and top-of-body hand around the ankles; (d) placing both arms between thighs; and (e) various combinations of lower and upper limb pretzeling in side lying.

Pretzeling can also be done with the child in various sitting positions. The principle remains the same, that is, placing body parts in various and unusual postures until countermovements and body righting are elicited. The clinician should also take advantage of the opportunity to name touched body parts during pretzeling maneuvers.

Figures 7.1, 2, and 3 show examples of supine, prone, and side-lying pretzeling.

REFLEX CONDITIONING

All four neurotherapy orientations discussed in Chapter 4 include in their programs forms of reflex conditioning or facilitation. As one of the preparatory maneuvers discussed here, reflex conditioning is defined as the regular elicitation of various reflexes for the purposes of preventing any tendency toward fixed postures, maintaining and building muscle volume, allowing for physiologic relaxation, normalizing muscle tone and posture, and facilitating volitional movements through simultaneous stimulation of specific reflexes. From the standpoint of neurodynamics, reflex conditioning provides the system with numerous forms of sensory inflow, with opportunity for integration of these afferents at various levels of the CNS, with numerous forms of motor outflow, and with sensory feedbacks from all these movements. In short, it is central to neurotherapy. Reflex conditioning should be done at least once a day, preferably twice; and about 20 reflexes should be stimulated, each for about five minutes. Special attention should be paid to affected limbs so that they are guided to participate in the

Fig. 7.1. Examples of supine pretzeling

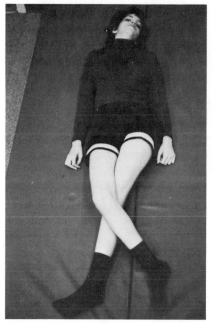

cross leg

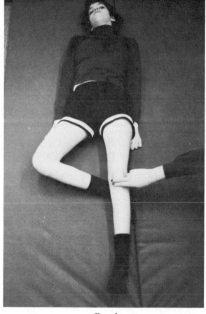

flex leg

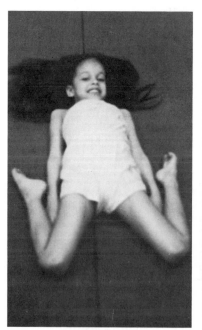

bend legs

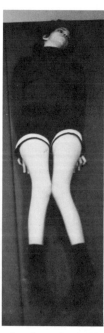

hands-under-butt

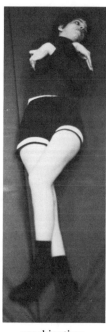

combination

Fig. 7.2. Examples of prone pretzeling

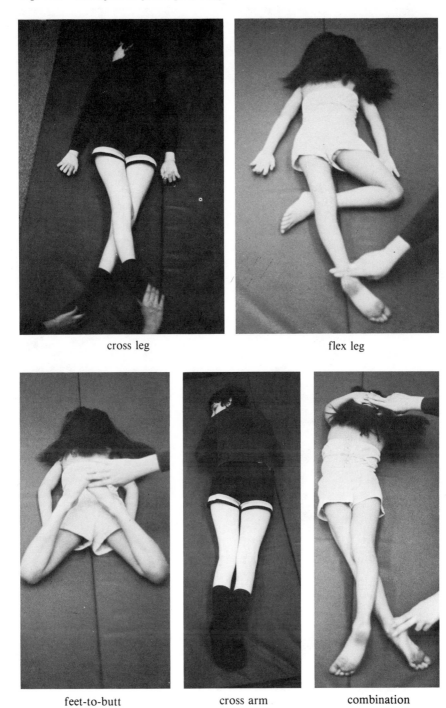

cross leg flex leg

feet-to-butt cross arm combination

Fig. 7.3. Examples of side-lying pretzeling

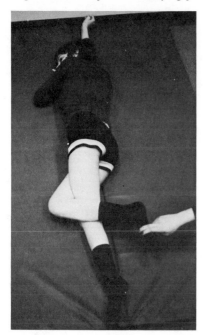

cross leg

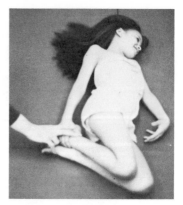

feet-to-butt

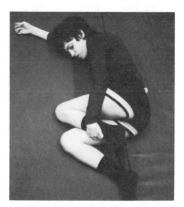

hands-to-ankles

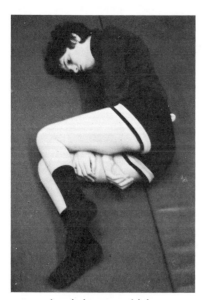

hands-between-thighs

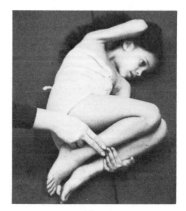

combination

expected movements and postures as much as possible. Such guidance is provided by timed placing, holding, extending, flexing, abducting, and adducting, and so on, of the affected limbs. Reflexes should be stimulated in accordance with the law of developmental direction, and, consequently, are presented here under the categories of eye, head, trunk, arm, hand, leg, and foot reflexes. Unlocking reflexes and synreflexive maneuvers are also described.

Eye Reflexes

Eye-tracking movements and eye-closure reflexes should be stimulated.

Eye-tracking movements are stimulated first. In back, elbow, or sit postures, eye-tracking movements are elicited by passing a finger through the visual field in a horizontal, vertical, oblique, and rotatory manner. To ensure differentiated eye movements, the head may be stabilized. Or, lift the child by the trunk, have him fixate on some point, and rotate his body from side to side and in an upward and downward fashion; corresponding eye movements should be observed.

Eye-closure reflexes are stimulated by blowing into the child's face or through McCarthy's reflex, that is, via a sudden tap of the supraorbital ridge, the glabella, or the margin of the orbit.

Head Reflexes

Head reflexes to be elicited include protective and vegetative movements and righting reactions.

Head protective reflexes are stimulated by steadily and carefully dorsiflexing or ventroflexing the head until reflexive countermovements are sensed. Similar counteracting responses may be elicited by flexing the head with an ear-to-shoulder movement. If present, nasocephalic and auriculocephalic reflexes should also be stimulated. These head avoidance reflexes are stimulated by applying "annoying" stimuli to the nostrils and ear lobes, respectively.

Head vegetative reflex, or the rooting reflex, is stimulated by applying a touch stimulus to the cheeks or perioral area. If present, head movement in the direction of the stimulus is the expected response.

Head righting reflexes and head control are critical to all body movements since the head leads all such movements; head righting and control is also essential to the development of equilibrium reactions. On-head righting reactions of the various types, that is, labyrinthine, body, and optical righting reactions, should be stimulated. Examples of the stimulation of such on-head righting reactions follows:

With the child in prone, the clinician lifts the child's shoulder girdle from in front or from behind the child and extends the spine and hips. The expected response is head righting and arm-support-forward. Or, with the child's chest on a roll, his spine in extension, and with his arms extended and abducted, head righting may also be facilitated.

With the child in supine, the clinician places her thumbs in the child's palms, facilitating grasping, then slowly pulls the child into sitting while simultaneously flexing the child's arms and bringing the hands toward the mouth. Reversing the maneuver by slowly lowering the child back to supine is also done. Both maneuvers facilitate head righting and control activities.

With the child in sitting, that is, lap sitting or sitting against the thigh of the clinician's flexed leg, extension of the trunk and neck, and consequently the head, may be facilitated by extension, abduction, and outward rotation of the arms.

With the child held free in the air and blindfolded, the clinician may move the child through prone, supine, and erect-angular positions, thus stimulating on-head righting activities. Gentle rocking in each of these positions may facilitate the desired reactions.

Elicitation of some on-head righting reactions from supine and in sitting is illustrated in Figure 7.4.

Trunk Reflexes

Primary sitting, bowing, dorsal, superficial abdominal, and lumbar reflexes, and body-on-body righting reactions are stimulated.

Primary sitting movements are elicited by placing the first and second fingers of each hand between the thumbs and forefingers of the child and stimulating the grasp reflex, then providing a lifting action eliciting trunk flexion, and, finally, the sitting position.

Bowing movements may also be stimulated in some young infants. The appropriate stimulus is extension of the lower limbs and pressure on the thighs. Trunk flexion into sitting may be marked by some side-to-side sway during the flexion movement.

Dorsal reflex elicitation causing trunk erection is effected by cutaneous stimulation over the erector spinal muscles.

Superficial abdominal reflexes may be stimulated by applying light strokes over each of the four abdominal quadrants with a blunt point such as a key or an orange stick with the individual in a supine position (Lenman, 1976, Ch. 5). Brisk contraction of the underlying muscles is the expected response.

Tonic lumbar reflexes may be stimulated by rotation of the trunk. Tendencies for arm flexion and leg extension on the side toward which the trunk rotates is the expected response.

Body-on-body righting reactions may be elicited in supine and prone positions. With the child in supine, the clinician flexes one leg and crosses it over the extended opposite leg. The maneuver should first cause the hips to rotate and then the shoulder girdle. Segmentation of body rotation is facilitated by holding one shoulder briefly while rotating the hips.

Fig. 7.4. Stimulation of on-head righting reactions

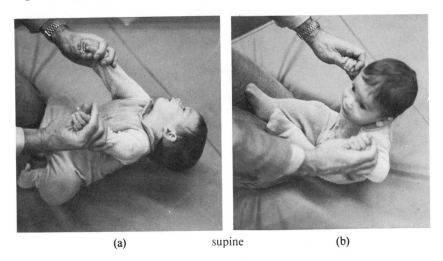

(a)　　　　　supine　　　　　(b)

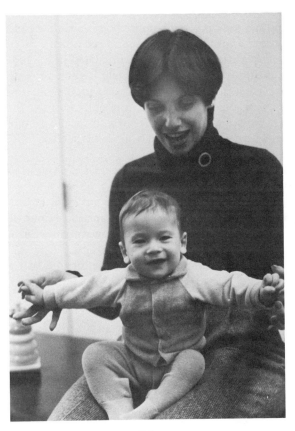

sitting

With the child in prone, and with arms upwardly extended, the clinician holds one arm by the wrist and with the arm gently rotates the shoulders, which is followed by the hips.

Elicitation of the body-on-body righting reaction and the dorsal reflex are illustrated in Figure 7.5.

Arm Reflexes

Reflexive arm movements to be stimulated include upper limb movement, arm-support-forward reaction, placing reaction of the arm, and arm walking.

Upper limb movement is stimulated with the child in prone and by placing the arms alongside of the trunk. Arm flexion and movement upward to an upper trunk supporting posture is the expected response. Such arm movements may be facilitated by applying pressure to the back of the head or to the palms of the hands.

Arm-support-forward is also stimulated from the prone position. With the child in a fully extended posture, raise the child at the level of the ankles, knees, or hips and then move the upper body toward the ground. The expected response is a protective extension of the arms.

Placing reaction of the arm may be stimulated in the on-fours or erect positions. In the on-fours position, the child is guided toward an elevation on the surface like a step and moved forward until an automatic limb raising and downward placing occurs. In the erect position the back of the child's hand is pressed against the edge of a surface like a table top; the expected response is a raising of the limb above the surface followed by a supporting extension of the arm.

Arm walking is stimulated by placing the child in prone in position for the upper limb movement reaction. Following upper limb movement, the child's body is raised above the floor by the ankles or knees, then a gentle forward movement of the body should elicit an arm-support-forward movement, and, finally, arm reciprocation or arm walking. Such arm walking should be stimulated forward and then backward.

Elicitation of the arm-support-forward reaction and arm walking are illustrated in Figure 7.6.

Hand Reflexes

Reflexive hand flexion (grasp reflex) and hand extension (avoiding response), finger flexion, and Darwinian reflexes are elicited.

Hand flexion-extension movements, the grasp reflex and the avoiding response, respectively, could be elicited in an alternating fashion. With the child in prone, the hand extension response is elicited by extending the arm and wrist and stimulating the dorsum of the hand; the hand flexion response is stimulated by flexing the arm and wrist and stimulating the

Fig. 7.5. Stimulation of trunk reflexes

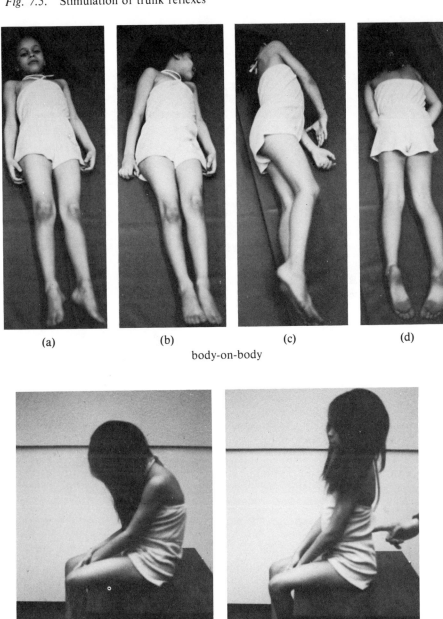

(a)   (b)   (c)   (d)

body-on-body

(a)   dorsal   (b)

Fig. 7.6.   Stimulation of arm reflexes

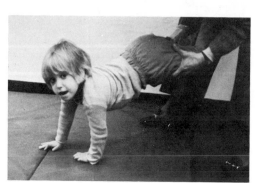

arm walking

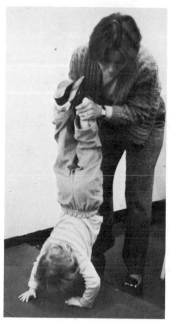

arm-support-forward

medial border of the palm. The maneuver should be done rhythmically and in an alternating fashion. It should also be done when possible in elbow and sitting postures. Tickling the palm, or the palmar reflex, may also elicit hand flexion.

Finger flexion reflexes (Lenman, 1976, Ch. 5), when present, are elicited by supporting with the clinician's own fingers the child's flexed fingers and tapping the child's fingers with the clinician's fingers. Slight flexion of the child's fingers is the expected response. Another finger flexion reflex is the Hoffman reflex. Again, if present, it is elicited by flicking downward the child's index or middle finger with the clinician's finger and thumb. The expected response is flexion of the child's thumb.

Darwinian reflex, or the grasp and hang tendency in young infants, may be elicited by stimulating the palms of the child's hands with both the clinician's index and middle fingers held together and horizontally. Once grasp is elicited the child may be slowly raised as far as possible off a surface, for example, head, trunk, and, if possible, the entire body.

Leg Reflexes

Among the leg reflexes that are stimulated are the leg automatisms (flexion, extension, magnet, cross reflexes), reinforced crawling, leg support reactions, placing reaction of the leg, primary walking, and hopping reactions.

Leg automatisms including spinal flexion, extension, and cross reflexes and the femoral and magnet reflexes are stimulated. Tonic flexion of the lower limb at all joints with dorsiflexion of the ankle and toes may follow the application of various stimuli such as the noxious stimuli of pinching or scratching the bottom of the foot; or the sudden flexion of the toes; or pressure applied to the ball of the foot; or the lateral compression of the foot. The extension reflex is elicited by applying noxious stimuli to the foot with the leg in the flexed position; a tap on the patellar tendon also elicits the "kick reflex" in the supine position. Extension of the knee and flexion of the foot may also be stimulated via the femoral reflex elicited by scratching the skin of the upper part of the front of the thigh. The cross movement is elicited by placing one leg in the flexed position and quickly flexing the other. A reciprocal extension pattern is stimulated by rapid and rhythmical alternation of leg flexion. The magnet reflex (Prechtl, 1977, p. 42) is stimulated by applying light pressure to the soles of the feet of the semi-flexed legs causing the legs to "follow the pressure" and to extend. Such leg automatisms may be stimulated in the supine position but preferably are done with the child in prone.

Reinforced crawling is stimulated with the child in prone. Pressure is applied to the soles of the child's extended legs eliciting flexion movements. It does not differ from leg flexion movements in prone when stimulated in alternating fashion as described under leg automatisms.

Leg-support reactions or the positive and negative supporting reactions are stimulated with the child held in the air in the erect position. In this position, the balls of the child's feet are tapped against a surface. The expected response is tonic extension or the pillar reaction of the legs. Cessation of the stimulation should result in diminution or loss of extensor tone.

Placing reaction of the leg is stimulated by pressing the instep of the foot against the edge of a surface, like a table. The expected response is leg flexion raising the leg above the surface followed by leg extension or a body-supporting movement.

Primary walking is elicited by holding the child erect in the air and moving the feet across a surface or a floor. The expected response is a series of steplike or walking movements.

Hopping reactions are stimulated by holding the child erect and moving him forward, sideways, and backward. The expected response is automatic movements of the legs to support the body as it is displaced in space.

Elicitation of leg support and placing reactions is illustrated in Figure 7.7.

Foot Reflexes

Among the foot reflexes that are stimulated are ankle clonus and the plantar responses (flexor and extensor).

Fig. 7.7. Stimulation of leg reflexes

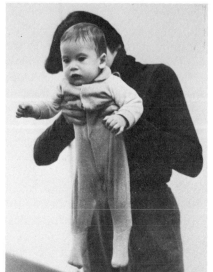 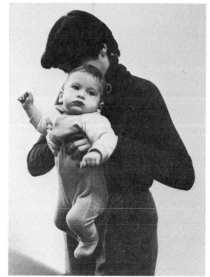

positive support   negative support

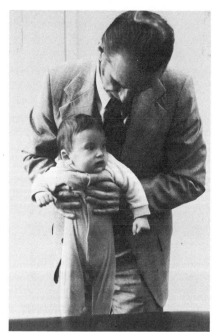

(a)   lower limb placing   (b)

Ankle clonus, if present, is stimulated with the knee flexed and by rapidly applying pressure on the foot to dorsiflex the ankle.

Plantar responses of various kinds may be stimulated. The flexor plantar response is elicited by application of firm pressure to the outer surface of the sole with a blunt point such as a key, orange stick, or end of an open paper clip. Starting from the heel the stimulus should move forward along the lateral margin of the sole toward the base of the little toe and then across to the base of the great toe. The expected response is flexion of the great toe usually accompanied by flexion of the other toes. Depending on the age or status of the child, the stimulus may elicit the extensor plantar response (Babinski's sign) with dorsiflexion of the great toe and outward fanning and dorsiflexion of the other toes.

Other plantar responses that could be stimulated are Chaddock's sign marked by dorsiflexion of the great toe when a large C is impressed around the outer malleolus at the ankle; Oppenheim's sign characterized by extension of the great toe upon progressive distal pressure by the clinician's thumb on the tibia; Gonda's sign marked by extension of the great toe upon forcible plantar flexion of the fourth toe; Rossolimo's sign reflected by flexion of the toes upon percussion of the ball of the foot; and Bechterew's sign manifested by flexion of the toes on percussion of the dorsum of the foot (Forster, 1973, pp. 19–20).

Unlocking Reflexes

If the child's hands, arms, or legs show extremes of tonus and posture that seriously limit movement, some of Fay's "unlocking" maneuvers could be tried.

Unlocking the spastic hand is done with the child in prone, face turned to the opposite shoulder, and by placing the hand in the palm-up position over the buttocks. The maneuver could result in opening of the fingers. If not, the clinician should apply passive manipulation of the fingers and wrist that should result in finger opening. Active opening of the fingers should then be encouraged.

Unlocking the spastic arm is done with (a) the child in prone, face turned toward the elbow elevated to the level of the shoulder cap with the thumb of the hand at the level of the teeth and (b) the hand and wrist then being drawn downward, outward, and backward and rotating the forearm until the hand assumes the palm-up position over the buttocks. The maneuver should be repeated slowly and rhythmically for a number of minutes.

Unlocking spastic legs is done with the use of the Marie Foix reflex in the prone or supine positions. To elicit the Marie Foix reflex, the toes are bent downward and pressure is simultaneously applied to the ball of the foot. The expected response is knee flexion and relaxation of leg adduction. (For greater details on the application of this maneuver, see the paleoreflex orientation in Chapter 4.)

Unlocking maneuvers of the arm, hand, and leg are illustrated in Figure 7.8.

Synreflexia

A number of reflexes emerge sequentially or in chainlike fashion and involve various combinations of body parts. Among these are various spinal and brainstem reflexes that combine to form different crawling patterns, and the Landau, Schaltenbrand, and chain-in-prone reactions that contribute to body extension-flexion patterns.

Crawling patterns, such as the homologous, homolateral, and cross-pattern types, are stimulated through eliciting various spinal-brainstem reflex combinations, similar to Fay's pattern-movement exercises. Chaining these spinal automatisms and tonic reflexes into functional movement patterns should be considered one way of facilitating their integration by higher sensorimotor integration centers. Depending on the neurophysiological development of the child, the clinician should stimulate crawling patterns in the following sequence: homologous, homolateral, cross-pattern.

Homologous crawling activity is stimulated by alternation of head flexion and extension in prone, stimulating the symmetrical tonic neck reflex so that head extension is accompanied by upper limb extension and head flex-

Fig. 7.8. Unlocking reflexes

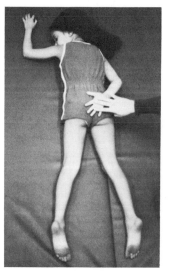
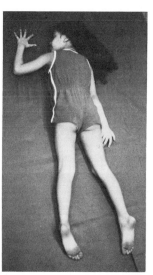
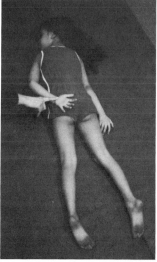

unlocking hand   (a)   unlocking arm   (b)

Fig. 7.8. Unlocking reflexes (continued): unlocking leg

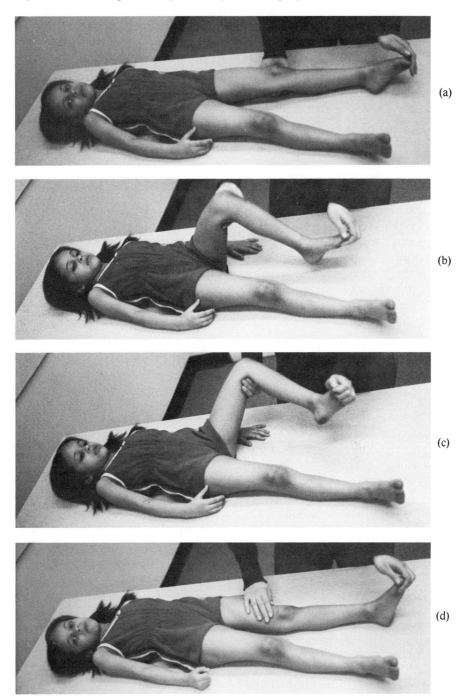

(a)

(b)

(c)

(d)

ion by upper limb flexion. Such tonic neck reflex activity should, in turn, facilitate the spinal automatism of bilateral flexion-extension movements of the lower limbs. The synreflexic chain sought then is head extension, arm extension (pulling limbs), and leg flexion (pushing limbs), followed by head flexion, arm flexion, and leg extension. If the chain is active, rhythmical head extension-flexion activity should result in homologous crawling. The presence of degrees of atrophy or dystrophy of the pattern may require that the clinician and an assistant impose the pattern until it becomes functional.

Homolateral crawling activity, which is a more advanced form of crawling, is stimulated by alternation of head lateralization to the right and to the left in prone, stimulating the asymmetrical tonic neck reflex, so that head lateralization to the right is accompanied by right limb extension and left limb flexion and vice versa. Such tonic neck activity should, in turn, facilitate the spinal automatism of associated extension-flexion movements of the lower limbs. The synreflexic chain sought then is head lateralization to the right eliciting upper limb extension—lower limb flexion on that side (pulling limbs) and the opposite movements on the left side (pushing limbs). A reversal of the pattern is manifested with the head lateralized to the left. If the chain is active, rhythmical head lateralization to the right and then to the left should result in homolateral crawling, or serialized head, neck, upper limb, trunk, and lower limb movements. If head lateralization alone does not elicit the chain response, the clinician and an assistant impose the pattern until it becomes functional.

Cross-pattern crawling activity, which is the mature pattern, is stimulated by alternating head rotation, which, in turn, may stimulate the long spinal reflexes characterized by forward thrusting of one set of diagonal limbs and backward thrusting of the opposite set of diagonal limbs. If the chain is active, rhythmical head rotation should result in cross-pattern crawling. Again, if the response is not elicited by head rotation, the pattern is imposed by the clinician and an assistant until it becomes functional.

To facilitate the integration of the synreflexic patterns by higher sensorimotor integration centers, the child should be encouraged to participate in voluntary initiation and production of the reflexive patterns as attempts are made to stimulate them reflexly.

Body extension patterns, such as in sitting and standing, are stimulated through eliciting the Landau, Schaltenbrand, and chain-in-prone reactions. Such reactions contribute to body extension and flexion movements required for bipedal sitting and standing patterns.

The Landau-Schaltenbrand reactions are stimulated with the child held in the air in the prone position and supported by one hand in the abdominal-thoracic region. The Landau reaction is manifested when the on-head righting reaction causes head righting which, in turn, stimulates tonic extension of the trunk and legs. If body extension is lacking or sluggish, running a finger down the spine, or eliciting the Perez reflex, may facilitate it. The

Schaltenbrand, or the reverse of the Landau reaction, is manifested when the righted head of the child is physically flexed which, in turn, results in flexion of the trunk and legs. The Landau reaction may be considered as preparatory to a standing pattern, while the Schaltenbrand may be viewed as preparatory to changing extensor-standing patterns to flexor-sitting patterns. Landau-Schaltenbrand reactions should be elicited in alternating fashion over a period of time, for example, five to ten cycles each time.

The chain-in-prone reaction is stimulated by placing the child in prone on a table and moving the child's head and trunk forward over the edge of the table until only the pelvis remains supported by the table. The clinician holds the child in the area of the upper thighs. The chaining phenomenon begins with the on-head righting reaction which, in turn, stimulates body-on-body righting reactions involving the neck, arms, trunk, pelvis, legs, and feet. The response is manifested by upward arching of the head and trunk, simultaneous raising and sideways stretching and flexing at the elbows of both arms, and extension of the legs. Depending on the child's reaction, different degrees of forward extension of the body over the edge of the table should be attempted, the goal being extension to the level of the pelvis.

Elicitation of the crawling pattern, and the Landau, Schaltenbrand, and chain-in-prone reactions is illustrated in Figure 7.9.

SUPPLEMENTARY TECHNIQUES

During pretzeling or reflex conditioning movements a number of tactile-proprioceptive techniques may be used to affect muscle tone, posture, and movement. The techniques may increase or reduce tone, increase general sensory stimulation, excite additional motor units, or encourage more normal or correct abnormal sensory feedbacks. They are discussed under the heading of toning, posturing, and movement techniques.

Toning Techniques

Stroking, tapping, kneading, rocking, bouncing, slapping, shaking, stretching, and compressing techniques may all be used to influence the type of muscle tonus displayed by a child.

Stroking or tapping quickly may increase tonus, and when applied to back muscles, for example, may help the child with trunk extension. Slow stroking and tapping may have the opposite effect.

Bouncing the child's buttocks on the floor, in a long sitting or tailor-sitting posture, by holding onto the child's hands and extended arms and alternately raising and lowering the child's trunk, may contribute to more normal head and trunk extension. A similar result may be accomplished by placing the child on the lap, facing toward or away from the clinician, and by bouncing the child on the knees.

Fig. 7.9. Synreflexive movements

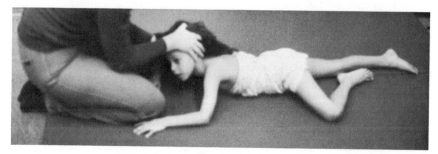

crawling pattern

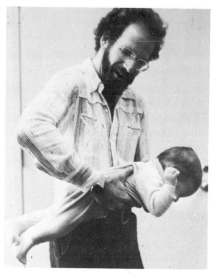

Landau reaction

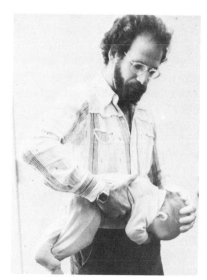

Schaltenbrand reaction

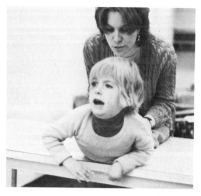

(a)

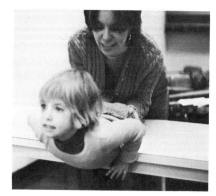

(b)

chain-in-prone reaction

Shaking a hypertonic limb or organ may reduce muscle tone if done slowly and rhythmically. Sudden and rapid shaking may accomplish the opposite effect.

Rocking in prone or supine in an up and down or front-to-back manner provides otolithic stimulation and reduces tension. Similar tension reduction may be accomplished in front-to-back and side-to-side rocking in sitting or standing.

Traction-compression maneuvers may be carried out in prone or supine, sitting, or in a hanging position. Stretching an individual by steady and measured pulling of the hands and feet should result in a counteracting increase in muscle tonus. Traction, through hanging (phyletic trace behavior), from a bar or from the clinician's hands, first with both hands and then with either hand for progressively longer periods of time may also prove useful to many children. The potential benefit from this activity is derived from the experience of total body weight bearing with fully extended limbs and from grasp functioning of the hands.

Compression maneuvers on lower or upper limbs results in cocontraction or body-weight supporting tonus. Downward pressure on the head or shoulders should also stimulate counteracting body extensor tone.

Posturing Techniques

Normal posturizing of body parts or the provision of corrective feedbacks is discussed here as posturing techniques.

Head posturing activity is done by tactile clues from the extended middle or index finger of each hand of the clinician. Head droop toward the chest would elicit from the clinician the word "crooked" and the normal front-to-back posturing of the head, with one middle finger placed on the forehead and the other on the nape of the neck, followed by the word "straight." Head droop toward the shoulder would also elicit from the clinician the word "crooked" and the normal side-to-side posturing of the head with one middle finger placed on the temple and the other on the opposite side of the neck, and the word "straight."

Trunk posturing activity is also done by tactile clues from the extended middle fingers of the hands. Forward chest droop is counteracted by pressure from one finger on the middle of the sternum and pressure from the other in the lumbar area resulting in the desired sitting or standing posture. Again, the word "crooked" should be uttered before the posturizing maneuver and the word "straight" following it. Sideways chest droop is adjusted by the application of finger pressure on the side of the upper thorax and on the opposite side of the waist.

Posturizing maneuvers with accompanying verbal reinforcement can be applied also to arms, hands, and legs.

Head and trunk posturing techniques are illustrated in Figure 7.10.

Fig. 7.10. Posturing techniques

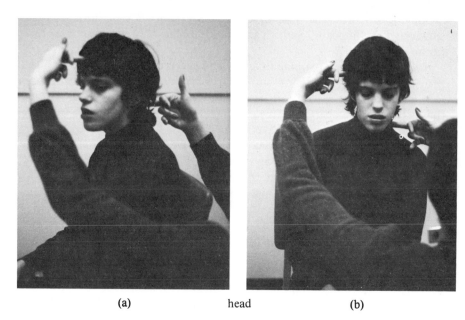

(a)   head   (b)

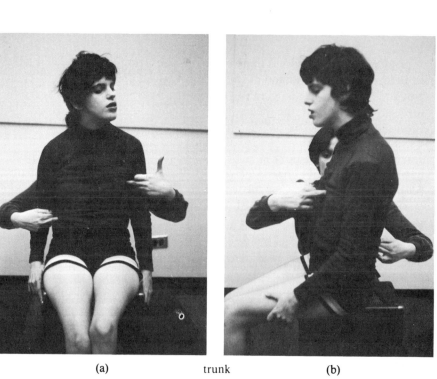

(a)   trunk   (b)

Movement Techniques

Imposing movement patterns, eliciting countermovements, and facilitating or inhibiting movements through various reinforcement techniques are described here as movement techniques.

Imposing movements and thus generating new feedbacks may be done whenever desirable movement patterns are absent in the child. Such techniques have been referred to variously as motokinesthetic techniques, passive movement work, patterning, and so on.

Imposition of homolateral and cross-pattern crawling movements was recommended by Fay and his followers. Similar maneuvers may be carried out in a creeping posture, where a clinician may guide or advance one set of upper and lower limbs in a homolateral or cross pattern and then return them to their starting position; this is then followed by advancing the other set of limbs and then returning them, and so on. The maneuver is described as static creeping and may be done by one clinician or by two. New and corrective feedback stimulation may be achieved through the maneuver.

Such imposition of movement, or more accurately of sensory feedback, may be done in any position and with all organs, including the speech organs.

Eliciting countermovements describes techniques designed to stimulate protective forms of automatic movements within the child.

Pushing a child in supine or prone forward by applying pressure to the soles of the feet could cause automatic extension of the lower limbs and reciprocal movements of the upper limbs. Applying pressure on a child's shoulders to move him along the floor may also cause automatic arm and leg movements.

Rolling the child over two or three times to the right and to the left should also elicit automatic head, arm, trunk, and leg movements.

Pulling the child by the arms or legs may also result in automatic head movements and arm, trunk, and leg movements.

Countermovements may also be stimulated by slow steady extension of the jaw, spreading of the lips, or by pushing or pulling the tongue. In each case, a point in the range of the maneuver triggers the countermovement.

Facilitating and inhibiting movements describes techniques designed to reduce excessive movements, to stimulate new movements, or to increase the range and direction of movement.

Inhibition of involuntary movements may be attempted through the technique of "fencing." The technique describes a procedure whereby involuntary movements of an involved limb may be reduced by limiting the space in which the limb is allowed to move; the space is delimited by the clinician's hands and the child is supposed to keep from touching either hand with his involved, oscillating part—the procedure may reveal that the range of oscillation of the child's body part does not have to be as great.

Facilitating new movements or increasing the range and direction of movements may be achieved by the application of various techniques already described under pretzeling, reflex conditioning, and supplementary techniques, and also by the motor unit orientation techniques of resistance, stretch, mass movement patterns, and reversal of antagonists (see Chapter 4).

BODY-IMAGE FORMATION

The last preparatory maneuver to be described is body-image formation. Adequate body-image development depends to a certain degree on the integration of sensory inflow resulting from moving normally. Body-image development is important to sensory-perceptual-symbolic maturation.

To the extent that pretzeling, reflex conditioning, and supplementary techniques have resulted in sensory-integrative-motor experiences, the phenomenon of body-image formation has been served. More specific techniques for body-image development are also recommended. Hand-body exploration accompanied by verbal reinforcement should be conducted in prone, supine, and sitting positions. The maneuvers are carried out following the law of developmental direction.

Assuming the child is unable to, or has difficulty in freely moving his hands, both the child's hands and then one at a time are directed by the clinician to the various body parts. While the hand(s) is in contact with various parts, the clinician accompanies the hand exploration with speech describing the parts and appropriate to the child's level of development. The maneuvers are carried out in the following sequence: (a) head—top, front, back, and sides, (b) face—ears, eyes, nose, mouth, chin, (c) neck—front, back, sides, (d) arms—shoulders, upper arms, elbows, forearms, wrists, palms, and fingers, (e) chest, (f) stomach, (g) buttocks, and (h) legs—thighs, kneecaps, shins, feet, and toes.

Listening Movements

Techniques for eliciting basic listening movements are identified under the headings of protective, listening, and tuning reflexes.

PROTECTIVE REFLEXES

The extensor startle reflex (Moro reflex) and the eye-closing (cochleopalpebral), eye-opening, and mouth-opening reflexes are seen as automatic, protective movements in response to loud, unexpected, or unfamiliar sounds.

Extensor Startle Reflex

The extensor startle reflex should be elicited with the child in the functional prone position. Since the reflex may be interpreted as a stabilizing movement in the prone position, the child should be placed in prone and then unexpected, unfamiliar, or loud sounds, or combinations of these factors, should be introduced. Depending on the maturity level of the child, the reflex may be stimulated repeatedly without apparent accommodation. The integration of this early reflex through daily stimulation is marked by adaptation of the reflex to repeated stimulation and eventual replacement by the more mature flexor startle pattern.

Eye Closing-Opening and Mouth-Opening Reflexes

Closing or opening reflexes of eyes and mouth in response to loud, unexpected, unfamiliar, or uncomfortable sounds are usually dependent on the distance the sound source is from the individual. Closer stimuli are more likely to elicit closing responses while more distant effective stimuli are more likely to elicit opening responses. Since these responses usually accompany the extensor-flexor startle behaviors, it may not be necessary to stimulate them separately.

Cry Reflex

Reflexive crying in response to loud, unexpected, unfamiliar, and/or uncomfortable sounds is integrated by the child via daily, graded presentation of effective auditory stimuli. Accommodation is judged by the lessening effectiveness of the stimuli in producing crying behavior.

LISTENING REFLEXES

Some of the earliest signs of true listening behavior are body stilling and cessation of suckling, or some other behavior, in response to soft, soothing, or interesting sounds such as human voices. Since such passive listening is precursory to active listening (reflected by preverbal and verbal replies to stimuli), passive listening behavior should be intentionally stimulated every day by the use of novel human vocalizations—made novel by shifting pitch, loudness, quality, and time factors. Also, exposure to various types of music—melodic, rhythmic, and so on—as well as to interesting environmental sounds such as a watch tick, running water, and so on should be planned.

TUNING REFLEXES

Auditory tuning reflexes refers to involuntary automatic responses to sound, such as changes in respiration, heartbeat, and hormonal flow, that tend to enhance listening behavior.

During attempts at eliciting listening reflexes the clinician should periodically feel the abdominal-thoracic area for respiratory shifts and listen for changes in heartbeat in response to certain sounds. Stimuli that effect such changes should be identified and periodically used on a daily basis.

Speech Postures

All techniques described under the section on preparatory maneuvers contribute to the development of basic speech postures. Specific stimulation of certain elemental, tuning, and stabilizing reflexes and reactions is also required in order to elicit, establish, and maintain back, elbow, sit, and stand speech postures. Especially appropriate discussions on facilitating various desired reflexes and reactions have been provided by the Bobaths (Bobath, K. and Bobath, B., 1964; Bobath, B., 1967) and these should be consulted. Primary and older forms of each of the major speech postures are described and pictorialized in Chapter 2. Only primary forms and methods of eliciting them are described here. All four primary forms should be stimulated once or twice a day and each movement-to-posture sequence should be repeated five to ten times. Also, whenever there is low, high, or intermittent tone, or limitations in speed, range, and direction of movement of various parts of the body, appropriate techniques of reflex conditioning and supplementary techniques described under preparatory maneuvers must be combined with the techniques described here.

BACK PATTERNS

Back-pattern speech postures are the first to be established.

Primary Form
The primary form of the back-pattern speech posture is characterized by head in alignment with the body with head and trunk in a semireclining posture, limbs gently flexed and abducted, and hands brought together and to the mouth. Such a posture allows for hand-to-mouth exploration and is conducive to reflexive vocalization.

Method of Elicitation
Elicitation of the back-pattern speech posture involves starting from a prone position, effecting a movement sequence through the stimulation of certain elemental righting reactions, and stabilizing the primary back pattern through stimulation of supine-lying balance and support movements.

Starting position in prone is designed to facilitate roll over into supine. The starting posture is characterized by face downward, neck, trunk, and legs extended, right arm in a gently extended posture above the head, with the left arm in a flexed push-off position at about the level of the face.

Movement-to-posture sequence is done through the facilitation of elemental neck, body-on-body, and on-head righting reactions. The clinician is positioned at the child's head, placing one hand under the chin and the other at the back of the head. The clinician then gently extends and rotates the head until the shoulder girdle follows, then the push-off limb is activated, and the pelvic girdle follows, and finally, roll over on the back is accomplished. Once roll over is accomplished, the clinician should stimulate the top of the head with a roll or wedge to elicit on-head righting in supine and trunk raising to the semireclining, back-pattern speech posture. Facilitation of body-righting reactions from the head is used in children with fair to good head balance and mild involvement of the arms and trunk, while facilitation of body-righting reactions from the shoulder girdle is used in children with substantial involvement of the neck and trunk. Depending on the clinician's position or the involvement of the child, shoulder girdle facilitation is done by placing the hands under the child's armpits or over the shoulders.

When parts of the movement sequence lag, the clinician should physically facilitate the movement. Accordingly, the eventual goal is to facilitate the movement with the least assistance from the clinician and, finally, without any assistance. Selective application of resistance to parts of the sequence should improve tone and movement, and segmentalization of movement is facilitated by timed resistance of the shoulder girdle and then the pelvic girdle.

Stabilization of the back-pattern posture is achieved through the facilitation of equilibrium reactions in the semireclining supine position. The child's hands may be placed on his feet, calves, or knees of his semiflexed legs and then he may be tipped gently sideways. Two responses are acceptable: a balance reaction where he may resist being tipped to the side and right himself toward the midline or a support movement where he may reach out with his limbs in a stabilizing movement. Such balance or support reactions should be stimulated following each movement sequence that leads to the assumption of the back-pattern posture.

If displacing the child's center of gravity through gentle tipping does not elicit balance and/or support reactions, the clinician should physically facilitate them until they are stimulated.

Figure 7.11 shows the starting position, and the beginning of the movement-to-posture and stabilization maneuvers for the back-pattern speech posture.

Fig. 7.11. Stimulation of back-pattern speech posture

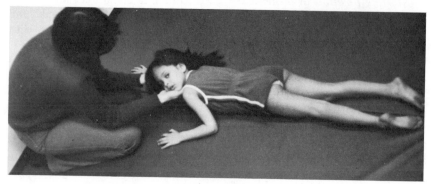

starting position

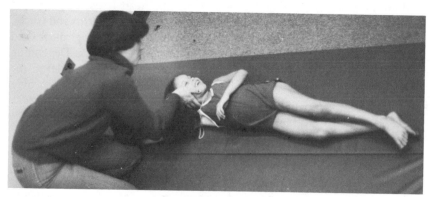

movement-to-posture

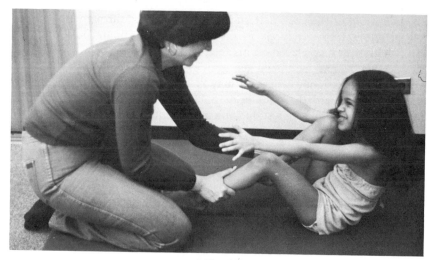

stabilization

ELBOW PATTERNS

Elbow-pattern speech postures are established next. Unlike back patterns, which are established first, elbow patterns are used much less frequently with time.

Primary Form

The primary form of the elbow-pattern speech posture is characterized by excellent head balance, good support of the upper body with upper limbs and hands, good extension of the neck and trunk, and extended abducted and outwardly rotated lower limbs. Elbow patterns result in expansion of auditory and visual perceptual fields and unilateral exploratory movements of the hand and are associated with more developed preverbal vocalization.

Method of Elicitation

Elicitation of the elbow-pattern speech posture involves starting from a supine position, effecting a movement sequence through stimulation of certain elemental righting reactions and tuning reflexes, and stabilizing the primary elbow pattern through stimulation of on-elbows balance and support movements.

Starting position in supine is characterized by the child on his back, the right arm outwardly extended somewhat above the level of the shoulder with the wrist rotated and the hand in contact with the surface, and the left leg flexed and crossed over the extended right leg.

Movement-to-posture sequence is done through the facilitation of elemental body-on-body and on-head righting reactions and of tuning Landau and chain-in-prone midbrain reactions. The clinician is positioned at the child's head; she or he places one hand on the back of the head and the other under the chin (or under the shoulders, if the shoulder facilitation technique is used). The head is then gently flexed forward and simultaneously rotated toward the right until the shoulder girdle follows and the child turns to his side. Rotation of the head continues with gradual extension of the head and spine as the body assumes the prone position. Once roll over is achieved, the clinician continues to apply a gentle, lifting action under the chin, thus further extending the head and facilitating the arm-support-forward response until the child assumes the on-elbows pattern.

The elbow pattern speech posture is tuned or primed through stimulation of the Landau and the chain-in-prone position reactions. The Landau reaction may be stimulated by—

1. holding the child free in the air in the prone position with the support hand in the abdominal-thoracic region and the stabilizing hand gently placed on the back. If the on-head righting reaction, which, in turn,

should stimulate spine and leg extension, does not occur, the child may be gently shaken or the head tapped. Physically raising the head with upward pressure applied under the chin or running the finger down the spine (Perez reflex) may also facilitate the desired body extension.

2. placing the child across the lap in the extended prone position with abducted and outwardly rotated lower limbs. Gentle extension of head and spine may result in increased extensor tone of the trunk and legs.

3. placing the child on a surface in a prone position and applying pressure on the sacrum. This may result in on-head righting, arm-support-forward, and extension of the spine reactions.

Chain-in-prone reaction is stimulated by placing the child on a plinth in the extended prone position and with abducted and outwardly rotated lower limbs. The child is slowly pushed toward one end of the plinth, until the head extends over the edge, and then the arms, and, finally, the trunk up to the pelvis. On-head righting, flexion and winglike posturing of the arms, and upward arching of the trunk is the expected response. Depending on the development of the reaction, only the head may be extended over the edge, then the arms, and, finally, progressively more of the trunk up to the level of the pelvis.

Stabilization of the elbow-pattern posture is achieved through facilitation of equilibrium reactions in prone, side lying, and on-forearms.

Prone equilibrium reactions are stimulated with the child on a prone-supine lying tilt board. With the child in the fully extended prone position, arms extended alongside the trunk, legs outwardly rotated, the board is tipped at a measured rate in order to elicit the reaction. Upward arching of the body toward the raised side and extension and abduction of the limbs in balance and support movements is the expected response.

Side-lying responses are elicited with the child in a modified fetal position with the under arm in a gently flexed position above the head. The upper arm is pulled by the clinician to raise the trunk from the surface, stimulating on-head righting and an arm-support-sideways response of the under arm.

On-forearms equilibrium reactions are facilitated with the child on forearms and with the clinician positioned in front of the child. The clinician gently pushes the child's shoulders from side to side, eliciting balance and support reaction tonus in the arms.

Figure 7.12 shows the starting position and the stabilization maneuver for the elbow-pattern speech posture.

SIT PATTERNS

Sit-pattern speech postures are the first erect form and are the most frequently used speech postures.

Fig. 7.12.   Stimulation of elbow-pattern speech posture

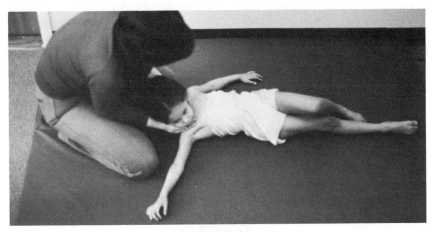

starting position

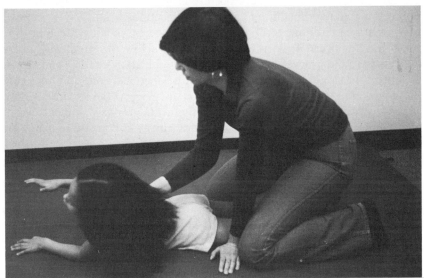

stabilization

Primary Form

The primary form of the sit-pattern speech posture is characterized by excellent head balance, an extended spine, flexed hips, and extended knees. Side-sitting postures as well as long sitting postures are considered primary forms. Sitting postures bring still further expansion of auditory and visual perceptual fields and increased exploratory activity of the hands. Primary talking may have reached the true echolalia stage.

Method of Elicitation

Elicitation of the sit-pattern speech posture involves starting from a supine position, initiating a movement sequence through stimulation of a chain of elemental righting reactions, resulting in a sitting posture, and stabilizing the posture by stimulation of arm-support and arm-balance reactions.

Starting position in supine is the same as the starting position for the elbow pattern, since the sitting posture is achieved via the complete rotation pattern that brings the child from supine into prone lying.

Movement-to-posture sequence includes the same maneuvers described under the elbow-pattern sequence that results in the child rolling over from supine into prone lying. Once the child is in prone, upward pressure is applied bilaterally in the pelvic area facilitating the assumption of the creeping position. Once in the on-fours position, a backward-sideways guiding movement brings the child into side sitting and then into long sitting.

Sitting is also tuned through elicitation of Landau and chain-in-prone reactions.

Stabilization of the sit-pattern posture is accomplished through stimulation of on-fours and in-sitting equilibrium reactions.

On-fours equilibrium reactions are facilitated by rocking the child forward and backward from the waist or from below the shoulders, or by pushing the child sideways from the hips or shoulders. The force and degree of movement should be measured to elicit balance reactions and not cause the child to fall. Equilibrium reactions that are prerequisite for creeping are elicited by raising one leg or arm and gently rocking forward and backward, and then by raising an arm and leg simultaneously and gently rocking forward and backward.

Arm-support reactions forward, sideways, and backward in sitting should be stimulated. In long sitting, the child's trunk should be brought forward; the thighs well flexed, abducted, and externally rotated at the hips; and with the hands brought to the feet. Gentle forward pushing at the back of the head or shoulder should elicit an arm-support-forward reaction. Arm-support sideways reaction may be stimulated by extending and abducting one arm and gently pushing the child toward the opposite side, thereby facilitating the extension of the arm on that side. The clinician can also be positioned on the side to which the support movement is desired. By extending the child's fingers and wrist with one hand and using the other hand to control the elbow and shoulder, the child can be pulled toward the side while his hand and arm are gradually lowered in a support movement. Arm-support-backward reaction is similarly facilitated with additional attention being paid to extension of the dorsal spine and shoulder.

Arm-balance reactions should also be elicited in long and side sitting. In long sitting, the child's body is held lightly at the sides of his trunk and slowly tipped to one side; the expected response is on-head righting and extension and abduction of the limbs opposite to the side of weight transference. Also in long sitting, one leg, and then later both of the child's legs, may be held below the knees, lifted, and then bent toward the trunk; the legs should be abducted and outwardly rotated. The expected balance response is arm extension and forward movement of the arms and upper body to prevent falling backward. In side sitting, with arms in nonsupporting positions, the child is required to maintain his balance while the clinician shifts both legs to the opposite side.

Figure 7.13 shows movement-to-posture and stabilization maneuvers for the sit-pattern speech posture.

STAND PATTERNS

Stand-pattern speech postures herald the maturation of the speech brain to the true talking level.

Primary Form

The primary form of the stand-pattern speech posture is characterized by the independent assumption of free standing, that is, standing without assistance from prone or supine lying. Standing postures represent the maximum expansion of the child's auditory and visual perceptual fields and usually co-occur with the onset of true speech.

Method of Elicitation

Elicitation of the stand-pattern speech posture involves starting from a supine position, initiating a movement sequence through stimulation of a chain of elemental righting reactions culminating in a standing posture, and stabilizing the posture by stimulation of various equilibrium reactions in standing.

Starting position in supine is the same as the starting positions for the elbow and sit-speech postures since the first phase in achieving a stand-pattern speech posture is to stimulate roll over from supine into prone lying.

Movement-to-posture sequence includes the same maneuvers described under the sit-pattern sequence that brings the child to the quadrupedal or creeping position. From this position, continued upward pressure applied bilaterally to the pelvic region should result in extension of the knees and legs into the simian stance, and then gentle forward pressure applied to the area of the lower trunk region should facilitate standing. Or, from the quadrupedal position, upward pressure is gently applied under the chin (or shoulders), further extending the head and dorsal spine, and facilitating the on-knees position; then, gentle pulling of the head forward by holding one hand at the back of the head and the other under the chin should facilitate the half-kneel and, finally, the standing position.

Fig. 7.13. Stimulation of sit-pattern speech posture

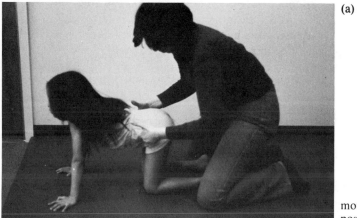

(a)

movement-to-posture

(b)

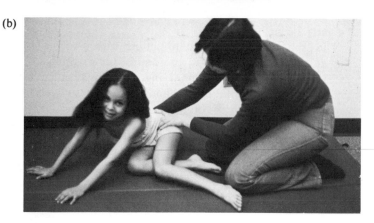

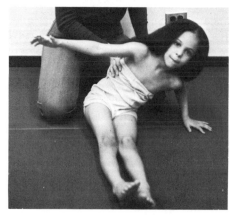

stabilization

Tuning for the stand-pattern sequence includes eye-movement lead and head movement lead reactions; that is, stimulating upward eye rotation and upward head rotation prior to facilitating kneel-standing, for example. On-head righting and body extension patterns, associated with the Landau and chain-in-prone reactions, also serve as tuning reactions for standing patterns.

Stabilization of the stand-pattern posture is accomplished through stimulation of equilibrium reactions at the intervening postures from on-knees through standing.

On-knees equilibrium reactions are stimulated sideways by lightly holding the child at the sides of the chest and gently rocking the child from side to side; the expected response is abduction and extension of the limbs opposite to the side of weight transference. On-knees equilibrium reactions are stimulated backward by gently pushing backward with an outspread hand against the sternum; the expected response is a forward movement of the head, arms, and trunk. On-knees equilibrium reactions are stimulated forward by gently pushing forward in the area of the lumbar spine; the expected response includes a backward movement of the head and arms. Whenever balance is lost by the child during stimulation of on-knees equilibrium reactions, the clinician should provide counterbalancing or counterpoising pushes or taps to assist the child in regaining balance. Such losing and regaining of balance activities corresponds with the concept that body progression, whether it be creeping, knee-walking, or walking, is a matter of sequentially losing and regaining balance.

Half-kneel equilibrium reactions are stimulated by having the child assume the half-kneel position first with his right knee serving as the support knee and then his left knee. The clinician holds the standing knee in each instance and the opposite hip and gently moves the child forward, sideways, and backward. The expected response is balance reactions of the head, arms, and trunk. Again, whenever needed, counterbalancing taps, pushes, and holds are provided by the clinician to assist the child in maintaining balance.

Various standing equilibrium reactions are stimulated:

1. Upper-body standing reactions are stimulated with the child in a well-balanced standing position. The clinician holds the child above the knees and gently pushes the child's thighs forward, sideways, backward and, finally, in a rotatory fashion. The expected response is a mobilized pelvis, and balance movements of the trunk, arms, and head.
2. Sideways standing reactions are stimulated with the child in a well-balanced standing position. The clinician holds the child by her hips and shifts the child's weight from side to side. The expected response

is extension and abduction of the limbs opposite to weight transference.

3. Step-position standing reactions are stimulated with the child standing well balanced with one foot in front of the other. The clinician then pushes the child backward with pressure applied to the sternum and forward with pressure applied to the back. The expected response is balance movements of the knees, pelvis, trunk, arms, and head. Similar maneuvers are carried out with alternation of the front and back foot with one foot serving as front foot at least three times.

4. One-leg standing reactions are stimulated with the child standing on one leg with the clinician positioned behind the child holding the other leg by the ankle at a right angle and providing further support by holding the opposite hip. The clinician then moves the child gently in a forward, sideways, backward, and a rotatory fashion. Again, the expected response is balance movements of the knee, pelvis, trunk, arms, and head.

5. Hopping reactions are stimulated with the child in a well-balanced standing position. The clinician is positioned behind the child and holds the child under the arms at the sides of the trunk. The child is then moved briskly in forward and backward directions eliciting hopping or stepping movements. The child is also moved sideways eliciting cross-over stepping movements.

Figure 7.14 shows movement-to-posture and stabilization maneuvers for the stand-pattern speech posture.

Hand Movements

Basic hand movements that contribute to the development of the symbolic and adjunctive gestural movements comprising hands talk are categorized under protective, progression, and vegetative reflexes. In preparation for the use of hands-talk movements, these reflexive hand movements should be stimulated.

PROTECTIVE REFLEXES

Arm-support-forward, sideways, and backward and arm-balance reactions are the protective movements to be stimulated.

Arm-Support Reactions

Of particular interest in eliciting arm-support reactions as background for hands-talk movements is the first phase of the support movement, that is, limb extension and hand and finger extension.

Fig. 7.14. Stimulation of stand-pattern speech posture

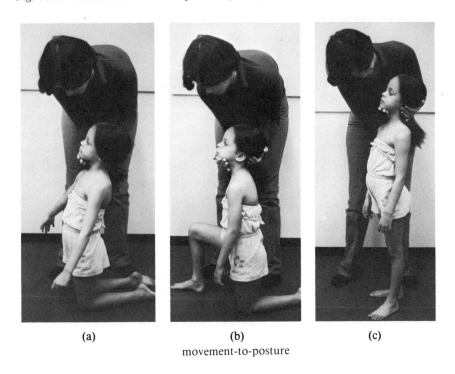

(a)   (b)   (c)

movement-to-posture

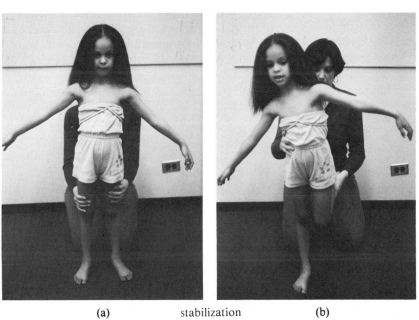

(a)   stabilization   (b)

With the child in prone lying, the clinician, who is situated behind and to the side of the child, grasps the shoulders and lifts them backward and upward. The expected response is arm and hand extension in a supportive movement.

With the child in side sitting, the clinician holds the child by one arm extended and outwardly rotated at the shoulder and forearm, and pulls or pushes the child forward, sideways, diagonally, or backward. Arm and hand extension in a supportive movement in the various directions is the expected response. To better control the support movement, the clinician can also hold the elbow, wrist, and hand of the support limb in an extended pattern and pull the child in various directions while gradually lowering the extended hand toward the support surface.

With the child in stool sitting, the clinician can also facilitate sideways support movements by extending and abducting the control arm and pushing the child sideways. Backward support movements are facilitated by extending the child's dorsal spine.

With the child in the on-knees position, the clinician holds the shoulders from behind and slowly lowers the child forward and downward. The one-arm version is done by holding one arm in an extended, abducted, and outwardly rotated fashion and pushing the body downward with it in various directions in order to elicit movements from the support arm.

Arm-Balance Reactions

The arm-balance movements characterized by limb extension and abduction opposite to the side of weight transference are also considered important background relative to hands-talk movements.

Arm-balance reactions should be stimulated in sitting, kneeling, and standing positions.

Examples of arm support and balance reactions are shown in Figure 2.5.

PROGRESSION REFLEXES

Arm progression reflexes include upper limb movement, upper limb placing, arm walking, and quadrupedal hopping activities.

Descriptions of the manner of stimulating most of these reflexes are provided in the arm-reflexes portion of the reflex conditioning section of this chapter. The portion on eliciting various hand reflexes is also pertinent to this discussion.

Examples of arm walking and upper limb placing are shown in Figure 2.6.

VEGETATIVE REFLEXES

Arm-hand vegetative reflexes include hand-to-mouth movements in general, as well as hand-to-mouth feeding activity; both activities should be stimulated.

Hand-to-Mouth Movements

Hand-to-mouth activity may be facilitated in side lying, supine lying, and sitting positions.

With the child in side lying, in a symmetrical pattern with the shoulders moved forward, the hands are brought together and to the mouth.

With the child in supine lying, the child's feet and hands are brought together and both are brought forward to the mouth. Also, the child may be pulled into sitting while simultaneously flexing the arms and bringing the hands to the mouth.

With the child in long sitting with abducted legs, well-flexed hips, and hands to feet, the hands may then be brought to the child's mouth.

Hand-to-Mouth Feeding

Hand-to-mouth feeding movements should be encouraged by placing the child's hands around the breast while suckling, by placing the child's hands around the bottle while suckling, or by placing cookies or biscuits in the child's hand and guiding it to the mouth.

Also, whenever the child is being spoon fed, the feeder should feed in such a way that the child's right hand is grasping the spoon or at least is being guided to move along with the spoon as it is brought to the child's mouth.

An example of hand-to-mouth feeding is shown in Figure 2.7.

Speech Movements

Basic speech movements that contribute to the development of skilled speech movements are categorized under protective, emotional, and vegetative reflexes, and reflexive vocalization. Whenever appropriate, all such basic movements should be stimulated.

PROTECTIVE REFLEXES

Among the protective reflexes to be stimulated are the glottic closing-opening reflexes, sneeze-cough reflexes, jaw-jerk-palatal reflexes, and lips-tongue protective movements.

Glottic Closing-Opening Reflexes

Reflexive head and neck extension and glottic opening are protective against interference with breathing. Such a glottic opening reflex may be stimulated by periodically occluding the child's nostrils by pinching them closed with the fingers. Reflexive glottic opening may also be "heard" during the inspiratory phase of vigorous crying.

Reflexive head and neck flexion and glottic closing are protective against the inspiration of noxious inhalants. Pungent odors such as those associated with vinegar or ammonia may elicit reflexive glottic closing.

Sneeze-Cough Reflexes

Reflexive sneezing serves the purpose of clearing the nasopharyngeal area of foreign matter, while reflexive coughing serves the purpose of clearing the laryngopharyngeal and oropharyngeal areas.

Reflexive sneezing may be triggered by soap powder, other harmless powdery material like pepper, and by stimulating the nostril area with a wisp of cotton.

Reflexive coughing may be elicited by inhaling pungent odors such as those associated with ammonia, vinegar, horseradish, and so on.

Jaw-Jerk-Palatal Reflexes

Reflexive jaw-jerk may be viewed as protective against excessive mandibular extension and consequent jaw injury. The jaw jerk may be elicited by the clinician placing the index or middle finger of one hand across the mental prominence of the mandible and briskly tapping the finger with the ends of the middle three fingers of the other hand. Another jaw-closing reflex can be stimulated by slowly and steadily extending the child's jaw until the tendency for jaw closing is sensed. Such maneuvers should serve to counter the habitual open-mouth posture or jaw droop frequently observed among children with cerebral palsy.

The palatal reflex may be viewed as not only important for creating negative or positive intraoral breath pressure required for suckling and swallowing but as protective against intrusion into the nasopharynx by foreign bodies. Reflexive velar elevation may be evoked by touching or stroking the velar raphe with a Q-tip. Activation of the reflex should contribute to more normal velopharyngeal closure and consequent reduction in the tendency for hypernasality among the cerebral palsied.

Lips-Tongue Protective Movements

Protective lip spreading may be summoned by slow and steady lateral compression of the lips. As soon as the clinician senses the lip countermovement, the compression maneuver should be terminated. Similarly, protective lip puckering may be stimulated by slow and steady spreading of the corners of the lips.

Protective tongue protrusion may be evoked by the use of chemical stimuli such as bitter substances placed on the tongue tip or blade—for example, touching the tongue tip with a slice of lemon or other foods known not to be liked by the child. Also, slowly and steadily pushing the child's tongue tip and blade back into his mouth with the clinician's finger or tongue depressor may also elicit a counteracting movement of the tongue.

EMOTIONAL REFLEXES

Among a number of other contributions to developing speech, cry, smile, and laugh reflexes contribute to the development of appropriate emotional color during speech. Daily excitation of these behaviors with emphasis on smile and laugh reflexes by parents, clinicians, and friends of the child should be planned. Numerous forms of movements, faces, noises, and touches constitute the appropriate stimuli.

VEGETATIVE REFLEXES

Among the vegetative reflexes to be stimulated are those associated with breathing and eating.

Vegetative Breathing

Goals in improving vegetative breathing include deepening breathing cycles, normalizing bpms, and stimulating thoracic participation in respiration. Techniques for stimulating respiration may be categorized under inspiratory reflex and inspiratory facilitation techniques and are based on the creation of oxygen need and on changes in intrathoracic air pressure.

Inspiratory reflex maneuvers include four techniques: evoking the yawn reflex by having the clinician simulate a deep yawn in the child's visual field, restricting the child's airway, having the child hold his breath or exhaust his breath, and by the application of chest-press or back-press techniques.

With the child in a back-pattern speech posture, the clinician may pinch the child's nostrils closed with his fingers, or he may ask the child to close his mouth, or he may hold the child's mouth closed, or he may hold the child's mouth closed and also press closed one nostril. The latter form of inspiratory restriction is the one most likely to trigger an inspiratory reflex. The child may also be asked to hold his breath for as long as possible, or to exhaust his breath by breathing out for as long as possible; both techniques may also evoke an inspiratory reflex. Or, the inspiratory reflex may be evoked by the application of downward pressure in the abdominal-thoracic area at the end of a regular expiratory phase, thus entering the child's expiratory reserve volume.

With the child in an elbow-pattern speech posture, all the aforementioned techniques may be repeated, except for the chest press. In the elbow pattern, the back press technique is used by applying downward pressure in the lumbar area at the end of an expiratory phase.

Again, except for the chest and back press techniques, all the other inspiratory reflex techniques may be used in sit- and stand-pattern speech postures.

Inspiratory facilitation maneuvers include four techniques: the arm lift (modified Silvester method of artificial respiration), leg roll, accordion, and butterfly techniques.

1. The vegetative arm-lift technique is done with the child in supine lying and with the clinician kneeling behind the top of the child's head. The clinician grasps the child's lower forearms and crosses them in parallel fashion over the child's lower chest. He then rocks forward until his arms are fully extended and exerts steady downward pressure facilitating expiration. Near, or at the end of the expiratory maneuver, the clinician quickly rocks backward and simultaneously extends and abducts the child's arms above the level of the child's head facilitating inspiration. The cycle should be repeated 12 to 20 times per minute.

2. The vegetative leg-roll technique is done with the child in supine lying either on a mat or plinth and with the clinician at the child's feet or at his side. The clinician grasps the child's shins, flexes and abducts the legs, and presses them toward the child's axillae, thereby displacing the viscera upward, stretching the diaphragm, and facilitating expiration. At the end of the expiratory phase, the clinician quickly extends and brings the legs downward, returning them to their original position and facilitating inspiration. A rhythm similar to normal vegetative breathing should be imposed. A variation of the leg-roll maneuver is done during the inspiratory phase by holding the shoulder girdle, and when the knees are about level with the waist, moving both legs toward one side, thus rotating the pelvis, returning both knees to the center position, and, finally, returning the legs to their original position.

3. The vegetative accordion technique is done with the child in a side-lying, semiflexed position, preferably on a plinth, and with the clinician facing the child and being positioned near the child's waist. The clinician holds the back of the child's neck with one hand, the shins with the other, pushes the child into maximum flexion, and facilitates expiration. At the end of the expiratory phase, the clinician quickly places the neck hand under the chin, and the shin hand on the calves, extends the child to the original position, and facilitates inspiration. A rhythm similar to normal vegetative breathing should be imposed.

4. The vegetative butterfly technique is done with the child in stool sitting and with the clinician positioned behind the child. The clinician places the child's clasped hands on the back of the child's head, abducts the child's elbows, and extends his head and dorsal spine, thus facilitating

inspiration. At the end of the inspiratory phase, the clinician quickly adducts the elbows, flexes the child's head and spine, and brings the head, arms, and shoulders down between abducted knees and facilitates expiration.

Examples of arm lift, leg roll, accordion, and butterfly maneuvers are shown in Figures 7.15, 16, 17, and 18.

Eating

Improvement of early eating movements, such as positioning for, and transporting, grasping, manipulating, preparing, and swallowing of foods should contribute to the development of skilled speech movements.

These early eating movements are considered a first-level integration and elaboration of feeding reflexes, that is, they reflect at least a semivoluntary use of these patterns. Accordingly, when semisolid or solid food is first introduced into the infant's mouth, reflexive movements associated with breast or bottle feeding may be observed and the infant appears to be "suckling" rather than "eating" the food. Integration of these basic

Fig. 7.15. Inspiratory facilitation maneuvers: arm-lift technique

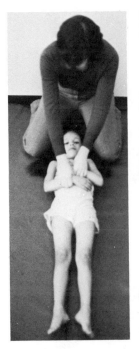 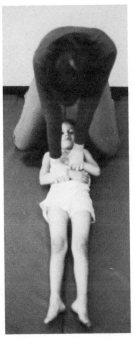 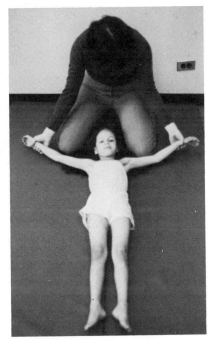

arms cross   arms press   arms spread

Fig. 7.16. Inspiratory facilitation maneuvers: leg-roll technique

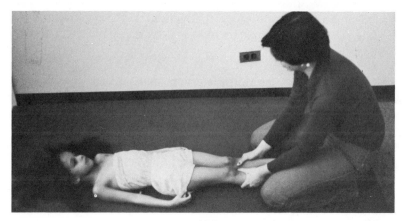

start

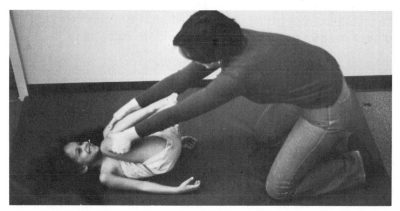

legs flex

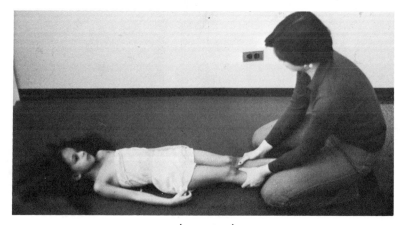

legs extend

Fig. 7.17. Inspiratory facilitation maneuvers: accordion technique

Fig. 7.18. Inspiratory facilitation maneuvers: butterfly technique

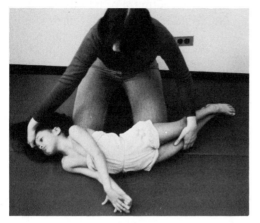

inflow

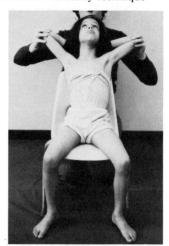

inflow

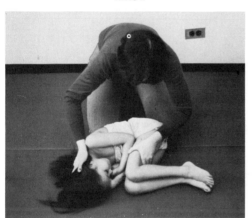

outflow

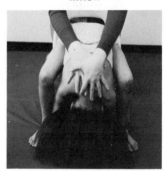

outflow

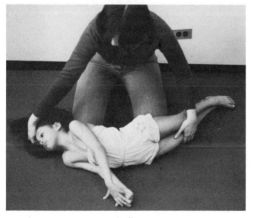

inflow

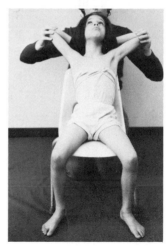

inflow

reflexes is observed when the child modifies rooting, lip, mouth-opening, tongue, biting, suckling, chewing, and swallow reflexive movements into movements more appropriate to the processing and ingesting of solid foods.

Improvement of eating movements is done through (a) the stimulation of the chain of feeding reflexes and (b) the facilitation of actual eating activity.

Feeding reflexes to be stimulated include the rooting, lip, mouth-opening, tongue, biting, suckle, chewing, and swallow reflexes. Stimulation of these reflexes should be done if their dysintegration is of the atrophic form; if dysintegration is of the dystrophic or hypertrophic form, techniques to facilitate their integration into mature eating movements should be employed. Since methods of stimulating feeding reflexes and descriptions of expected responses are found in the "Vegetative Reflexes" section of Chapter 2, these are not repeated here; however, comments pertinent to therapeutic stimulation of these reflexes are offered. Meader (1940) was one of the early workers to recommend the stimulation of feeding reflexes such as sucking, chewing, and swallowing in therapy for certain speech problems. Natural stimuli should be used to stimulate these reflexes such as a finger, nipple, part of a biscuit or a cookie, or a pretzel stick. Also, if the reflexive movement is not evoked, it should be imposed by the clinician until the reflex emerges or the movement can be voluntarily accomplished by the child.

When stimulating the rooting reflex, which is a head-turning reflex toward a food source, the stimulus should be brought into the upper- or lower-face visual fields and side-face visual fields. More direct stimulation should also be applied such as stroking or tapping the upper and lower lips, corners of the mouth, or cheeks. The clinician first seeks appropriate head turn toward the stimulus—up, down, to the right, and to the left. Head turning may also be accompanied by other parts of the feeding chain such as lip and mouth opening and tongue orientation toward the stimulus. If stimulation for rooting triggers the entire feeding chain, that is, lip movement, mouth opening, biting, tongue movement, suckling-chewing, and swallowing, the clinician has accomplished more than if only part of the chain was stimulated.

When stimulating the lip reflex, characterized by lip movements, closure, and pursing as in preparation for or during eating (such movements are seen in older individual who are anticipating eating some favorite food like ice cream, a pickle, or steak), the middle of the lips may be touched or tapped with the stimulus or the upper or lower quadrants of the lips may be stroked. Successful lip stimulation may evoke the reflexive links following lip activity, that is, mouth-opening, biting, tongue, suckle-chewing, and swallowing, and this should be sought.

When stimulating the mouth-opening reflex, the stimulus should be brought into the visual field from different directions and moved toward the mouth. If necessary, the middle of the lips may be touched, lightly pressed, or the clinician may move the stimulus gently on the lips. Successful stimulation of mouth-opening may trigger the consequent reflexive links of biting, tongue movement, suckle-chewing, and swallowing, especially if the stimulus is allowed to enter the mouth.

When stimulating biting, or mandibular grasping, touch or slight pressure is applied to the incisor-gingival areas. Movements of the stimulus may facilitate the grasping response. Elicitation of biting may stimulate the consequent reflexive links of tongue movement, suckle-chewing, and swallowing.

When stimulating the tongue reflex, characterized by protrusion-retrusion or lateroflexion movements in response to touch or pressure stimuli, the stimulus is applied to the tip or blade to elicit tongue protrusion (part of suckle) or the lateral margins of the tongue to stimulate tongue lateroflexion (part of chewing). Consequent reflexive links include suckling or chewing movements and swallowing.

When stimulating the suckling reflex, which represents a feeding chain in itself composed of lip, mouth-opening, grasping, tongue movement, and swallowing activities, the stimulus may be brought into contact with the lips, gingiva, tongue tip and blade, or hard palate. Gentle movements of the stimulus facilitate suckling.

When stimulating the chewing reflex, the stimulus is touched or pressed in the incisor-gingival or molar-gingival areas. Rubbing the molar teeth may also stimulate chewing movements. The consequent reflexive link is swallowing.

When stimulating the swallowing reflex, which is the ultimate reflexive link in the feeding chain, visceral or somatic forms may be observed, depending on the age and condition of the child. Anticipatory swallow may be stimulated whenever an attractive food stimulus is brought into the visual field and such anticipatory swallowing is present to varying degrees throughout life. Adequate stimuli for swallowing include coughing, sneezing, and hiccoughing, and touching and stroking the palate, fauces, back of the tongue, and posterior pharyngeal wall. Other techniques for stimulating swallow include (a) directing a stream of water or other liquid from an eye dropper past the velum and (b) inserting a straw well back into the child's mouth and periodically blowing gentle puffs of air into the child's oropharynx. About two reflexive swallows per minute for about 10 minutes a session and two or three times a day should contribute to the reduction of drooling secondary to hypoactive swallow reflex.

Examples of the elicitation of some of these reflexes are displayed in Figure 3.3.

Eating movements to be facilitated include head and body positioning toward the food source, a number of intermediate processing movements, and, finally, swallowing. It is during work on the facilitation of eating movements that integration of the chain of feeding reflexes are facilitated. Among the early advocates of feeding therapy to improve speech movements were Meader (1940), Palmer (1947), and Westlake (1951). Continued interest and development of feeding therapy as an adjunct of speech therapy and in the treatment of dysphagia is manifested by the accumulated literature in the area (e.g., see Blanchard, 1964; Bosley, 1965; Mueller, 1972; Larsen, 1972; Griffin, 1974; Davis, 1978; Sheppard, 1978). The recommendations for facilitation of eating movements here are eclectic and are based on experience, observation, and many of the views of the above-mentioned workers. The nine factors to consider in a program of facilitation of eating movements are nursing, positioning, protecting, priming, transporting, grasping, manipulating, preparing, and swallowing.

1. Nursing as a factor in the facilitation of eating movements—Whenever possible mothers of children suspected of, or diagnosed as having cerebral palsy, should be encouraged to nurse their babies. Nursing facilitates the emergence of the chain of feeding reflexes; provides milk that affords excellent nutrition, unique immunological protection, and reduces the chances of the infant contracting various diseases and conditions; provides maternal heartbeat, voice, and facial stimulation; and is the prototype for future face-to-face communication. If, because of the degree of involvement of the child, nursing does not provide sufficient nourishment, supplementary bottle feeding should, of course, be provided. The brain-involved child needs the various benefits of nursing much more than the normal child, even when "nourishment" from nursing is other than food nourishment.

   Along with nursing is the desirability for eating therapy to be conducted whenever possible by parents and other family members. The clinician should begin the work, demonstrate the techniques, observe progress of the mother and family in carrying out the techniques, assign the techniques, and periodically check family progress with the techniques.

2. Positioning as a factor in the facilitation of eating movements—Numerous workers (e.g., Mueller, 1972; Davis, 1978; Sheppard, 1978) stress the importance of proper positioning in eating therapy. Some of the benefits to be derived from proper positioning, in addition to facilitating eating, may include facilitation of integration of tonic neck and labyrinthine reflexes, and a consequent increase in body-part differentiation and symmetry, and a reduction in chances of food aspiration. By positioning here is meant not only the final eating position, but also the child's ability to adjust and orient the body toward the food source. At least three speech postures, with

some modifications, serve as eating postures—the back-pattern, elbow-pattern, and sit-pattern postures. Since eating and speaking may be concomitant functions, eating and speaking postures should share common features. Correspondingly, whenever possible, eating and speaking should be stimulated together.

a. Back-pattern eating postures are used for young infants or severely involved children. The basic pattern is head somewhat flexed and in good alignment, hands capable of being brought together and to the mouth, and lower limbs partially flexed and abducted. The classic back-pattern eating position is the lateral position with the child across the mother's lap and with his head cradled in the crook of the mother's arm. The frontal position is where the child is positioned on the lap vertically in front of the mother or clinician. The position is facilitated by having the feeder seated in front of a table with feet on a stool or roll, and with the child placed on a pillow or wedge that spans the lap and edge of the table. To ensure adequate flexion of the head an additional small roll or pillow may be placed under the child's neck. To ensure adequate adduction of the shoulders, and flexion and symmetry of the arms, the child's hands are brought forward and together in the midline. To ensure adequate flexion and abduction of the lower limbs, the child's legs may be abducted around the feeder's waist or the child's feet may be placed against the feeder's abdomen.

In either of the back-pattern postures, the feeder should periodically, and in a measured way, unbalance the child's position just before the next feeding maneuver in order to excite within the child automatic adjustment movements as the food source approaches the child. As necessary, the automatic adjustment movements should be facilitated by the feeder.

b. Elbow-pattern eating postures are used to facilitate the child's reaching and grasping movements while being fed (hand-to-mouth feeding) and to assist with special eating problems. For example, Bosma (1960, 1963) recommended the prone feeding position for children with serious suckling and swallowing problems and functional retrusion of the mandible. The basic pattern is extension of the head, neck, and trunk; upper limb support of the extended upper body; and extension, abduction, and outward rotation of the legs. Across-the-lap positions may be achieved in at least two ways (Mueller, 1972): the child may be placed across an asymmetrical lap formed by the clinician crossing her legs in a way designed to slant the child's body upward at various angles; or the child may be placed across an asymmetrical lap formed by the clinician placing one leg on a small stool or a roll.

To satisfy the adjusting criterion of the elbow-pattern eating postures, and after postures are established, the clinician should periodically, as she brings the food source into the child's visual field, unbalance the lap postures in various ways and to various degrees. The unbalancing maneuver is done to stimulate body adjusting movements on the part of the child, so that he may receive the food most efficiently.

c. Sit-pattern eating postures represent mature eating postures and should be used as soon as possible. The basic pattern is erect sitting with good head and neck balance, extended spine, and flexed hips. Slight neck and shoulder flexion and full hip flexion are desirable. Depending on the status of the child, at least two sitting positions may be used: lap sitting and chair sitting. In lap sitting the child is placed across the lap with well-flexed hips, knees somewhat abducted, and with one of the clinician's arms around the child's back. Flexion in the child's hips and knees may be increased by the clinician raising one of her legs and creating an asymmetrical lap. In chair sitting, the child is positioned with slightly flexed neck and shoulders, with elbows at right angles, hips fully flexed, knees somewhat abducted, and feet on the ground.

To satisfy the adjusting criterion of the sit-pattern eating postures, and after the postures are established, the lap position may be periodically unbalanced in measured fashion, or the food may be placed in front of the child in such a way as to require the child to make orienting movements and body adjustments in order to obtain the food most efficiently.

Back-pattern, elbow-pattern, and sit-pattern eating postures and three-finger cradle manuevers are shown in Figures 7.19, 20, and 21.

3. Protecting against aspiration, choking, and undesirable foods as a factor in the facilitation of eating movements—Some workers (e.g., Sheppard, 1978) stress the importance of the presence of the gag reflex in patient selection for swallowing therapy.

Certainly, clinicians involved in eating therapy should be concerned about the presence of oral protective reflexes. For example, does the child demonstrate reflexive mouth closure when undesirable objects approach the mouth?; or reflexive tongue protrusion when something undesirable or bitter enters the mouth?; or reflexive sneeze, cough, palatal, and pharyngeal reflexes when undesirable or unwanted materials have entered further into the oral and nasal cavities?

Protective mouth closure and tongue protrusion may be stimulated with foods known to be undesirable to the child. Such activities must be done within as pleasant an "exercise atmosphere" as possible. The manner of eliciting the protective sneeze, cough, and palatal reflexes has already been discussed.

Fig. 7.19. Back-pattern eating posture

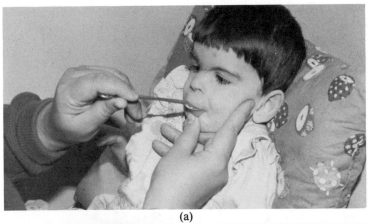

(a)

frontal
position

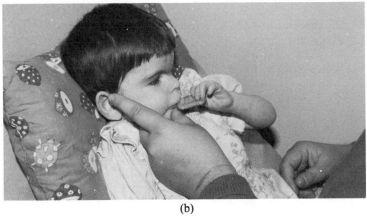

(b)

Fig. 7.20. Elbow-pattern eating posture

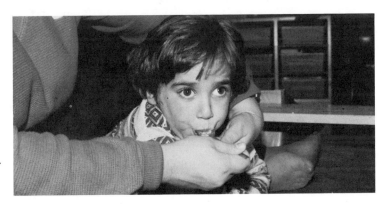

Fig. 7.21.   Sit-pattern eating postures

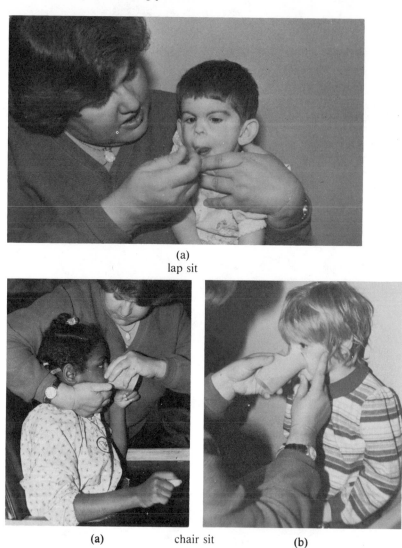

(a)
lap sit

(a)   chair sit   (b)

Courtesy of United Cerebral Palsy of New York State and of New York City and of Leslie Davis.

Another protective procedure is to ensure that the mouth is free of any unswallowed morsels following each session of eating therapy. Also, it should be remembered that a general flexor pattern tends to facilitate swallowing and protect against aspiration.

4. Priming of orofacial muscles as a factor in the facilitation of eating movements—Pre-eating ("natural priming") movements of jaw, lips, tongue, and swallowing are frequently observed in individuals who are

about to eat. The concept of "muscle priming" here encompasses the sensory stimulation techniques of Rood (Stockmeyer, 1967) and the desensitizing techniques of the Bobaths (Mueller, 1972; Davis, 1978).

Improvement of neck stability and laryngeal control and jaw and lip activity may be gained through the application of special sensory stimulation to the neck, jaw, and lip muscles. For example, pressure applied to the top of the head and to the mandibular joint may contribute to stability of the head and mandible, while quick touch and tapping of lip and jaw muscles may facilitate their mobility.

Reduction of sensitivity in chest, shoulders, neck, face, and oral areas is the other form of muscle priming. Intended or inadvertent stimulation of the chest, neck, face, and oral areas in some children with cerebral palsy may trigger various involuntary movements including startle movements. Tolerance of stimulation and eventual adaptation may be attained gradually (a) by daily handling by the clinician and parents and then self-handling by the child of sensitive chest, neck, face, and oral areas and (b) by the clinician stimulating affected areas and resisting any associated involuntary movements. Stimulation of the chest, shoulders, neck and face areas may include touching, tapping, stroking, and kneading. Stimulation of the facial area with wash cloths and soft toys followed by stimulation of the oral area with soft toys was also suggested as desensitizing techniques (Davis, 1978).

Some specific techniques for normalizing facial and oral area sensitivity were described by Mueller (1972). What has been called in Chapter 2 a three-finger cradle posture is used as a jaw, lip, tongue control maneuver in back, elbow, or sitting positions. In the frontal position, three-finger cradle, I is formed by the clinician's thumb under the child's lower lip, the index finger on the cheek, and the middle finger under the chin and across the soft tissue; in the side position, the clinician's arm is around the back of the child's head and three-finger cradle, II is formed by the thumb across the cheek, the index finger under the lower lip, and the middle finger under the chin across the soft tissue.

The routine for normalizing orofacial sensitivity, which should be done regularly before eating, includes the imposition of the three-finger cradle position to allow for head control, cheek control, jaw and lip closure, and control of tongue protrusion. Then with the jaw in a symmetrically closed position (a) the outer gums on one side are firmly stroked a few times (three or four times) stimulating saliva production, and (b) the upper lip below the nose is pressed with the index finger facilitating lip closure and until swallowing of the saliva occurs, or the lip closure and subsequent swallowing may be facilitated by lightly stroking the lower lip, pulling it out and allowing it to close on the upper lip. The stroking-swallowing procedure is repeated for the inside gums on both sides of the mouth, the palate on the midline and lateral areas (front-to-back stroking), and the tongue (front-to-back stroking). The stroking maneuver in each case should be followed by quick removal of the stimulating finger and closure of jaws and lips to avoid a gag reaction and to facilitate swallowing. The desensitizing technique, in short, is composed of repeated stimulation of saliva production and facilitation of swallowing.

5. Transporting of food to mouth in hand-to-mouth fashion, or self-feeding, as a factor in the facilitation of eating movements—One of the important goals in eating therapy is the transition from rooting feeding, where the child depends on a feeder to bring the food to the child's mouth, to self-feeding, where the child transports food to the mouth independently. "One of the basic developmental problems of the human infant is to use his hands adaptively to grasp food and to manage implements for conveying food through the short but troublesome route from hand to mouth" (Gesell and Ilg, 1937).

Depending on the child's level of development, the food-transporting sequence to be stimulated is hands-suckling, and hands-holding of bottle, hands-guiding of spoon, and hands-playing with food. Transporting techniques may be employed in all three eating postures.

Hands-suckling (about one month) in the normal infant may be viewed as a precursory form of "self feeding." Accordingly, during eating therapy, even during the rooting-feeding stage, the clinician should routinely bring the child's hands together and to the mouth. Such a maneuver may precede rooting-feeding or may be periodically employed during rooting-feeding therapy.

Hands-holding of the bottle (about 5 or 6 months) or breast during suckling may also be considered a pre-self-feeding behavior. Clinicians and parents should routinely place the child's hands around the bottle or encourage breast holding and kneading during suckling.

Hands-guiding by the infant of the feeder's hand and spoon to the infant's mouth (about 8 or 9 months) represents an important pre-self-feeding stage. The clinician or parent should place the child's hands and then hand, preferably the right (which may mean that the feeder feeds with the left hand depending on the feeding position used) in a grasp position first on the feeder's hand and later on the stem of the spoon. As much feeding as possible should be done with the child's right hand in the food-transport position and sensing the food-transport movement.

Hands-playing with food (about 9 to 12 months) and spoon represents the stage immediately prior to self-feeding. Feeders, therefore, should provide opportunity for and facilitate such play during portions of the actual feeding time.

Self-feeding (15 to 24 months) movements, when developmentally appropriate, and whether associated with spoon, solids, or cup, should be imposed and guided by the feeder to provide appropriate stimulation and corrective feedback in instances where the movements remain incomplete or anomalous.

6. Grasping of the food source as a factor in the facilitation of eating movements—At least three types of food grasping may be recognized: lip(s) grasping, tongue grasping, and teeth grasping.

Lips or lip grasping is manifested by nipple grasping, cup grasping, and straw grasping.

a. In nipple grasping (breast or bottle) the nipple is placed between the lips and lip puckering and holding is facilitated through use of one of the three-finger cradle maneuvers. In the event of a tendency toward tongue protrusion, or hypertrophied tongue reflex, upward pressure by the flat of the middle finger of the cradle against the root of the tongue should reduce or help integrate the tongue movement.

b. In cup grasping, the rim of the cup is placed on the lower lip. The cup should be plastic so that by squeezing the rim a convenient spout can be formed. Also, the jaws should be approximated through the use of the three-finger cradle maneuver. The rim of the cup is then placed on the lower lip and small amounts of liquid are periodically introduced into the mouth—the cup remains on the lower lip during swallowing.

c. In straw grasping (plastic tubing) the tube is placed between the lips like in nipple grasping. Straw grasping follows the development of good cup grasping. With good jaw position and with the tube between the lips, lip sucking should be stimulated. Biting is avoided by not allowing the tube between the teeth.

Tongue grasping is manifested in spoon grasping and grasping of solid foods. Using one of the three-finger cradle maneuvers, mandibular opening is controlled by the clinician's middle finger under the child's chin; mandibular lateralization is controlled by the clinician's index finger; and initial mandibular opening, chewing movements, mandibular closure, and gentle head flexion is controlled by the flat of the clinician's thumb on the chin below the lower lip.

a. In spoon grasping, the child's mandible is first gently closed via the three-finger cradle maneuver. An appropriate size spoon with a small amount of food on the end of the bowl is brought to the mouth. Then partial mandibular opening is facilitated and the spoon is placed on the anterior tongue and downward pressure is applied facilitating lip closure and encouraging integration of tongue protrusion and bite reflexes. As lip closure begins, the spoon is quickly withdrawn and the mandible closed until swallowing occurs. Tongue pressure and mouth closure procedures contribute to the integration of the forward suckle movement of the tongue.

b. In solid food grasping, the same maneuvers described for spoon grasping are performed except that a morsel of food is placed on the anterior tongue, the lips are closed, and chewing movements are facilitated.

Teeth grasping is used with foods requiring a "biting off" action. Again, maneuvers similar to lip and tongue grasping are performed except the food is placed between the teeth and a biting movement facilitated.

7. Manipulating of the food source as a factor in the facilitation of eating movements—Manipulating is defined here as the capacity of the child to adjust the position of the nipple, spoon, morsel, cup, or straw so as to grasp the food source properly and then to prepare it appropriately, that is, suckle or chew it. Manipulating work follows grasping work, since its purpose is to facilitate grasping of a difficult-to-obtain food source. Lip and tongue manipulating movements are stimulated.

Lip manipulating is stimulated by placing the nipple partially between the lips or off center. Adjustive lip movements of reaching and lateralizing are sought and may be facilitated by appropriate use of a three-finger cradle maneuver. Similar adjustive lip movements may be stimulated by incomplete insertion or lateral placement of a cup or straw.

Tongue manipulating is stimulated by incomplete insertion or displacement of the bowl of the spoon on the anterior tongue and by touch stimuli to lateral margins of the tongue. Voluntary tongue reaching and lateral movements are sought. Various other tongue manipulating movements are stimulated by placing chewable morsels in different parts of the mouth, for example, the palate, lips, and buccal areas.

8. Preparing of the food as a factor in the facilitation of eating movements—Preparing is defined here as the eating movement immediately preceding swallowing. In the case of liquids and semisolids, it represents the tongue suckle movement in obtaining milk from the bottle, the upper- lip suckle movement to obtain liquid or semisolids from the spoon, and the lips-suck movement to obtain liquid from a straw. Preparing, relative to liquids and semisolids, is simply drawing the food into the oral cavity to prepare it for swallowing. In the case of solids or morsels of food, it represents chewing movements.

Tongue-suckle preparing of liquids from the nipple is facilitated by adjusting the holes in the nipple and by gentle in-out and rotatory movements of the nipple.

Lips-suck preparing of liquids from the straw is facilitated by holding the end of the straw first above the level of the mouth and then releasing the liquid, and then progressively decreasing the angle until the straw is at the level of the mouth, and, finally, at the level below the mouth or the level requiring suck activity. Resisted sucking and having the child suck thickened liquids contributes to suck-preparing ability. Intraoral negative pressure for suck-preparing is facilitated by tapping the labial muscles to improve lip closure and by applying pressure on the top of the head to improve velopharyngeal closure.

Upper-lip suckle preparing of liquids and semisolids from the spoon is facilitated by use of the three-finger cradle maneuver. Through the maneuver, the jaw is allowed to extend appropriately, the bowl of the spoon is placed on the anterior tongue, and then the bowl is gently pressed downward and held until the lips move to take the food.

Upper-lip suckle preparing of liquids from a cup is facilitated by the three-finger cradle maneuver, forming a spout in the plastic cup, placing the rim on the lower lip, and allowing the child to take small sips at regular and appropriate times. To discourage head extension and "gravity drinking" during cup drinking, the nondrinking side of the cup may be trimmed to allow space for the child's nose as he drinks up. Also, upper lip movement may be stimulated by giving the child thickened liquids to drink.

Chew preparing of morsels is facilitated by the three-finger cradle maneuver, especially by the finger below the lower lip that initiates mouth opening and controls rotatory chewing movements. Placing morsels between the molars or gums facilitates chewing movements. Foods suggested as transition foods to a solid food diet include graham crackers, pieces of peeled fresh fruit, cubes of chicken, diced vegetables, and hard bread crusts (Davis, 1978).

9. Swallowing of the food as a factor in the facilitation of eating movements—Since swallowing is the ultimate stage in the ingestion process, it is facilitated by attention to all the aforementioned factors as well as by attention to special sensory stimuli and food characteristics such as temperature, taste, and texture.

Swallowing coordination, of the somatic type, is facilitated by use of the three-finger cradle maneuver and the stimulation of saliva production, and hence also contributes to the control of drooling. Once the jaw is in a symmetrical and closed position (three-finger cradle maneuver), the outer gums on one side are stroked firmly a few times causing saliva production, then lip closure is accomplished through the application of horizontal pressure across the upper lip with the other index finger or using this finger to stroke the lower lip and stretching it into closure, and, finally, maintaining mouth closure until swallowing occurs. Any tendency for tongue protrusion during swallowing is suppressed through upward pressure at the root of the tongue. Swallowing is elicited a number of times, but each time a different oral area is rubbed (front to back) to stimulate salivation—the inside gums, anterior and posterior parts of the palate, and the tongue. Other stimuli used to stimulate the swallow reflex include the introduction of a stream of liquid via an eye dropper into the oropharynx or puffs of air by blowing through a straw inserted into the oropharynx.

Swallowing is also facilitated by appropriate selection of food characteristics such as taste, temperature, and texture (Sheppard, 1978). Of course, foods characterized by temperature, taste, and texture preferred by the child are more "swallowable." Mildly sweet, mildly salty, and warm chewable foods usually facilitate swallowing. Foods that tend to thicken saliva, such as milk and milk products, and that are strong tasting tend to inhibit swallowing.

Finally, the eating process is composed of a sequence of automatic movements that, for the sake of exposition, may be divided in various ways. Here the sequence used consists of positioning, protecting, priming, transporting, grasping, manipulating, preparing, and swallowing. Overlap in the stages are evident especially in the last four stages; however, the process was divided in this way because it allowed for the application of certain therapeutic techniques.

Also, some general guidelines that should be kept in mind regarding eating therapy are: (a) It should be done as quickly as possible by parents and other family members. (b) The speech communication opportunities afforded during eating therapy should be fully exploited. (c) The transition from arm and lap feeding to chair feeding should be made as quickly as possible. (d) The transition from bottle, to spoon, to cup, to finger feeding should be made as soon as possible. (e) At each stage of the therapy, the child should be provided with only that amount of assistance that is absolutely necessary and all efforts at self-feeding movements should be encouraged and facilitated.

REFLEXIVE VOCALIZATION

Among the forms of reflexive vocalization to be stimulated are movement vocalization, hand-to-mouth vocalization, and happy-play vocalization.

Movement Vocalization

Movement-associated vocalization is explained on the basis of reflexive glottic closing for purposes of developing intrathoracic breath pressure required to facilitate certain movements. Two classes of such movements are manifested in struggle and work efforts.

Struggle-movement vocalization may be elicited from the child when the clinician resists the child's attempts to raise his head from prone or supine lying, or his attempts to roll over, or to sit up. The child's efforts to resist being pulled or pushed along the floor may also stimulate struggle-movement vocalization.

Work-movement vocalization may be elicited from the child when the clinician creates tasks for the child that require lifting, pushing, pulling, squeezing, pressing, striking, kicking, throwing, and swinging—for example, the use of push-pull and squeeze toys and the use of balls for throwing or kicking.

Hand-to-Mouth Vocalization

Hand-to-mouth vocalization may be observed in infants during teething, eating, and playing.

Teething vocalization may arise from the discomfort felt by the child during this period and also from the hand-elicited focus on touch, pressure, and movement sensations from the lips and gingival area. The hand-elicited sensory focus should be facilitated by bringing the child's hands together and to the mouth during this period and encouraging associated vocalization.

Feeding vocalization may arise from the sensations felt by the child during feeding. For example, pleasant sensations from eating in general may elicit automatic vocalization, while lip holding during suckling may give rise to labial sounds, front-tongue movements during chewing may give rise to tongue-tip sounds, and back-tongue movements during swallowing may give rise to linguavelar sounds. Since the child may want to reexperience these vocalizations just prior to or after feeding, such hand-elicited vocalization should also be facilitated by bringing the child's hands together and to the mouth at these times.

Playing vocalization arises from the sound and sensory variations produced by the child's hands when they are in the mouth during reflexive vocalization. Because the presence of the hands in the mouth may increase the amount and variety of vocalization, the clinician should facilitate their presence during periods of reflexive vocalization.

Happy-Play Vocalization

Happy-play vocalization refers to the child's cooing behavior in response to pleasant sensations and to babbling behavior in response to pleasant sensations and the desire to play with sound-making per se.

Cooing and babbling are facilitated by instructing all those in the child's environment to produce extra amounts of sounds when the child is experiencing "good feelings," like when he is being bathed, powdered, dried, rubbed, fed, and rocked.

Theoretically, the stimulation of basic speech movements as described in this chapter should allow for the spontaneous emergence of skilled speech movements, however, since this may not always occur, or may only occur to various degrees, a discussion of techniques designed to stimulate skilled movements directly is presented in the next and final chapter on neurospeech therapy.

REFERENCES

Blanchard, I. Results of controlled presentation of food to three cerebral palsied patients. *Cerebral Palsy Rev.,* 25, 9–12 (1964).

Bobath, B. Motor development, its effect on general development, and application to the treatment of cerebral palsy. *Physiotherapy,* November, 1–7 (1971).

———. The very early treatment of cerebral palsy. *Devel. Med. Child Neurol.* 9, 373–390 (1967).

Bobath, K. and Bobath, B. Cerebral palsy, Part II: The neurodevelopmental approach to treatment. In P. H. Pearson and C. E. Williams (Eds.), *Physical therapy services in the developmental disabilities.* Springfield, Ill.: Charles C Thomas (1972).

———. The facilitation of normal postural reactions and movements in the treatment of cerebral palsy. *Physiotherapy,* August, 1–19 (1964).

Bosley, E. Development of sucking and swallowing. *Cerebral Palsy Rev.,* 26, 14–16 (1965).

Bosma, J. F. Disability of oral function in infant, associated with displacement of the tongue. *Acta Pediat.,* March (1960).

———. Oral and pharyngeal development and function. *J. Dent. Res.,* January–February (1963).

Davis, L. F. Pre-speech. In F. P. Connor, G. G. Williamson, and J. M. Siepp (Eds.), *Program guide for infants and toddlers with neuromotor and other developmental disabilities.* New York: Teachers College Press, Columbia University (1978).

Forster, F. M. *Clinical neurology.* St. Louis: The C. V. Mosley Company (1973).

Gesell, A., and Ilg, F. *Feeding behavior of infants.* Philadelphia: J. B. Lippincott (1937).

Griffin, K. M. Swallowing training for dysphagia patients. *Arch. Phys. Med. Rehab.,* 55, 467–470 (1974).

Larsen, G. L. Rehabilitation of dysphagia paralytica. *J. Speech Hearing Dis.,* 37, 187–194 (1972).

Lenman, J. A. R. The nervous system. In I. A. D. Bouchier and J. S. Morris (Eds.), *Clinical skills: A system of clinical examination.* London: W. B. Saunders Company, Ltd. (1976).

Meader, M. H. The effect of disturbances in the developmental processes upon emergent specificity of function. *J. Speech Dis.,* 5, 211–219 (1940).

Mueller, H. Facilitating feeding and prespeech. In P. H. Pearson and C. E. Williams (Eds.), *Physical therapy services in the developmental disabilities.* Springfield, Ill.: Charles C Thomas (1972).

Palmer, M. Studies in clinical techniques II: Normalization of chewing, sucking, and swallowing reflexes in cerebral palsy: a home program. *J. Speech Hearing Dis.,* 12, 415–418 (1947).

Prechtl, H. F. R. *The neurological examination of the full term newborn infant.* London: William Heinemann Medical Books Ltd. (1977).

Sheppard, J. J. Treatment of dysphagia-dysarthria. Unpublished Paper (1978).

Stockmeyer, S. A. An interpretation of the approach of Rood to the treatment of neuromuscular dysfunction. *Amer. J. Phys. Med.,* 46, 900–961 (1967).

Twitchell, T. E. Variations and abnormalities of motor development, *J. Amer. Phys. Ther. Assoc.,* 45, 424–430 (1965).

Westlake, H. Muscle training for cerebral palsied speech cases. *J. Speech Hearing Dis.,* 16, 103–109 (1951).

8

Neurospeech Therapy: Stimulation of Skilled Movements

SKILLED SPEECH MOVEMENTS arise as a function of the integration of basic movements and the establishment of stable speech postures. Skilled speech movements include early auditory-perceptual-motor activity as well as preverbal and verbal movements. Specific stimulation of skilled movements becomes necessary when there is delay or retardation in the integration of basic movements.

Listening Movements

Included in a program of stimulation of skilled listening movements is early detection and management of hearing disorders, selective inhibition of startle, and facilitation of localizing and speech perception. Procedures and techniques outlined here are in addition to those for stimulating basic listening movements described in Chapter 7.

DETECTION-MANAGEMENT OF HEARING DISORDERS

Part of any program of stimulation of skilled listening is early detection of the various kinds of hearing disorders that cerebral palsied children may

287

display, as detailed in Chapter 3. Early detection must be followed by swift medical and/or habilitation procedures. Whenever hearing aids are indicated, they should be fitted as quickly as possible. Reducing speaker-listener distance, raising voice level, and using auditory training units should also be considered wherever appropriate.

SELECTIVE INHIBITION

Indiscriminate startle to auditory stimuli is reflective of a lack of cortical participation in auditory processing. The ability of the infant to ignore familiar sounds while less familiar and even softer sounds may elicit startle is the "first sign of cortical function in relation to auditory stimuli" (Murphy, 1964). Integration of indiscriminate startle is attempted via adaptation and corrective feedback techniques.

Adaptation Techniques

By adaptation techniques is meant the "overpresentation" of familiar sounds each day. That is, environmental sounds that are common to the child's environment and that elicit startle should be introduced many more times than are necessary. For example, a door may be slammed, items may be dropped on the floor, and the child's name may be called loudly and unexpectedly.

Gradualism is also part of adaptation techniques. Exercise stimuli should be presented from progressively decreasing distances, with progressively increasing loudness, and with full warning to no warning.

Corrective Feedback Technique

If attempts at facilitating adaptation to indiscriminate startle are progressing slowly, the clinician may combine the startle stimuli with physical restraint of extensor or flexor startle patterns. As quickly as possible, the degree of physical restraint should be lessened.

LOCALIZING

Localizing of auditory stimuli is important to the processing of nonspeech and speech signals. Stimulation of localizing is attempted through on-effect and stimulating feedback techniques.

On-Effect Technique

By the on-effect technique is meant the use of interesting, novel, and changing stimuli to facilitate localization attempts by the child. Indoor stimuli such as the vacuum cleaner, hair dryer, TV, radio, electric shavers, and electric tools may produce on-effect and excite localizing attempts.

Outdoor stimuli such as airplane and motorcycle sounds, lawn mowers, sirens, and dog barking may also produce on-effects. Most important is the production of on-effect through the use of human voice; such on-effect may be facilitated by varying pitch, loudness, quality, and time factors of voicing.

The on-effect technique includes the factors of body position, and direction, distance, and loudness of stimuli. Exercise stimuli should be presented first with the child in back-pattern speech postures and then in elbow and sit patterns. Stimuli should be presented first from right-side and then left-side positions and first from below and then from above positions. Also distances from the stimuli should be progressively increased and loudness levels progressively decreased.

Stimulating-Feedback Technique

The stimulating-feedback technique describes the passive imposition of certain feedback associated with a movement that is not present, with the expectation that the imposed feedback will eventually stimulate the movement. For example, head roll in back postures, head lateralization in elbow postures, and head lateralization and flexion-extension in sitting postures should be initiated and guided in response to on-effect stimuli, when these movements are not spontaneously exhibited by the child. Eventually, stimulating feedback should hopefully provoke these movements, or at least degrees of these movements.

PERCEPTION

Facilitation of auditory perception includes attention to certain hygiene considerations, stimulation of listening attitudes, and perceptual exercises.

Auditory Hygiene

Auditory hygiene considerations are related to the concepts of "auditory atrophy" and "auditory rejection."

Atrophy, or the failing to develop or the wasting away of auditory interest in speech, may be related to (a) undetected or untreated acuity losses that make listening difficult and consequently discourage the child from listening and (b) unrewarded listening, that is, when listening does not help the child advance, gain something, or adjust to the environment. Both acuity loss and nonuseful hearing are sources of progressive lessening of listening interest.

Early hearing screening and vigorous habilitation programs contribute to reducing acuity-loss atrophy; while ensuring that when a child makes an effort to listen she will be reinforced in some way contributes to reducing unrewarded-listening atrophy.

Rejection, or voluntary disengagement of listening, may be related to (a) failure experiences associated with listening and (b) auditory anxiety associated with unpleasant experiences such as verbal punishment.

Success experiences associated with listening should be planned daily, such as requests that can be followed, questions that can be answered, and stories that are enjoyed by the child. Auditory anxiety can be kept to a minimum by ensuring that the child is not present when medical, psychological, schooling, and speech problems are discussed. Also, verbal discipline or punishment should be avoided or kept to a minimum.

In general, the clinician should discuss the concept of auditory hygiene with parents, clinicians, therapists, teachers, and physicians, and offer suggestions for ensuring it.

Listening Attitude

Listening attitude describes auditory stilling, searching, localizing, fixing, and tracking behaviors of the child. Such attitudes are developed in various ways.

Abundant use of pleasant voice by mother, father, and other family members during efforts to soothe or comfort the child and during feeding, bathing, and play periods should be encouraged.

Recognition by the child of parental and family members' voices through smile and localization responses should be stimulated. The recommended techniques for such stimulation include varying voice in ways that attract the child's interest, producing voice from different and novel directions and distances, combining voice with visual stimulation of various kinds (pictures, objects), and reinforcing responses through the use of word, smile, touch, and hug.

Response-to-name stimulation is done by having all those who relate with the child speak the child's name upon making face-to-face contact. Also, all the child's communicants should frequently use the child's name when telling stories, describing events in the environment, or describing the child's activities. Smiling, localizing, and other bodily movement responses to the sound of the child's name, on the part of the child, should be quickly and generously reinforced.

Response to simple utterances such as to "no" commands, greetings and goodbyes, and requests should also be evoked. "No" commands and "give me" games are facilitated through use by the clinician of physical guidance and gesture.

Perceptual Exercises

Perceptual exercises for span, discrimination, analysis, synthesis, sequencing, and imagery should be planned. Exercises should be graded for capacity and ability of the child.

Span is developed by having the child (a) point to or eye-localize a progressively increasing number of things named by the clinician; (b) repeat progressively longer words, phrases, or sentences; and (c) answer questions about progressively longer and more complex questions and stories.

Discrimination is developed by having the child (a) signal whether pairs of similar-sounding syllables, words, or phrases are the same or different and (b) identify the correct pair of similar-sounding names of pictures or objects uttered by the clinician.

Analysis is developed by having the child (a) identify component syllables of a word and (b) identify component words of a phrase or sentence.

Synthesis is developed by having the child (a) identify words from component syllables and (b) identify phrases or sentences from component words. In these tasks pauses between component syllables and words are made progressively longer.

Sequencing is developed by having the child (a) point to a progressively increasing number of things named by the clinician, and in the correct order; (b) execute a progressively longer series of simple instructions, and in the right order; and (c) unscramble out-of-order syllables of words, and words of phrases and sentences.

Imagery is developed by having the child (a) defer responses to various perceptual tasks for progressively longer periods of time until signalled by the clinician and (b) "hear" responses with their "mind's ear" before responding to various perceptual tasks.

Imitative Vocalization

Imitative vocalization, babble talk, or echolalia may all be considered terms for primary talking. Primary talking is viewed as a parallel phenomenon to primary sitting and walking. Primary talking specifically refers to the capacity in children for various forms of preverbal and early verbal replies to speakers. The forms of primary talking that are progressively integrated by higher speech centers are two levels of auto-echolalia and three levels of true echolalia.

AUTO-ECHOLALIA

The earliest vocal replies or echoes made to speakers by infants are to "pre-words," which are sounds and sound combinations that infants themselves make spontaneously. A second-order auto-echolalia is in response to sounds and sound combinations made by the speaker that are similar to the sounds made spontaneously by the child.

Stimulation of auto-echolalia should take place when infants are normally expected to engaged in spontaneous vocalization, for example, during and after feeding, bathing, or playing. The goal of the clinician or family member is to extend the auto-echolalia through eliciting the two levels of reply described.

TRUE ECHOLALIA

The first order of true echolalia or vocal reply made to speakers by infants is to sounds and sound combinations made by the speaker but which have not yet been made spontaneously by the child. A second order of true echolalia is to true words uttered by the speaker. A third order of true echolalia is the deferred repetition by the child of true words uttered by the speaker.

Stimulation of true echolalia is also done during periods when spontaneous vocalization is expected from the child. Also, efforts at true echolalia should follow successful stimulation of auto-echolalia.

Speech appears to arise then from a bank of automatic sounds and sound combinations that are progressively shaped into arbitrary speech symbols through the stages of auto- and true echolalia.

Speech Movements

Techniques for stimulating skilled speech movements are divided into sections on speech breathing and effector coordination.

SPEECH BREATHING

Cortical integration of reflexive breathing for speech purposes is manifested by neuroregulation that allows—

1. a voluntary initiation and cessation of breathing and a change in breathing rate and mode of inspiration;
2. a change in thoracic-abdominal movement relationships including increased thoracic participation and physiologic asynchrony whereby abdominal movements precede thoracic movements at the start of the expiratory phase;
3. a shift in I-fraction from about 40 percent to one of about 15 percent;
4. a shift from primarily a nasal to an oral mode of inspiration; and
5. multisyllabic babbling or multisyllabic speaking per breathing cycle.

Stimulation of more complete cortical integration of reflexive breathing is done through voluntary control exercises and inspiratory facilitation maneuvers.

Voluntary Control Exercises

Various voluntary control exercises may be used. Children may be asked to cease or to begin breathing upon command; to hold the breath for as long as possible; to deepen breathing; to hasten breathing rate; and then alternately to breath through the nose and through the mouth.

Increased proficiency in such voluntary manipulation of breathing would indicate the establishment of the kind of neuroregulatory control over breathing that is required for good speech breathing.

Inspiratory Facilitation Maneuvers

The inspiratory facilitation maneuvers for speech breathing are based on those described in Chapter 7 for vegetative breathing, but with certain intake and timing modifications.

The speech arm-lift, leg-roll, accordion, and butterfly techniques vary from the vegetative techniques in the following ways: (a) the expiratory phase is lengthened and voicing, either sustained vowels or syllable strings, is encouraged and stimulated during the procedure; and (b) the inspiratory phase is quickened so that its duration is approximately 10 percent of the duration of the respiratory cycle. Also, the mode of inspiration should be oral, and this can be facilitated by pinching the nostrils at the beginning of the inspiratory phase.

Such stimulating-feedback maneuvers should also contribute to the kind of neuroregulatory control over breathing required for speech.

EFFECTOR COORDINATION

The progressive integration and elaboration of primary talking into true talking is reflected by the increasing coordination of the respiratory, phonatory, resonatory, and articulatory effectors. Such increased coordination of the effector system is facilitated through stimulation of system differentiation, praxis, and diadochokinesia.

Differentiation

Differentiation of the effectors is facilitated through the use of certain conditioning and isolation maneuvers.

Conditioning maneuvers, designed to facilitate effector differentiation, are carried out in various speech postures and include—

1. flexing the upper trunk with front-to-back, side-to-side, and rotatory movements;
2. flexing the head with front-to-back, ear-to-shoulder, and rotatory movements;

3. stretching the mandible with passive extension and flexion movements and through elicitation of the jaw-jerk reflex;
4. stretching, shaking, and tapping upper and lower lips;
5. spreading and stretching the cheeks on either side by lifting the cheeks away from the dental arch with the thumb;
6. stretching the tongue by lifting it and bringing it over the lower incisors, shaking and stroking it, and eliciting push and pull counteracting reflexes; and
7. stroking and tapping the velum and eliciting palatal reflexes.

Differentiation goals are served when the clinician names the particular effector under treatment and when the clinician eventually asks the child to identify each effector following the conditioning maneuver.

Isolation maneuvers follow conditioning maneuvers and involve holding or stabilizing all major body parts except the effector to be differentiated. Once the hold has been imposed, sometimes with the aid of an assistant, the child is asked to move the isolated part. If he or she cannot, the movement of the part is assisted. Progress is marked by a reduction in the degree of hold by the clinician and by an increase in the degree of voluntary movement by the child.

1. Head isolation from the trunk is done first by passively ventroflexing and dorsiflexing the head, lateralizing it, and bending it in an ear-to-shoulder fashion while providing full hold of the arms, trunk, and legs. Then the child is asked to make the movements spontaneously without or with assistance while the hold is maintained. Then the movements are requested with progressive release of the hold until the hold is completely eliminated.
2. Larynx isolation from the head is done by requesting the child to produce vowels, strings of syllables, or words while the clinician provides full hold of the head. Full hold is provided with the clinician standing behind the sitting child, with the back of the child's head against the clinician's trunk and the sides of the child's head cradled between the hands of the clinician. Progressively less hold of the head is provided until the child can vocalize without associated head movement.
3. Mandible isolation from the head is done by standing behind the sitting child and passively extending and flexing the mandible while providing full hold of the head. Full hold is done by placing the hold-hand across the child's forehead and pressing the head against the clinician's trunk, while the move-hand carries out the mandibular movement. Then the child is asked to make the movements spontaneously without or with assistance while the hold is maintained.

Progressively less hold of the head is provided until the child can voluntarily extend and flex her mandible without associated head movement.

4. Lip isolation from the head is done similarly to mandible isolation except that the move-hand alternately protrudes and spreads the lips. The goal is isolated lip round and lip spread movements.

5. Tongue isolation from the head is done with an assistant providing head hold while the clinician physically lifts and brings the tongue out over the lower incisors and lifts the tongue tip to the upper lip. The goal is isolated tongue protrusion and elevation movements.

6. Mandible, lip, and tongue isolation from the head and from each other is the ultimate goal of effector differentiation. Eventually, the child should be able to open and close her mandible independently of the lips and tongue and with the lips and tongue in an at-rest state; to round and spread her lips, with the mandible in a half-open position, independently of the mandible and tongue and with the tongue in an at-rest state; and, finally, to elevate and depress the tongue tip alternately behind the upper and lower incisors, with the mandible in a three-quarters open position, independently of the mandible and lips and with the lips in an at-rest state. While the child progresses toward such intra-articulator differentiation, varying degrees of hold assistance to the at-rest articulators may need to be provided.

Effector differentiation is achieved when children are able to move their heads and the various articulators independent of the rest of the body and of each other. Depending on the individual child's involvement, varying degrees of such differentiation will be possible.

Praxis

Praxis is the ability to perform specific actions or movements. In terms of speech function, good laryngopraxis and articulopraxis are essential. Stimulation of effector praxis is done through stimulating-feedback and movement-facilitation maneuvers, and movement exercises.

Stimulating-feedback maneuvers are maneuvers that impose particular sensorimotor speech patterns upon the child's articulatory effector with the expectation that such imposed feedbacks will facilitate emergence of the respective movements. Accordingly, the child's articulatory organs are brought through the movements and points of contact associated with the production of various speech sounds for the purpose of generating therapeutic feedback.

1. The bilabial pattern of movement and contact is imposed by bringing the child's lips together with the fingers, holding the lips in contact,

and asking the child to blow open the contact. Bilabial implosion and explosion sounds may be facilitated by simultaneously pinching the nostrils and reducing the lip contact pressure.

2. The labiodental pattern of movement and contact is imposed by lifting the corners of the child's upper lip with the thumb and index finger of one hand and exposing the teeth. Then, with the middle three fingers of the other hand placed under the lower lip and the flat of the thumb placed under the chin for leverage, the lower lip is raised against the upper incisors. Finally, the child is asked to blow air through the teeth. Labiodental friction sounds may be facilitated by pinching the nostrils. Such a maneuver may first elicit an oral inspiration that the clinician should allow by releasing the labiodental seal. The seal should be quickly reestablished in time for the oral expiration phase through the labiodental contact resulting in labiodental friction. Such "labiodental speech breathing" should be imposed for a number of cycles.

3. The linguadental pattern of movement and contact is imposed by extending the mandible through use of one of the three-finger cradle maneuvers, bringing the tongue tip over the lower incisors with the other hand, gently flexing the mandible, and then requesting the child to blow through the teeth. Occlusion of the nostrils may be used to facilitate "linguadental speech breathing."

4. The lingua-alveolar pattern of movement and contact is imposed by gently flexing the mandible through use of one of the three-finger cradle maneuvers, applying upward pressure with the finger placed under the chin and thereby facilitating tongue tip to alveolar ridge contact, and asking the child to blow open the contact. Occlusion of the nostrils and sudden release of the mandible timed with the child's attempt at explosion are techniques used to facilitate "lingua-alveolar speech breathing."

5. The linguavelar pattern of movement and contact is imposed similarly to the lingua-alveolar pattern, except that the upward pressure by the chin finger is applied further back in the chin-neck angle, thereby facilitating tongue back to palate contact, and asking the child to blow or "cough" open the contact. Again, occlusion of the nostrils and sudden release of the mandible timed with the child's attempt at explosion is used to facilitate "linguavelar speech breathing."

All of the above maneuvers should be done in conjunction with appropriately timed audiovisual sound stimulation from the clinician so that the stimulating feedback contains all the important speech-sound sensory dimensions. Also, wherever possible, children should assist in or perform the maneuver themselves.

Movement-facilitation maneuvers are used when there are certain limitations in direction and range of articulatory movements. Among the neurofacilitatory techniques that may be used are resisted, associated, counter-, reversed, and reflex-movement maneuvers. Forms of these maneuvers are discussed under the various neurotherapy orientations identified in Chapter 4.

1. The resisted-movement maneuver describes neurofacilitation via the application of a challenging force to an intended movement. The expectation is that the force will excite a "marshalling effect" within the SCNS resulting in special innervation of motor units and hence more vigorous movement.

   Mandibular flexion or extension may be facilitated by the application of measured resistive pressure applied by the clinician's thumb on the child's mental prominence during efforts to flex the mandible and by the clinician's middle three fingers under the chin during efforts to extend the mandible. Lip rounding or spreading may be facilitated by the application of measured resistive pressure applied by the clinician's thumb and middle finger on the corners of the child's mouth during efforts to round the lips and by the clinician's thumb and middle finger on the child's cheeks during efforts to spread the lips. Tongue tip raising and lowering may be facilitated by the application of measured resistive pressure applied by the clinician's middle finger against the top of the child's anterior tongue during efforts to raise the tongue and by the flat of the clinician's thumb against the bottom of the child's anterior tongue during efforts to lower the tongue. Velar elevation may be facilitated by the application of resistive pressure applied by the clinician's hand on the crown of the child's head and then requesting the child to push against the pressure while he attempts to phonate /a/.

2. The associated-movement maneuver describes neurofacilitation via the stimulation of nonintentional smaller movements out of intentional larger movements, or the "overflow effect." Physiologically, associated movements may be observed when an individual is engrossed in activities such as writing, drawing, or threading a needle, and the effort is accompanied by varying degrees of associated head-cocking and lingual movements; or when children are asked to open their mouths widely, and the effort is accompanied by associated extension and abduction of the fingers of the hand (hand-and-mouth synkinesia). Pathologically, associated movements may be observed when a paralyzed individual attempts movement on the paralyzed side and the effort is accompanied by involuntary movement on the nonparalyzed side (imitative synkinesis); or when a paralyzed individual

initiates movement on the nonparalyzed side and the effort is accompanied by involuntary movement on the paralyzed side (spasmodic synkinesis).

Mandibular flexion may be facilitated by having the child begin from a thorax-flexed-forward position and requesting the child to attempt mouth closure as he extends his trunk into a normal position against measured resistance. Lip spreading may be facilitated by having the child begin from an arms-flexed-palms-out position and requesting the child to spread his lips as he extends his arms against the palms of the clinician who offers measured resistance. Lip rounding may be facilitated by having the child begin in an arms-extended position and requesting the child to round his lips as he pulls on the hands of the clinician who offers measured resistance. Lingual elevation may be facilitated by having the child begin from a chin-to-chest position and requesting the child to attempt to raise his tongue as he extends his head into a normal position against measured resistance.

3. The countermovement maneuver describes neurofacilitation via the introduction of a threatening movement requiring an opposing movement, or the "protective effect." Countermovements were discussed under the section of "Protective Reflexes" in Chapter 7. They are discussed here, because they may also be used when improvement in specific voluntary actions is needed.

Mandibular flexion may be facilitated by slowly and steadily extending the jaw until a counteracting flexor movement is elicited; lip rounding may be facilitated by slowly and steadily spreading the lips until a counteracting lip-rounding movement is facilitated; and tongue protrusion may be facilitated by slowly and steadily applying backward pressure on the anterior tongue with a tongue blade or finger until a counteracting forward movement is elicited. Care must be taken by the clinician with the extent and pressure used in the application of the therapeutic maneuver.

4. The reversed-movement maneuver describes neurofacilitation via the use of an opposite, facilitatory motion immediately preceding the intended, main motion, or the "coiled spring effect." Such reverse movements are seen in sports, for example, the backward preparatory raising of the arm and leg of the baseball pitcher that precedes his forward pitching movement. Similar preparatory and main action motions are seen in kicking a football, and hitting a baseball, golfball, and tennis ball. Preparatory and main action motions are also observed in work movements such as swinging an axe, hammer, or pick.

Mandibular flexion may be facilitated by having the child attempt to extend further the jaw against measured resistance and then attempt to close the jaw against measured resistance. Lip spreading may be facilitated by having the child attempt to round or pucker the lips further against resistance and then attempt to spread the lips against measured resistance. Tongue elevation may be facilitated by having the child attempt to depress further the anterior tongue against resistance and then attempt to elevate the tongue against measured resistance. Reversed-movement maneuvers may be carried out with resistance applied to opposite movements through the entire or through only parts of the range of motion, and to intended movements through the entire, parts, or none of the range of motion.

5. The reflex-movement maneuver describes neurofacilitation via the simultaneous stimulation of a reflex and a voluntary motion that are dependent on the same muscle group, or the "reflex conditioning effect."

  For example, velopharyngeal closure may be facilitated by having the child utter /a/ while the clinician simultaneously elicits the palatal reflex.

  Kabat, who is associated with the development of many facilitation techniques, as described in Chapter 4, stresses the importance of the simultaneous application of a combination of facilitating techniques in order to achieve maximum facilitation of target movements.

Movement exercises are used to ensure the full use of movement potential emerging from stimulating-feedback and movement-facilitation maneuvers. Praxic exercises of various kinds and sensor-awareness exercises are among those recommended.

1. Praxic exercises involve well-performed movements of the larynx, velopharyngeal closure mechanism, and the articulators.

  Laryngopraxic work describes the serial production of discrete on-off voicing. Emphasis is placed on the definition of voice onset and voice termination movements. Various vowels and diphthongs are used for the voice practice. An exercise unit is composed of ten cycles of series of ten phonations.

  Velopraxic work describes the serial production of distinct nasal and non-nasal sounds. Bilabial /mʌ-bʌ/, lingua-alveolar /nʌ-dʌ/, and linguavelar /ŋʌ-gʌ/ distinctions are used. An exercise unit is composed of ten cycles of series of ten bilabial, lingua-alveolar, and linguavelar distinctions. Nasal pinching simultaneous with production of the non-nasal syllable of the pair may be required at the beginning to ensure maximum nasal and non-nasal sound distinctions.

  Articulopraxic work involves the production of sets of two-syllable, three-syllable, and four-syllable combinations. Sets are composed of syllable combinations including bilabial, labiodental, lingua-alveolar, linguapalatal, and linguavelar sounds. An example of a two-syllable set with the lead syllable /bʌ/ follows:/bʌ-vʌ, bʌ-ðʌ, bʌ-dʌ, bʌ-nʌ, bʌ-lʌ, bʌ-dʒ, bʌ-ʒʌ, bʌ-rʌ, bʌ-gʌ/. An exercise unit consists of repeating each pair of the series five times. Other two-syllable sets should be arranged with other syllables serving as lead syllables. As the child progresses, three- and four-syllable sets should be developed. Sounds that the child cannot easily produce are excluded from the exercise sets.

2. Sensor-awareness exercises are composed of speech forms that are nonspontaneous, reduce rate, and amplify feedback from the effectors. Among the exercise forms used are hard-contact speech, exaggerated speech, slow-motion speech, and struggle speech.

Hard-contact speech emphasizes the pressure feedback from the articulators. The child is requested to increase the pressure between the lips when making bilabial sounds, increase the pressure between the lower lip and upper teeth when making labiodental sounds, increase the pressure between the tongue tip and alveolar ridge when making lingua-alveolar sounds, increase the pressure between the anterior tongue and palate when making linguapalatal sounds, and increase the pressure between the posterior tongue and the palate when making linguavelar sounds.

Exaggerated speech emphasizes the movement feedback from the articulators. When speaking, the child is asked to exaggerate the range of mandibular extension when making mandibular sounds, exaggerate the range of lip rounding and spreading when making lip sounds, and exaggerate the range of tongue elevation when making lingual sounds.

Slow-motion speech emphasizes movement feedback and also auditory feedback. When speaking the child is asked to maintain longer contacts for all stops and continuant sounds and to stretch out the vowels.

Struggle speech is characterized by the inhibition of one major articulator and the elicitation of compensatory movements within the others. Mandibular-struggle work is done by having the child speak while the child maintains the mandible in a closed position—thus stimulating compensatory movements of the lips and tongue. Labial-struggle work is done by having the child speak while the child maintains the lips in an open but immobile state—thus stimulating compensatory movements of the mandible and tongue. Tongue-struggle work is done by having the child speak while the child keeps his anterior tongue immobilized against the alveolar ridge—thus stimulating compensatory movements of the mandible and lips.

Diadochokinesia

Diadochokinesia represents the ability of the child not only to produce effector movements well but to produce them at certain minimum rates.

Following degrees of success with differentiation and praxis tasks, diadochokinesia tasks should be introduced. Laryngopraxic, velopraxic, and articulopraxic exercises are converted into laryngodiado, velodiado, and articulodiado exercises by adding the speed component. In addition to the speed or rate of the sets of exercises, duration (ten seconds or more) and rhythmicity of performance should also be emphasized.

Expressive Communication

Expressive communication represents any and all means that the child may possess for symbolic intercommunication. It should emerge spontaneously as a result of the intervention techniques and maneuvers described in Chapters 7 and 8. When direct stimulation of expressive communication is required or desirable, specific attempts at expanding body language, spoken language, and compensatory language are made. Also attention needs to be paid to the communispheral levels in which communication takes place.

BODY LANGUAGE

Body language includes hands and face talk and represents the normal "background language" for effector talking. Hands and face talk are viewed as tuners and facilitators of effector talk.

Hands Talk

Hands talk includes the use of hand movements for symbolic gestural and adjunctive gestural purposes.

Symbolic-gestural stimulation is done by developing communication tasks for the child that can only be resolved by the use of symbolic hand movements. For example, the child is instructed not to speak but to gesture "hello," "goodbye," "pick me up," "I want," "give me." More difficult nonspeaking communication tasks may also be developed; for example: "I want to eat," "I want a telephone," "I want my clothes." The exercises are designed to elicit idiosyncratic gestures, not formal ones.

Adjunctive-gestural stimulation involves the stimulation of supportive hand movements of a nonspecific nature frequently associated with running speech, and facilitatory hand movements of a more specific nature frequently associated with word-finding efforts during running speech. Such supportive and facilitatory hand movements may be stimulated through modeling and through encouragement of their use. Specific practice of their use may also be planned.

Face Talk

Face talk may also be stimulated by developing communication tasks for the child that can only be resolved by the use of facial expressions. For example, the child is instructed not to speak or to use hands but to express facially joy, sadness, boredom, fright, or contentment.

SPOKEN LANGUAGE

The use of spoken language is stimulated via the use of various biolinguistic techniques designed to stimulate vertical-lateral integration of the speech central nervous system (SCNS), and through opportunity for experiencing communicodramas.

Vertical-Lateral Integration

Techniques to stimulate vertical-lateral integration of the SCNS include speech brain oxygenation (SBO), speech brain lateralization (SBL), imagistic-symbolic looping, and speech emergence exercises.

Speech brain oxygenation is done by having the child take maximum inhalations through the nose and maximum exhalations through the mouth. Inhalation and exhalation phases should extend up to counts of ten each. Exercise units should begin with ten inhalation-exhalation cycles, three times a day, and increase daily up to thirty cycles, three times a day. Additionally, SBO work should precede all speech activities.

Speech brain lateralization describes techniques designed to stimulate right ear-left brain speech orientation. Among the techniques that might be used include having children speak while they place a finger into their right ear; while masking-level white noise is fed into the left ear; and while the voice is amplified and fed back into the right ear.

Imagistic-symbolic looping describes techniques designed for interhemispheral and intrahemispheral brain stimulation. The looping technique is composed of three basic steps: actual perceptual experience associated with an object, evocation of perceptual images associated with the perceptual experience, and association of the images.

For example, the child is presented with an object that has a number of sensory dimensions, like a banana. First, the clinician asks the child to "study" the banana with his eyes while the clinician utters its name, to study the banana with his hands while the clinician utters its name, to study the banana with his nose while the clinician utters its name, and, finally, to study the banana with his mouth (child allowed to take a bite) while the clinician utters its name. Second, the clinician removes the banana and asks the child to "see" the banana with his mind's eye, to "hear" banana with his mind's ear, to "feel" the banana with his mind's fingers, to "smell" the banana with his mind's nose, and, finally, to "taste" the banana with his mind's mouth. The child may be given a small piece of banana to eat after such successful perceptual evocation. Third, the child is asked to "see" the banana and "hear" its name, to "feel" the banana and "hear" its name, to "smell" the banana and "hear" its name, and to "taste" the banana and "hear" its name.

Since it is the imagistic-symbolic looping (I-S looping) that is important and not learning the name of some object or thing, it is more important for the clinician to collect objects that lend themselves to the looping technique than to use the technique to teach new words. I-S looping work should be done on a daily basis.

Speech emergence work refers to the theorized, progressive emergence of cortical speech from R-complex and limbic speech. R-complex, or ritual speech, includes social-gesture forms such as "hi," "bye," "all right," "I'm fine," and "OK"; and memorized forms such as nursery rhymes, prayers, counting, days of the week, and months of the year. Limbic, or emotional speech, includes recurring expressions of love, anger, fear, hatred, and so on. Cortical, or logical speech, includes descriptive, conversational, narrative, and persuasive forms.

The biolinguistic levels of ritual, emotional, and logical speech should be kept in mind by the clinician when stimulating the child's SCNS. All three levels are used by individuals throughout life, but there is, over time, a progressive integration and elaboration of ritual and emotional talk by the logical level. The emergence of the logical level of speech is facilitated in those children whose SCNS are dominated by ritual and emotional talk by use of the emergence technique. For example, if a child is using ritual speech in the form of counting or reciting nursery rhymes, the emergence of these forms into logical speech may be facilitated by (a) making environmental associations with various of the numbers uttered by the child such as "you said three, I see three chairs in the room," or "you said five, I see five children in the room," and so on and (b) asking questions or requesting elaborations on objects, people, or actions involved in a particular nursery rhyme being recited.

If a child is using emotional speech such as "angry or fear talk," the emergence of these forms may be facilitated by asking questions, providing clarifications, and, in general, involving the child in discussion relative to understanding his emotional utterances.

Communicodramas

The communicodrama technique refers to the creation by the clinician of sociocommunicative situations that require various functional uses of speech and which, therefore, make different demands on the SCNS. At least five functions of speech have been identified (Van Riper, 1963, pp. 2–11): speech as a means of formulating thought, transmitting information, social control, emotional expression, and self-identification.

An inner-talking communicodrama is developed by asking the child to imagine that he will be saying something very important to someone and that he must rehearse carefully in his mind what he will say; for example, asking his parents to go to Disneyland, explaining why he can't attend school that day, or justifying his need for a new pet. Once inner-speech rehearsal has occurred, the child should be given the opportunity to try out his talk with the clinician serving as the individual in question. The child should also be encouraged to use inner talking for solving problems and also just for fun.

An information communicodrama is developed by telling the child that you will pretend to be different people seeking information and that they are to provide the information. For example, the clinician may pretend to be a stranger and ask instructions on how to get from one part of the building to another, or a friend asking the child how he spent his summer vacation.

A control communicodrama is developed by telling the child that you will pretend to be his father, mother, brother, sister, doctor, or nurse. His job is to talk you into doing something for him, like getting you to bring him some food, or make a phone call for him, or make an excuse for him.

An emotional communicodrama is developed by having the child pretend that he has won lots of money or something he wanted very much, or that he is very angry about something, or frightened about something. He is supposed to tell the clinician all about it.

An identification communicodrama is developed by the clinician playing the part of a stranger and the child having to tell the clinician all about himself—his family, neighborhood, career goals, and so on.

COMPENSATORY LANGUAGE

In the interest of ensuring that each child actualizes all his potential for intra- and intercommunication, the clinician must be prepared to help the child employ modified speech and nonspeech forms of compensatory language. Among the reasons for employing compensatory language techniques are (a) to facilitate the development of spoken language and (b) to supplement or replace spoken language when it is proceeding slowly, is limited, or where there is little hope of attaining it.

Modified Speech

Forms of modified speech include those used as sensor-awareness exercises such as hard-contact, exaggerated, and slow-motion talking, as well as spell talk and topic talk, electronically treated speech, and synthetic speech.

Hard-contact, exaggerated, and slow-motion talking are voluntary forms of talking which slow rate, exaggerate consonants, and amplify sensory feedback, all of which should contribute to speech intelligibility.

Spell talk and topic talk are used in conjunction with the other forms and are ways to improve speech communication in cases of questionable understandibility. Children may be instructed to identify the topic of their utterance before beginning to communicate; for example, "I want to tell you about my family," or "about my school," or "about my pet." Once the topic is understood by the listener, then the child proceeds talking. The child must learn to identify new topics as the conversation shifts.

Spell talk refers to the child's willingness and readiness to spell aloud words with which listeners are experiencing difficulty.

Electronically treated speech require devices to be worn by the child that are designed to increase speech understandibility. At least two devices have been developed: the electronic speaking aid (National Institute for Rehabilitation Engineering, Pompton Lakes, New Jersey) and the Auditory Feedback Mechanism or AFM (Berko, 1965).

The electronic speaking aid basically amplifies and filters the child's speech and transmits the treated signal into a loudspeaker contained in the speech aid. Speech aids are individually constructed to provide the most intelligible output for each child.

The AFM also amplifies and filters the individual's speech, but then the treated speech is fed back to headsets worn by the individual. In Berko's experiment three types of feedback were used: accelerated, amplified feedback without band-pass filtering, accelerated, amplified feedback with high-band pass filtering, and accelerated, amplified feedback with low-band pass filtering. With adult athetotics, the high-band pass filtering produced the most understandable speech. In a later study, a trend for better speech among spastics was observed when their speech was treated by low-band pass filtering.

Synthesized speech, a different type of "modified speech," is still a speech form of compensatory language. Portable models of speech synthesizers are now commercially available (Phonic Mirror, H. C. Electronics, Inc.). The use of such synthesizers is limited by cost and by the child's physical and mental abilities.

Nonspeech Forms

Under nonspeech forms of compensatory language may be placed signal and code forms, symbol forms, and communication board forms. Such modes of communication are usually reserved for the more severely involved children. The choice of an alternate mode of communication depends on the voluntary movements available and the mental abilities and motivation of the child. Cooperation from the child's parents, family, teachers, clinicians, and therapists is also important. The use of nonspeech communication should not mean a cessation of speech therapy, especially since a number of studies have shown an increase in speech attempts and intelligibility accompanying such use (e.g., McDonald and Schultz, 1973; Beukelman and Yorkston, 1977). Since the topic of nonspeech communication is not directly related to neurospeech therapy concepts, this topic is only briefly discussed here.

Signal and code forms include the use of some simple yes-no system, audio-signalling, and Morse code.

1. A simple yes-no system of signalling may be devised such as the use of available hand, head, face, or eye movements by the child in response to expressed alternatives uttered by the speaker concerning needs, wants, and feelings of the child.
2. A portable audio-oscillator that emits a loud tone has been used with cerebral palsied children (Hagen, Porter, and Brink, 1973). Activation of the device is adjustable to suit the individual child. Children were taught four simple signals representing "I need help," "Yes," "No," and "See the list." The list contained information that the children wanted to communicate most often with respect to wants, feelings, people, and places. When the list was requested, information was then transmitted by the child by his giving yes-no responses to the series of available information. The system is relatively simple and can be used by severely involved children.
3. Morse code (Clement, 1961) has been used as a means of communication for severely involved children. The child must be capable of learning the code, and a decoder must be available for people in the environment. Depending on the movement ability of the individual child, dots and dashes may be transmitted by activation of an audio-oscillator, by different movements of the head, face, eyes, or by certain vocalization.

Symbol forms involve the learning and use of special symbols that represent sounds or words. Two symbol systems have been used with cerebral palsied children: Bliss Symbols and the Initial Teaching Alphabet.

1. Bliss Symbol Communication has been used effectively with certain severely involved children with cerebral palsy (Vanderheiden and Harris-Vanderheiden, 1976). A report has shown that the Blissymbolics not only has provided functional communication for nonverbal cerebral palsied children, but has also increased vocalization and verbalization in many children (Archer, 1977). The system was developed by Charles K. Bliss as a visual symbol system for nonoral individuals. The symbols represent concepts rather than specific words—some are pictorial; others are arbitrary. Depending on the child's ability, symbol vocabularies of up to 400 may be learned. Symbol display boards

may be adjusted to suit the child's ability for finger, hand, head, or eye-gaze pointing.

2. An electronic conversation board called the "Expressor" (Shane, 1972) was designed to facilitate the use of the Initial Teaching Alphabet (i/t/a). In the i/t/a system one symbol represents one sound, and if the child learns the 44 symbols he would be capable of producing any English word. As with other code or symbol systems, the child must be willing and able to learn the system, and also communication is slow and limited to those willing to learn the system.

Communication boards and materials include nonelectronic and electronic boards that may display letters, words, numbers, and pictures.

1. Nonelectronic communications boards and materials have been used with the cerebral palsied for some time (Westlake and Rutherford, 1961; McDonald and Chance, 1964). These materials should be developed on an individual basis in accordance with each child's needs and physical and intellectual abilities.

   Pictures and objects may be collected representing important needs of the child such as foods, family members, pets, and rooms of the house. The child is conditioned to contact the representative materials through some means of pointing or touching each time he desires to express a specific need.

   More organized forms of communication boards have been developed (McDonald and Schultz, 1973). Such boards may display numbers, letters, words, pictures, and sentences. To facilitate the learning of sentence structure, a column for articles, conjunctions, prepositions, and adjectives and adverbs may be added. Word spelling may be done by reference to letters displayed in the form of a typewriter keyboard; such displays should facilitate eventual typing potential. The advantages of such nonelectronic boards are their comparatively low cost and adaptability to individual ability levels.

2. Electronic communication boards are also available. An interesting one, developed by the Cerebral Palsy Communication Group at the University of Wisconsin, is called the Auto-Monitoring Communication Board or Auto-Com. Some of its features include operation that requires only limited pointing ability; activation that is sensitive to a lack of motion rather than specific motion; capacity to printout letters allowing the child to intracommunicate and to monitor and practice his communication; an accessory component that allows for printout of words, phrases, and sentences; a television read-out component; and interfacing with a typewriter. It is also expected that Auto-Com may be used in controlling a voice synthesizer. The experience of a severely involved 10-year-old cerebral palsied child with Auto-Com

was reported (Bullock, Dalrymple, and Danca, 1975). The child made progress in visual, perceptual, cognitive, and linguistic skills.

COMMUNISPHERAL RANGE

Whatever the mode of language used by the child—body, spoken, or compensatory—the clinician should aim to stimulate and expand the child's communispheral range. Of the four ranges recognized, that is, the intimate, personal, family, and public ranges, the first three are important for the cerebral palsied child.

Intimate Communisphere

The intimate or body-contact range of communisphere is experienced by the child when the child is nursed, bathed, dressed, and played with and hears large amounts of intimate talking. Such intimate talking is experienced throughout life during emotional episodes, dancing, and so on.

It is recommended that speakers in the child's environment take advantage of body-contact periods with the child and speak as much as possible, especially in the face-to-face position. The emphasis in the intimate communisphere is talking from the speaker to the child. Opportunity for reply from the child should be provided but is of secondary importance at this range.

Personal Communisphere

The personal or arms-length range of communisphere is experienced by the child in all the major speech postures—back, elbow, sit, and stand.

The child should experience arms-length talking (or distances up to 6 feet) as much as possible during each day. Such talking is facilitated when the speaker places his extended right arm on the child's left shoulder and the child's extended right arm on the clinician's left shoulder. Unlike the intimate range, this range is designed for interpersonal conversation, and the child is stimulated to reply as well as to initiate utterances.

Family Communisphere

The family or person-to-small-group range (about 6 to 12 feet) of communisphere is experienced by the child at the dinner table and certain play situations. The degree of development of the family range of communisphere is related to developments at the intimate and personal ranges.

The family range of communisphere is also to be experienced by the child as often as possible during the day, most appropriately, during the three daily meal periods and in group play situations. Unlike the intimate and personal ranges, this range is designed for more "talking to others" by the child and less "talking back and forth" or being "talked at by others."

It is clear that all three communispheral ranges should be experienced each day by the child, and the clinician should plan accordingly. On the matter of proportion of time spent within each range, it is recommended that the most time be spent in the personal range, then the family range, and, finally, the intimate range. Time of actual and/or attempted speech communication by the child each day, or total speaking time, should exceed an hour at first and eventually reach approximately one hour each in the morning, afternoon, and evening.

REFERENCES

Archer, L. A. Blissymbolics. A non-verbal communication system. *J. Speech Hearing Dis.,* 42, 568–579 (1977).

Berko, F. Amelioration of athetoid speech by manipulation of auditory feedback. Doctoral Dissertation, Cornell University (1965).

Beukelman, D., and Yorkston, K. A communication system for the severely dysarthric speaker with an intact language system. *J. Speech Hearing Dis.,* 42, 265–270 (1977).

Bullock, A., Dalrymple, G. F., and Danca, J. M. Communication and the nonverbal, multihandicapped child. *Am. J. Occup. Ther.,* 29, 150–152 (1975).

Clement, M. Morse code method of communication for the severely handicapped cerebral palsied child. *Cerebral Palsy Rev.,* 22, 15–16 (1961).

Hagen, C., Porter, W., and Brink, J. Nonverbal communication: An alternative mode of communication for the child with severe cerebral palsy. *J. Speech Hearing Dis.,* 38, 448–455 (1973).

McDonald, E. T. and Chance, B. *Cerebral palsy.* Englewood Cliffs, N. J.: Prentice-Hall, Inc. (1964).

McDonald, E. T., and Schultz, A. Communication boards for cerebral palsied children. *J. Speech Hearing Dis.,* 38, 73–88 (1973).

Murphy, K. Development of articulation and hearing. In *Learning problems of the cerebral palsied.* London: The Spastics Society (1964).

Shane, H. A device and a program for aphonic communication. Master's Thesis. University of Massachusetts (1972).

Vanderheiden, G., and Harris-Vanderheiden, D. Communication techniques and aids. In L. Loyd (Ed.), *Communication assessment and intervention strategies.* Baltimore: University Park Press (1976).

Van Riper, C. *Speech correction.* Englewood Cliffs, N. J.: Prentice-Hall, Inc. (1963).

Westlake, H., and Rutherford, D. *Speech therapy for the cerebral palsied.* Chicago: National Society for Crippled Children and Adults, Inc. (1961).

Concluding Comment

This book's journey into the concepts, principles, and methods of neurospeech therapy is done. To those readers who made the entire journey, and the many stops along the way, I trust the trip was interesting and informative. More importantly, it is the author's fondest hope that the sounds and sights of the journey have in some way added to the reader's capacity to enhance the speaking ability of children with cerebral palsy.

Index